Clinical Facial Analysis

Fabio Meneghini • Paolo Biondi

Clinical Facial Analysis

Elements, Principles, and Techniques

Second Edition

Springer

Authors
Fabio Meneghini, M.D.
Aesthetic and Maxillofacial Surgery
Padova, Italy

Paolo Biondi, M.D.
Maxillofacial Surgery
Forlì, Italy

ISBN 978-3-662-49992-1 ISBN 978-3-642-27228-8 (e-book)
DOI 10.1007/978-3-642-27228-8
Springer Heidelberg New York Dordrecht London

Softcover reprint of the hardcover 1st edition 2012

Printed on acid-free paper

Springer is part of Springer Science+Business Media (www.springer.com)

Acknowledgments

This text is dedicated to our patients.

We thank the medical and all patient care staff at Maria Cecilia Hospital and G.B. Mangioni Hospital. We also thank Massimiliano Crespi, Carol Grocott, David G. Smith, Edoardo Lombardi Vallauri, Giorgio Marconi, Sverre Klemp, Irmela Bohn, and Martina Himberger. A special thanks to Gabriele Schröder, for her confidence, from the very beginning, in a proposal for a book on clinical facial analysis.

Contents

Introduction: Facial Analysis – What, Why, When, and How

This book contains, in the rationale of the authors, some elements and principles of facial analysis, which are the immutable and universal component of the work, and some technical details, which are personal, debatable, and changing every day. The reader should retain the first and judge and improve on the latter.

Analysis: detailed examination of the elements or structure of something, typically as a basis for discussion or interpretation.

Elements: the rudiments of a branch of knowledge.

Principle: a general scientific theorem or law that has numerous special applications across a wide field.

Technique: a way of carrying out a particular task, especially the execution or performance of an artistic work or scientific procedure.

Taken from: *The New Oxford Dictionary of English*, Oxford University Press, 1998

What Is Clinical Facial Analysis?

Clinical facial analysis (CFA) is the method utilized by physicians for evaluating and judging the patient's face, to define its proportions, volume, appearance, symmetry, and visible deformities. It is based on direct examination, clinical photographs, and conventional and computerized x-ray imaging.

Clinical facial analysis is essential for many specialists, such as plastic surgeons, facial plastic surgeons, maxillofacial surgeons, ophthalmic plastic surgeons, otorhinolaryngologists, head and neck surgeons, cosmetic surgeons, orthodontists, rehabilitative dentists, and dermatologists, and, generally, for any physicians dealing with facial aesthetics and functions.[1]

Clinical facial analysis is not a particular phase of clinical practice or a moment during a patient consultation. It is the largest part of a professional life and a never-ending process. Furthermore, CFA is not separable from everyday activities and we should be able to analyze the face of the patient and, at the same time, answer his or her questions, or illustrate a procedure.

[1]Facial analysis is also important for many nonmedical professionals, such as hairdressers, eyeglasses designers, make-up artists, and aestheticians.

Clinical facial analysis is not delegable to other colleagues. Our findings, along with patient needs and requests, are the basis for treatment planning and the successive surgical treatment. Dealing with facial aesthetics, we are responsible for the overall process and not just a single aspect of it.

Facial surgery, as well as orthodontics and any "aesthetic" treatments, is a matter of rearranging things that already exist. Through CFA we can visualize, evaluate, and prioritize what exists.

How Do You Train and Develop the Skill for Clinical Facial Analysis?

You need situations where you can practice. Help other colleagues in documenting and analyzing new patients if you are a beginner.

As with any skill, daily practice is most important. Become obsessed with CFA. Read everything that is relevant. Talk with the experts and observe how they deal with difficulties. Feed your passion and, after time, accentuate your own distinctive approach and cultivate your unique style. But above all, practice. Practice in the real clinical activity and practice in your imagination.

The Spiral of Analysis

The never-ending process of CFA can be divided into four consecutive steps: the preoperative, the intraoperative, the early postoperative, and the late postoperative analysis. The final step, known as the follow-up, which concludes the process for a given patient or group of patients, is functional to the next preoperative step with a new patient, creating the positive spiral of analysis. This is probably the best self-teaching exercise we do (see Diagram). To create a positive spiral of analysis, one must respect the following rules:

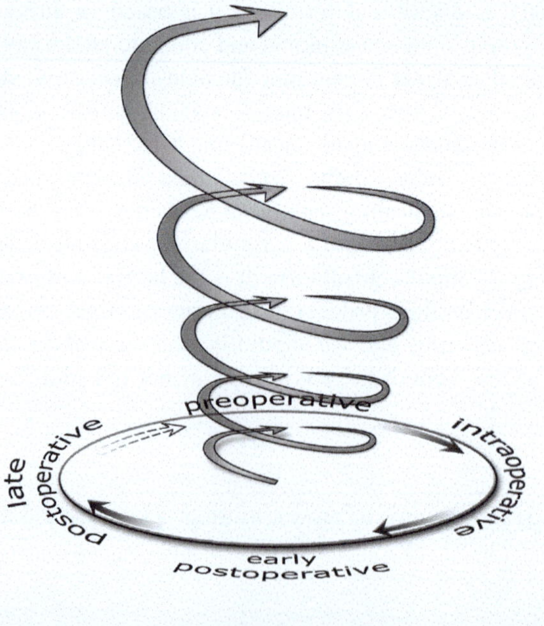

- Document with clinical photographs and written notes every new patient in the best way you can, whether or not he or she will be treated later.
- Continue to document during the intraoperative, early, and late postoperative phases utilizing, as a template, the initial materials to ensure the best comparative value to the clinical case.
- Continue to schedule the old patients about once a year to perform the late follow-up. Seeing the patient again, you are obliged to review the case immediately before and during the consultation. Nothing is so effective for your memory than reviewing the case with the patient himself.
- Collect and store the materials in the best way you can, remembering that you need these data as a working instrument.
- You need a spiral of analysis and only you are responsible for its continuous growth.

Time should not be seen as a line on a graph, running from left to right, but as in nature, running from spring to summer, autumn, and winter. To complete a cycle, one year for nature and a clinical case for facial analysis, all four "seasons" must be started and finished. Our experience is of more value if we can personally follow the entire cycle.

Sometimes, we explain to my patients the significance of the spiral of analysis as a component of the general process of continuing medical education of the physician.

Searching for a Flexible Method of Clinical Facial Analysis

A fundamental characteristic of our current approach to patient analysis is flexibility. Flexibility, at first, could be misinterpreted as lack of consistency, reproducibility, and control, but we need it for many reasons; the first of these is the unique experience of treating different patients with different problems that require a personalized approach.

The best way to guarantee consistency, reproducibility, and control is to have a rigorous method in the initial phase, introducing the flexibility only later on as the case analysis progresses. This means that, during the first consultation, we must collect basic and complete documentation for performing a thorough general facial analysis and after careful selection continue in a personalized manner.

Do Not Apply a Method of Analysis in a Linear Way

Like any diagnostic tool, the CFA may be misunderstood or inappropriately applied in a linear way. Sometimes our list of goals, in its logical and linear scale of priority, as dictated by the analysis, should be modified according to the expressed and "unexpressed" patient needs. Sometimes it is better to widen the treatment plan with one or more adjunctive procedures; sometimes a limited and minimally invasive procedure is all our patient wants. Sometimes the linear application of CFA in a treatment plan leads to technically difficult surgery, to time-demanding treatments (multiple steps!), or to unstable results.

To avoid or limit these problems, we need to be constantly vigilant against false logic derived from linear application of CFA.

The Four Main Components Involved in Facial Aesthetics

Four main components are involved in facial aesthetics:

- The soft tissue quality
- The soft tissue quantity
- The soft tissue dynamics
- The supporting skeleton

Problems related to the quality of the soft tissue involve mainly the skin color, texture, elasticity, phototype, stains, superficial wrinkles, and scars. Also the characteristics of the hair, eyebrows, eyelashes, lips, the color of the iris and sclera, and the makeup play different roles in what we perceive as the quality of facial surface.

Problems related to the quantity of the soft tissue are the relative thickness and spatial distribution of the single components, such as fat, muscles, glands, mucosa, and skin.

Problem of the soft tissue involve the activity of mimic and skeletal musculature. Also the head posture, sustained by isometric muscular activity, plays a major role in the perception of different facial units by the observer.

The supporting skeleton is the outer bony skeleton, the nasal and ear cartilage, and the anterior teeth. A particular supporting tissue structure in the face is the eye globes, whose dimension and spatial position greatly affect aesthetics.

In Chaps. 4, 5, 6, 7, 8, 9, and 10, much effort is dedicated to examining all aspects of the facial aesthetic, identifying the specific role played by these four main factors.

The Three Error Groups

Problems with patients can be divided into three main categories:

- Errors in patient selection
- Errors in preoperative analysis
- Errors in technical execution

Errors in Patient Selection

Errors in patient selection occur, for example, when a patient is too interested in the detail of his face and cannot see the whole picture; when a woman decides to rejuvenate her lips surgically to satisfy her husband; or when a boy wants Brad Pitt's nose.

For an in-depth study of the argument, some suggested reading is provided in Chap. 15.

Errors in Preoperative Analysis

Errors in CFA produce errors in planning and treatment, with undesirable outcomes. Results come from analysis!

There are three basic preoperative facial analyses: the doctor's initial one, the patient's initial one, and the definitive preoperative one, resulting from cooperation between the patient and the doctor. The main goal of this book is to help the reader to avoid errors in all three analyses.

Errors in Technical Execution

After the thorough preoperative work in the office is done, the final step is the realization of the planned treatment. Although this book does not describe surgical, orthodontic, or cosmetic techniques, Chap. 12 is dedicated to intraoperative and postoperative analysis, a powerful way to identify technical errors in order to avoid them in the future.

The Appearance-Changing Treatments

Frequently a change in facial appearance is the main request of the patient, as in aesthetic surgery, aesthetic medicine, and many orthodontic cases. In others, a functional problem is the main concern, as in severe nasal airway obstruction, severe dental malocclusion, and upper lid ptosis. Also in the latter situations a thorough facial analysis is mandatory because:

- The original condition is correlated, more or less, with an aesthetic problem.
- The treatment of the functional problem almost always leads to changes in facial appearance.
- These patients are likely to focus more on changes in appearance than on altered function after the treatment [1].

These three points must be explained and exhaustively discussed in the preoperative consultations, as described in the next chapter.

Reference

1. Heldt L, Haffke EA, Davis LF (1982) The psychological and social aspects of orthognathic treatment. Am J Orthod 82:318–328

Approaching the Patient for Direct and Photographic Facial Analysis

1

Contents

Only by walking behind him shall I discover where he is going!

This chapter discusses how to approach a new patient. The ideal room – with three separate areas dedicated for the interview, clinical examination, and clinical photography – is described in detail.

The first consultation is divided into various steps: entrance, interview, direct clinical examination, photographic documentation, and final communication. The successive preoperative consultations are also considered.

1.1 The Single Room Concept

The communication between patient and doctor, the direct clinical examination, and the taking of clinical photographs require three dedicated areas of the office. After a variety of experiences, we strongly favor concentrating all three areas in the same room. Figure 1.1 shows the plan of the room in my current office.

1.1.1 The Interview Area

For the initial and successive consultations, most of the time is spent in the interview area. A large table, with a lateral extension for the computer, the printer, a plant, and the telephone, is centered under a diffuse, but not too intense, light; care is taken to avoid any visual obstruction preventing

F. Meneghini, P. Biondi, *Clinical Facial Analysis*,
DOI 10.1007/978-3-642-27228-8_1, © Springer-Verlag Berlin Heidelberg 2012

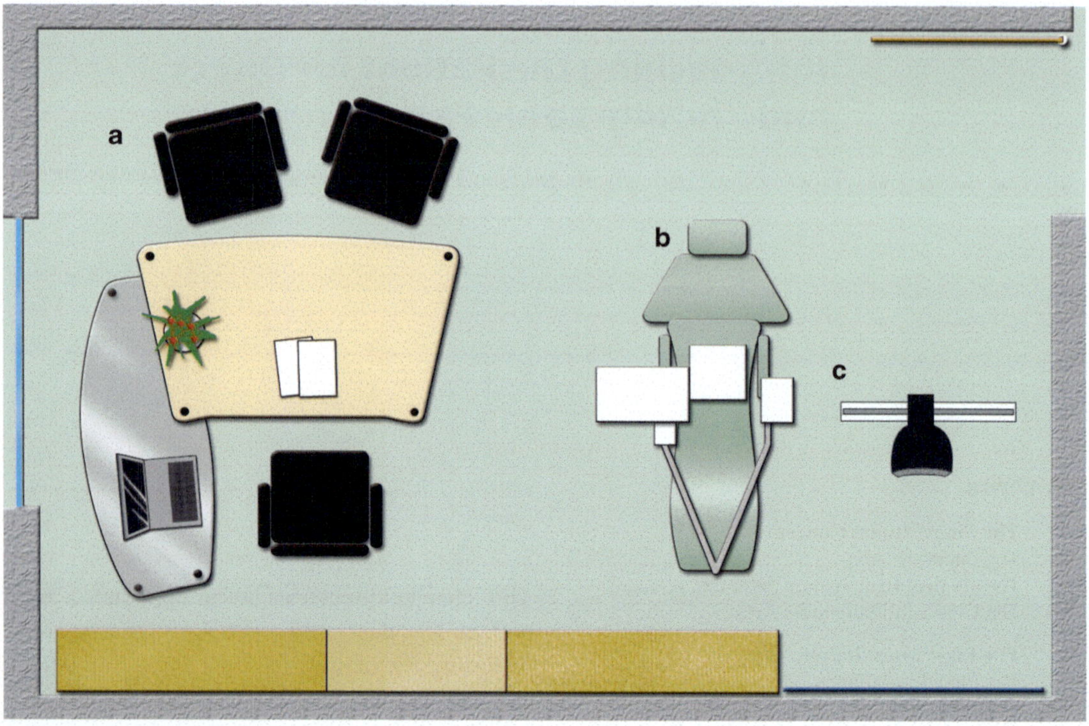

Fig. 1.1 Plan of the room in my current office with the three areas dedicated to interview (**a**), clinical examination (**b**), and clinical photographs (**c**)

eye contact. Adequate extra space around the table is needed when other colleagues and accompanying persons are attending the interview.

When sitting down around the table, the distance between the doctor and the patient is about 110 cm (Fig. 1.2). Only in one of the successive consultations, when we discuss the clinical photographs and the treatment plan in detail, does the doctor sit beside the patient, reducing the distance to about 60 cm (Fig. 1.3).

1.1.2 The Clinical Examination Area

A modified dental chair and two different lighting systems occupy the central area of the room, which is dedicated to the clinical examination.

The main characteristics of the chair are:

- It is adjustable in height and inclination. As I remain in a standing position during direct clinical examination, I can elevate the chair in order to have my eyes at the same height as the patient's eyes so that I may help him to maintain the natural head position[1] (Fig. 1.4).
- Instead of the original dental instruments, there is a small plane support useful for holding a facial mirror, a camera, a ruler, or other small objects.
- It is equipped with a vacuum tube and an air-compressed tube.
- It is easily adjusted to the Trendelenburg's position.One large, ceiling-mounted lighting system produces a diffuse and intense white light. This is preferred for the external examination due to the complete absence of dark shadows.

The other lighting system is adjustable and produces an intense light beam that is very helpful for the anterior nasal and intraoral examination.

[1]See Sect. 3.1.

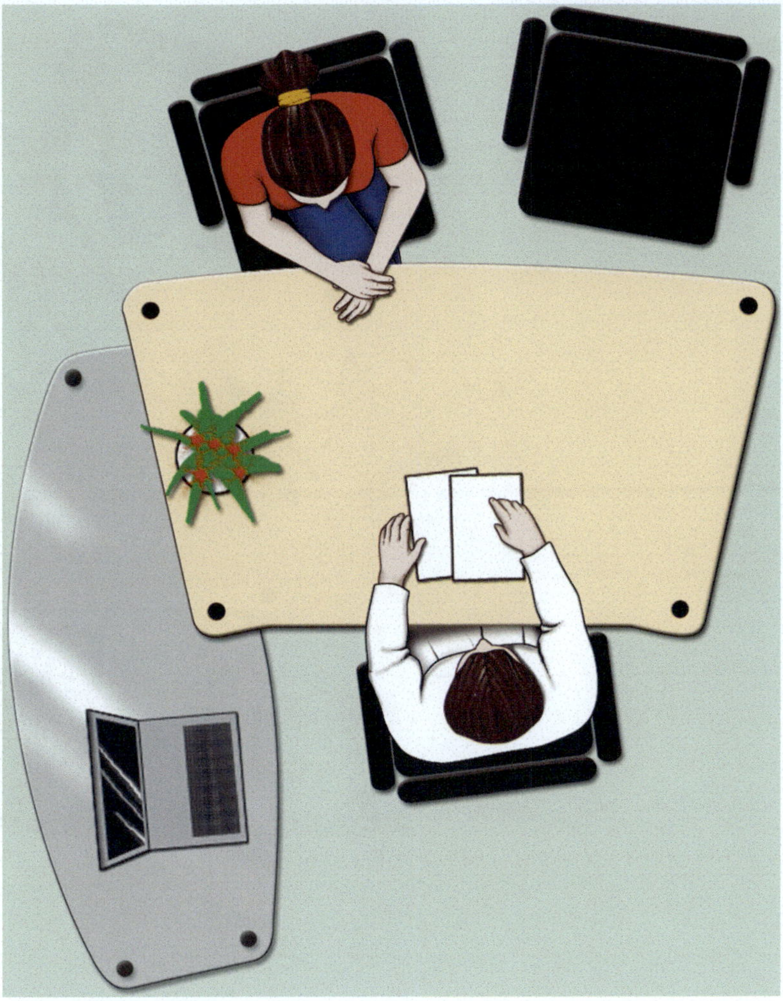

Fig. 1.2 During the initial interview and successive communication, the patient is seated opposite the doctor (the distance between them is about 110 cm)

There is enough space around the chair to see the patient's face from any view point and at any distance.

When the patient is seated in the examining chair, the mean distance between the doctor and the patient is about 60 cm (Fig. 1.4).

1.1.3 The Clinical Photography Area

The space for clinical photography is rather limited and occupies a corner of the room. The lighting equipment and technique for capturing the images are described in Chap. 2, whereas Chap. 3 illustrates how to acquire a complete set of clinical facial photographs.

1.2 The First Consultation Approach

1.2.1 The First Ten Minutes

The first 10 min spent with a new patient is the most decisive in establishing the best line of communication. In that brief period of time, personal impressions about each other are created and are

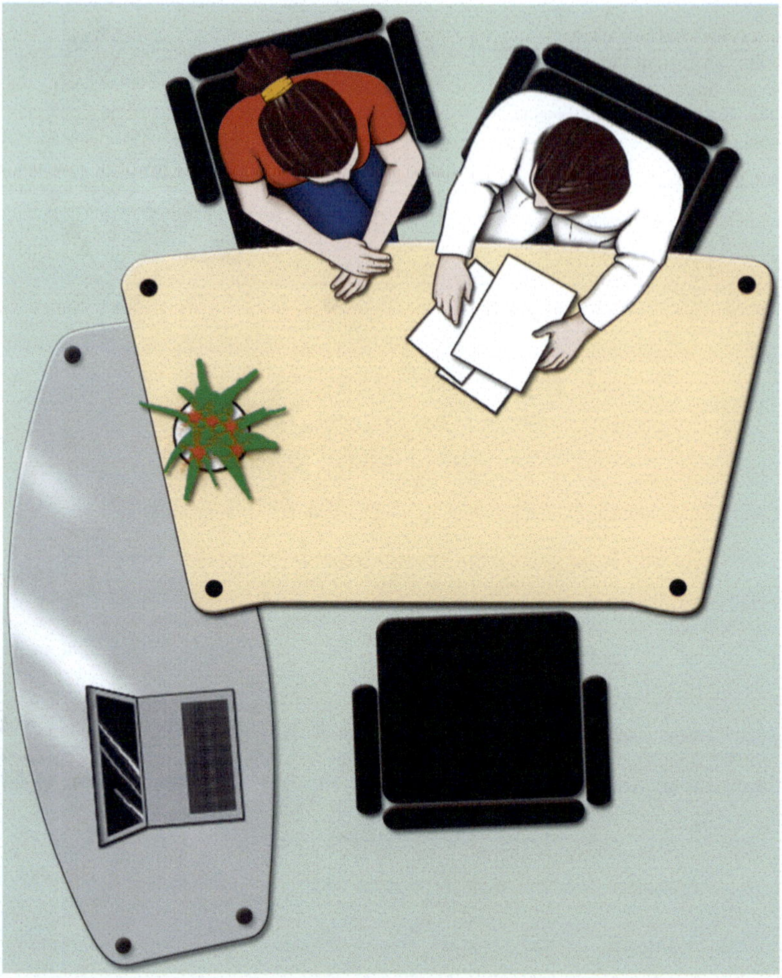

Fig. 1.3 Only when discussing the clinical photographs and the treatment plan in detail is the doctor seated beside the patient, reducing the distance to about 60 cm

later changed only with great difficulty. So, exceed patient expectations on their initial consultation.

1.2.2 The Entrance

When I meet a new patient, I need to know in advance a few important facts. She has had two contacts with my staff before: the first, a telephone call for the booking, a few days earlier, and the second, at the entrance to the office, a few minutes before. These are two perfect occasions to ask her:

- Her name, address, and telephone number
- The most suitable day and time for her consultation
- The reason for the consultation
- Which of my patients, friends, or colleagues referred her to my practice (I must reward this person soon!)

This knowledge will allow me to direct the approach and the information toward her needs.

Also, the patient needs to know in advance something about the competence, care, and specializations of my practice, and the first telephone contact should be an important opportunity to offer these, as well as some other information.

When the nurse introduces the patient and the accompanying persons into my room, I am in another workroom, and I come in after a few seconds. I prefer this more dynamic type of introduction rather than the other, where the doctor is

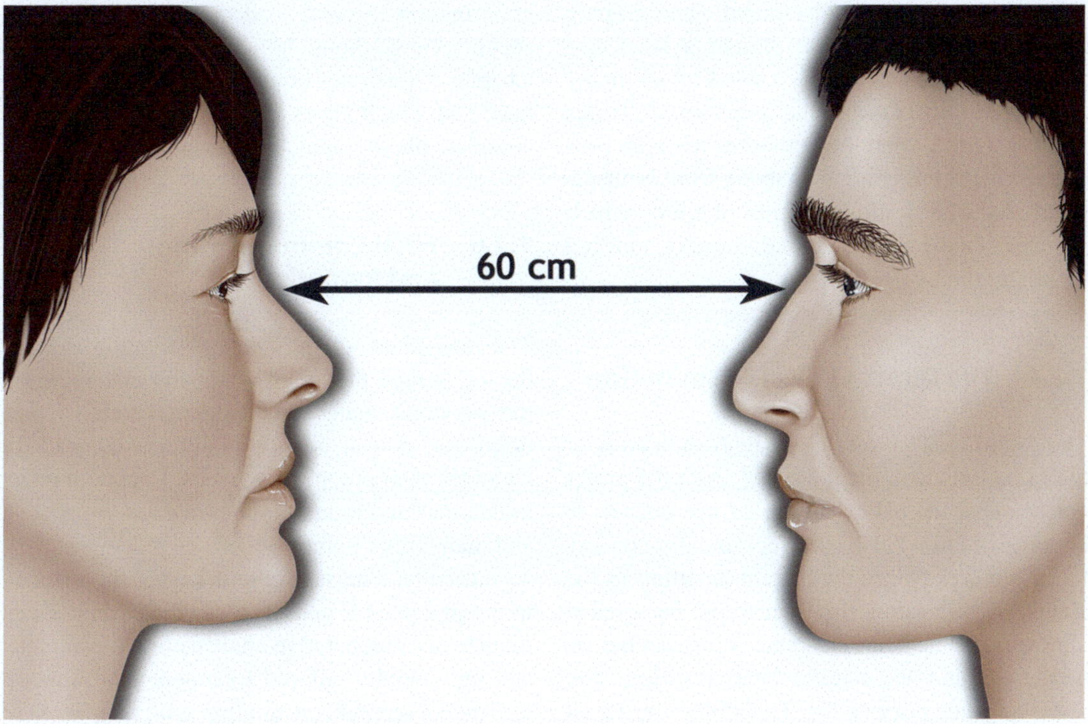

Fig. 1.4 During the clinical facial examination, the doctor's eyes should be at the same height as the patient's eyes, and the distance between them is about 60 cm

waiting, sitting in a relaxed position on his chair. In this manner, I greet the patient with a handshake, smile, and introduce myself before sitting in front of her [4].

1.2.3 The Interview

I have learned to ask questions to establish a rapport. Even if my secretary has informed me that the next person requested a consultation because she has a nose that she considers to be too large and I am a rhinoplasty surgeon, I start by asking "What is the main reason you are here today, Mrs. Smith?"

My open questions concentrate on the patient's concerns, and I want to remain focused on that aspect, resisting the temptation to interrupt the patient in this early phase if she is still talking.

The next step is to help the patient organize and dictate her personal patient's priority list, her way of communicating problems, needs, wishes, and expectations. I write this down personally in an itemized way to make the order of importance given by the patient clear at every point. Avoid "translating" into strict medical language everything she says and be sure not to suggest undetected problems at this time.

Beginning with this fixed scheme, I avoid any improvisation in the first 10 min, which means loss of control and insecurity in the patient's eyes. As Tardy and Thomas [6] pointed out, "… two relative strangers proceed to make judgments about each other: the patient about whether she can have unqualified confidence in the surgeon consulted, and the surgeon about whether a favorable outcome is likely to be achieved that will result in a satisfied and happy patient."

The interview continues in order to obtain information about general health status, taking of aspirin and other drugs, allergies, previous medical, and surgical treatments and to offer detailed information about the successive direct clinical examination and clinical photographic documentation. I give the patient a brief and clear explanation as to why I need to ask many of the questions. During the interview, I always say that an important objective for me is to produce an in-depth clinical analysis from both the functional and aesthetic points of view, which serves as a basis for an individually tailored treatment plan.

1.2.4 The Direct Clinical Examination

The "unofficial" direct clinical examination of the face starts with the interview, even if I prefer not to make the patient aware of my interest in her nose or chin. I also avoid commenting on any facial features before the patient is sitting in the chair. After elevating the chair to put her eyes at almost the same height as mine, I instruct her on how to obtain the natural head position, and reviewing her priority list, I examine the facial features. I always give her a facial mirror, which helps in communicating ideas and points to each other.

The direct examination continues with some maneuvers, which I carry out utilizing a pair of examining gloves; these are specific to the clinical case (e.g., palpation of the nasal dorsum and tip in rhinoplasty patients to explore the length of the nasal bone and the resilience of the cartilaginous skeleton). Intranasal and intraoral examinations are mandatory in almost every case; to reassure and obtain the consent of the patient, I never forget to inform her about what I am doing.

Again, also in this more "practical" step of the consultation, I must resist the temptation to interrupt the patient when she is telling me something she thinks is important.

1.2.5 The Clinical Photographic Documentation

The taking of clinical photographs must be performed after the interview and the direct examination in order to decide which series of specific views should be added to the basic one. Chapter 3 illustrates how to position the patient's head and which views should be taken to obtain complete photographic documentation.

1.2.6 Final Communications and Remarks

The final phase of the first consultation is conducted around the table, as for the interview. In the previous stages, my listening activity was dominant; now it is time to inform the patient about the next preoperative steps, treatment plan, indications and limits of the procedure proposed, and many other points.

Basically, I must decide if I want this patient in my practice [3] and, if this is the case, if I can finalize my preoperative analysis into a complete and individually tailored treatment plan now or schedule a second consultation with the patient.

When dealing with facial aesthetics, I am cautious about putting a right profile view into the monitor of my personal computer to show, in a spectacular way, how I could cut the nasal hump and project the chin. Moving quickly on to a definitive treatment plan requires two conditions: a doctor with long experience and a well-motivated "ideal" patient. Often, I favor giving information about the feasibility of the treatment, and, if it is appropriate, I give the patient a take-home brochure with an overview of the surgery recommended, reserving the discussion on the optimal treatment plan for the next visit.

The last phrase before the final greeting is "Please read the brochure and write down any questions for the next consultation."

1.3 The Time Spent in Organizing the Next Consultation

Ideally, the patient is scheduled for her second consultation 1 week later, in order to give her time to complete the preoperative instrumental examinations requested (e.g., CT or plan radiograms). I prefer not to exceed 10 days because even if I have several methods to review in my mind, waiting longer is counterproductive, both because the patient forgets what has been discussed and it prolongs her psychological stress.

In each case, this time is necessary for me to organize the clinical images and data collected and to debate the feasible treatment options. The main steps are:

- For each photographic view, select the best image, optimize its contrast and brightness, and print it. For the right profile view, I also enlarge and print a life-size copy.
- Confirm or partially modify and enrich the findings obtained with the direct clinical examination and also perform the analysis on photographs.
- Perform the dental casts and the cephalometric analysis if necessary.
- Create the doctor priority list and review the patient priority list.
- Create an ideal provisional treatment plan and any other viable alternatives to it.

The doctor priority list is the itemized list of findings (not only problems!) obtained in order of importance. In this way, positive aspects like a beautiful and proportioned nose or a healthy facial skin are also detected and reported as things that need to be conserved. This step is made easier by utilizing the checklists discussed in Chaps. 5, 6, 7, 8 and 9, which are also available on Springer Extra Materials (extras.springer.com).

1.4 The Second (and Successive) Consultation Approach

The successive preoperative consultations are quite different to the first for two reasons. First, I do not need a standard and sometimes rigorous approach because, knowing the person, her problems and needs, it is time to personalize the approach. Second, my previous role of "listener" should move into a new and more active one of the surgeon, who produces the best treatment plan for the patient.

Immediately before meeting the patient, I review the patient priority list, the doctor (my) priority list, the provisional treatment plan, and all the documents collected or developed and the instrumental exams delivered by the patient. To show and explain my findings and treatment purposes, I sit alongside the patient and utilize extensively her clinical photographs.

1.5 How to Enhance Patient/Physician Communication

Good communication is vital for a constructive patient/physician relationship as well for the clinical facial analysis. How well you explain your ideas and understand the needs of the patient directly influences all your successive work. The cornerstones of communication are:

- Greet your patient with a handshake, and sit down in front of her during the consultation.
- Listen, really listen to your patient. Listen to understand. Listening requires us not only to hear what the other person is saying, but to comprehend it as well. Improve your ability to listen by videotaping yourself and note how many times you mistakenly stop the patient when she is talking to you.
- Maintain eye contact. Be sure to look directly at the patient and to any accompanying person.
- Smile and offer reassuring comments such as "I understand," "Okay, right," "Yes." Echo what she has said to show you are paying attention.
- Utilize some visual tools to explain the relevant aspects of the treatment. A high percentage of what we remember, we recall because we associate it with images.
- Use general and simple examples to reinforce your ideas.
- Avoid excessive pessimism and unrestrained optimism in delivering any information.
- Review the main points before the end of the consultation. Repetition is the doctor's way of emphasizing crucial points, and it is not necessarily redundancy.

- Work cooperatively with your staff to further enhance communication.
- Do not forget to communicate the positive aspects of your work as well as your commitment in doing it [1, 2, 5].

1.6 The Single Operator Concept

All patients want a coordinator and a leader to approach their problems and feel negatively toward different people conducting the assessment and the planning. The single operator concept emphasizes the importance of your patient being followed by you in all the main clinical steps with the ideal coordination of information and activity with the medical team and office personnel.

If you need to consult a more experienced colleague or a different specialist, you must directly organize, present, and actively coordinate the meeting, to underline the importance and the support you continue to give the case.

References

1. Bernard S (2001) Communication in health care. In: The Health Care Communication Group (ed) Writing, speaking, and communication skill for health professionals. Yale University Press, New Haven
2. Casella PJ (2001) Speaking for success. In: The Health Care Communication Group (ed) Writing, speaking, and communication skill for health professionals. Yale University Press, New Haven
3. Daniel RK (2002) Rhinoplasty. An atlas of surgical techniques. Springer, New York
4. Guastamacchia C, Tosolin F (1997) Gestione della pratica professionale odontoiatrica. Masson, Milan
5. Rohrich RJ (2001) The market of plastic surgery. Cosmetic surgery for sale – at what price? Plast Reconstr Surg 107:1845–1847
6. Tardy ME, Regan Thomas J (1995) Facial aesthetic surgery. Mosby Year Book, St Louis, p 148

2 Lighting Techniques for Clinical Facial Photography

Contents

Several times we have observed my colleagues getting annoyed because of a less-than-perfect result obtained with the latest high-ended camera. What are the weak points in clinical facial photography? The principal variables are the type of camera, the quality of the lighting, the lenses, the film (or the CCD), the background panel, patient positioning, and camera positioning (framing) during the photographic shoot. Additional important steps are film developing and printing, as well as picture storage.

After years of direct experience and commitment, I am convinced that the most demanding aspects of clinical photography are patient lighting, the topic of this chapter, and patient positioning and framing, which is discussed in Chap. 3.

2.1 Lighting Techniques for Clinical Facial Photography[1]

The taking of clinical photographs, to record and to utilize during surgery, is an essential part of the activities of every professional practice or facial surgery department. The narrowness of the office, the cost of the equipment, and a vague lack of time do not constitute excuses for less precise patient documentation.

To obtain the best quality and consistency of results, many suggest the use of a professional lighting system composed of two or more flash

[1] Adapted from [5]

F. Meneghini, P. Biondi, *Clinical Facial Analysis*,
DOI 10.1007/978-3-642-27228-8_2, © Springer-Verlag Berlin Heidelberg 2012

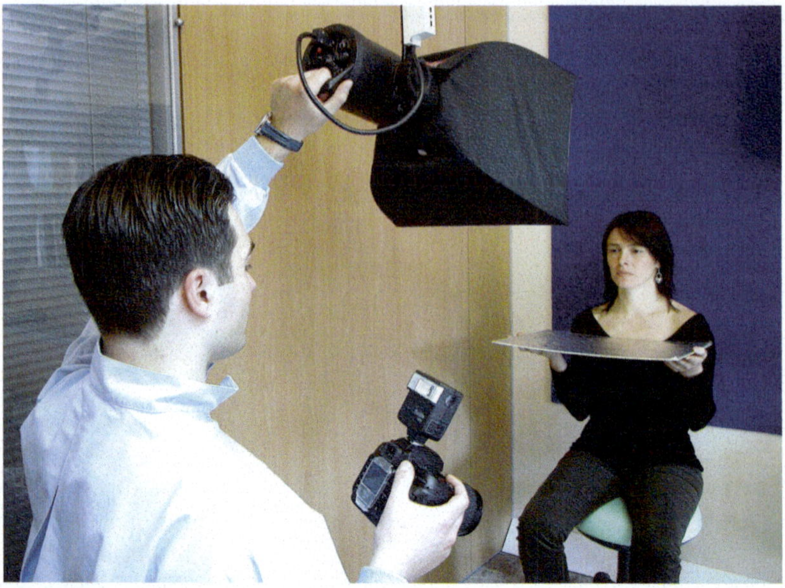

Fig. 2.1 Photographic set. The patient holds, with her hands, a small rectangular reflecting panel positioned horizontally against the chest, just under the collarbone. The operator easily adjusts the monolight vertically and horizontally

units. Thus, an entire room or a large part of it should be permanently reserved for this use.

In the past 8 years, I have utilized a system of lighting based on a unique source of light (monolight flash), which is ceiling-mounted in a corner of a room also dedicated for other activities, with good results. This chapter presents a description of the key technical points and the rationale for using single-light equipment. All the clinical facial photographs that illustrate this book have been obtained utilizing this lighting system.

2.2 Equipment and Technique

The studio lighting equipment consists of a single professional flash (System 300 professional compact flash by System Imaging Ltd, UK), which is ceiling mounted on a straight rail parallel to the background panel. The total length of the rail is 0.95 m. The distance of the flash unit from the background is fixed at 1.6 m. A pantograph (Friction Pantograph 3250 by I.F.F., Calenzano–Firenze) holds the monolight and allows unrestricted vertical adjustment. A rectangular 0.75 × 0.35 m soft box (75 Light Bank by System Imaging Ltd, UK) fits on the flash unit, softening and diffusing the light. An alternative smaller and more practical soft box, 0.4 × 0.3 m (Chimera Lightbanks, Boulder, Colorado, USA), has also been utilized during the past 5 years.

The distance from the monolight to the subject is fixed (about 1.1–1.2 m), so each photograph is taken at the same F-stop of 16 with 100 ISO films.

The lighting is directed toward the subject in all views, maintaining the flash unit at a higher level. The rectangular soft box is held in a horizontal position.

In order to eliminate the problem of shadows on the submental region and under the nasal base, the patient holds, with her hands, a small rectangular reflecting panel of 0.35 × 0.7 m (Fig. 2.1). This panel is positioned horizontally against the chest, just under the collarbone.

The ceiling-mounted rail allows the adjustment of the monolight to a side or central position (Fig. 2.1). It easily follows the rotation of the subject from the frontal to oblique and lateral views. Figure 2.2 shows the basic positions of the flash unit used in the different views to achieve the best results. An important rule is to maintain the subject's position close to the background panel itself in order to avoid the need for an adjunctive flash unit to light the background panel.

For a routine set of photographs consisting of full-face portraits and closeup views, I use the 105 mm Micro-Nikkor lens.

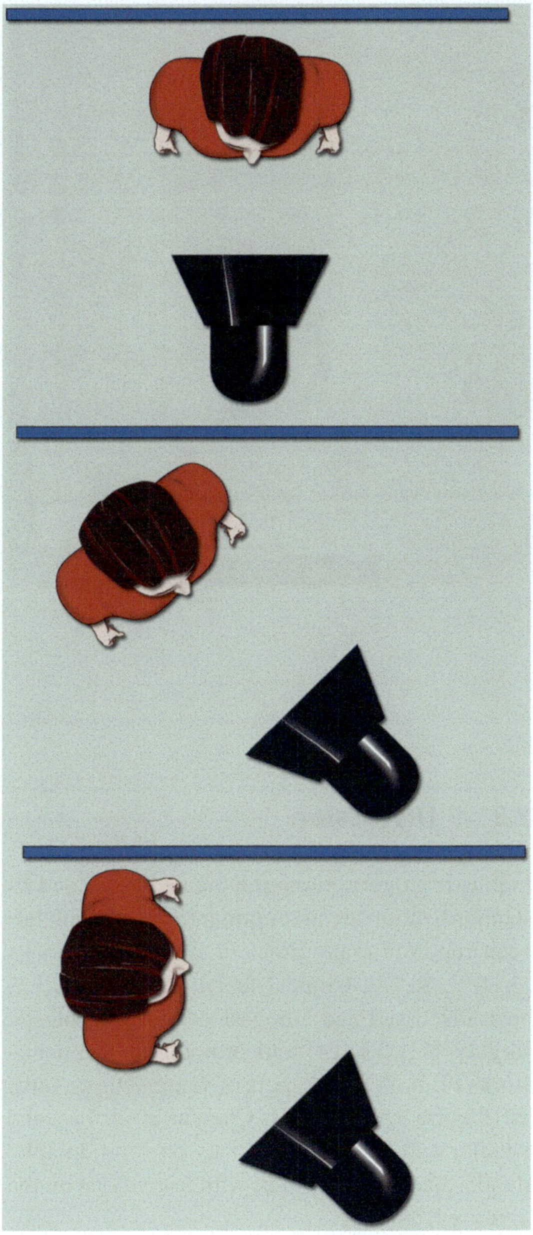

Fig. 2.2 The three main patient/monolight positions utilized to capture the various facial views

I personally do not use a camera tripod for stability because of the very short time of light emission by the flash unit; focusing is done by moving the camera back and forth. A camera tripod also interferes with the positioning of the monolight and the patient's head. In almost every case, I directly help the patient during positioning, touching her chin with my hand (Fig. 2.3). On the other hand, a viewfinder grid screen is highly recommended to help the surgeon orient the camera precisely.

To avoid using a direct wire connection to the monolight, a small on-camera electronic flash, oriented in a reverse direction, gives the input to the built-in slave unit of the main flash.

The space reserved for clinical photography in the room is rather narrow, as illustrated in Fig. 1.1 of the previous chapter.

Due to the combination of movements permitted by the pantograph and the ceiling-mounted rail, the flash unit can be easily positioned high up, near the ceiling and on the left wall of the room when not in use to leave space for other activities.

The blue background panel, 0.95 m wide and 1.10 m high, is made from a sheet of plastic material for outdoor use. An advantage of this panel is that it is washable without running the risk of losing or changing the color.

The patient and I sit on rotating stools with rollers. The chairs are easily adjusted in the vertical position in order to maintain the subject and the camera at the same height during the capture of the images.

I usually take my clinical photographs personally, without the aid of an assistant, and the entire procedure requires no more than 5 min. For better efficiency and to save time, I follow a specific sequence:

- I ask the patient to meet me in the photo area, turn on the monolight, instruct her on how to use the reflecting panel correctly, and adjust her height on the stool, close to the blue background panel.
- I pick up my camera, turn on the small on-camera electronic flash, and set the standard time/diaphragm couple of 1/125 s–F16 with the monolight adjusted to full-power light emission.
- I shoot the frontal view first, with the patient and the flash unit oriented, as in Fig. 2.2 (top).
- I position the patient's head for the extended and basal views and take the photographs. The position of the monolight remains unchanged.
- I position the patient for the right oblique views, taking care to maintain her close to the blue background panel. The monolight is oriented, as in Fig. 2.2 (central), and the photos are taken.
- I position the patient for the right profile view, taking care to maintain her close to the blue background panel, and shoot the photo.

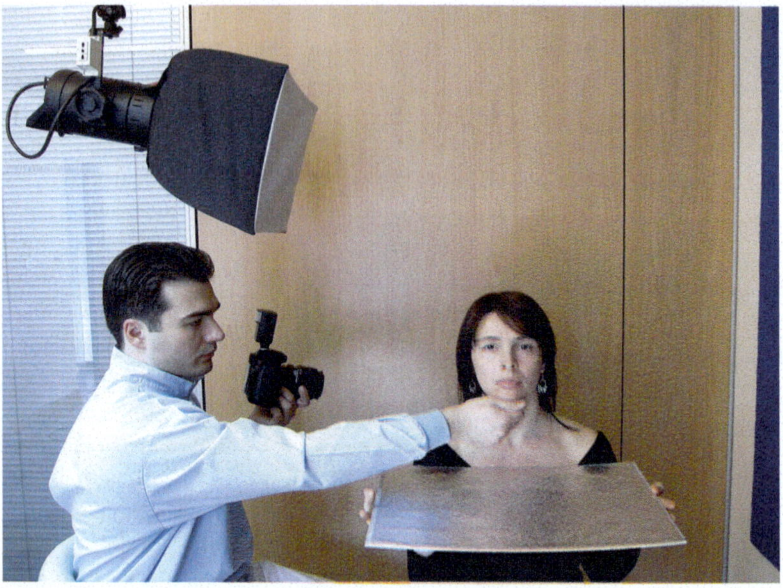

Fig. 2.3 Positioning of the patient's head

The position of the flash unit remains unchanged, as depicted in Fig. 2.2 (bottom).

- I repeat the two latter steps for the left oblique and profile views, orienting the patient's head and the monolight consequently.

During the procedure, I help the patient to assume a relaxed face and no smile, if indicated. For each view, I systematically take at least two shots to reduce the possibility of photos with the eyes closed and generally to ensure a better choice of photos later.

Currently, this lighting equipment is also used with a digital camera (Fujifilm digital camera FinePix S1 Pro) mounted with the 105 mm Micro-Nikkor lens. The quality of the imaging is fairly good, but, in this particular case, the distance between the camera and the subject for a full-face portrait, using the 105-mm lens, is increased to 1.5 m, due to the reduction of the sensitive area of the CCD compared with the sensitive area of the conventional 35-mm film.

Chapter 3 shows a complete set of clinical facial views using the equipment and technique described above.

2.3 Discussion

In plastic surgery, photographic technique and its standardization are an important topic, which has been reported many times in articles and books [3, 4, 7, 8, 15]. Clinical facial photography has been discussed and emphasized in facial plastic surgery [11, 12, 14] and orthodontic published works [1, 6, 9]. The papers of some authors, such as Ellenbogen et al. [4], Claman et al. [1], and Sandler and Murray [9], focus on reproducible, standardized photographs, with less advice on the lighting technique.

Other authors, such as Zarem [15], warn of the poor results obtained with an on-camera single flash or a ring-light flash. The on-camera single flash creates sharp shadows on the subject and background, so many facial details and contours are, unfortunately, lost. A system using a ring-light flash mounted on the frontal element of the lens reduces the problem of shadows on the subject but produces flat, unrealistic images and frames the subject with a dark halo.

The reported literature recommends having professional studio lighting in a dedicated photo room in order to obtain images of the highest quality.

DiBernardino et al. [3] recommend the use of two or more flash units and present a diagram in which two main lights at 45° angles to the subject are combined with two additional background lights, again at 45° angles, to eliminate shadows in the background. Daniel et al. [2] advise the occasional use of an additional light placed overhead to accentuate the hair and highlight certain areas.

Many authors [2, 10, 11, 13] have investigated lighting techniques for facial photographs in rhinoplasty patients. Daniel et al. [2] and Staffel [11], in particular, report their observations on the effects of different positioning of the two main lights on the nasal tip. Both articles point out that any changes in lighting produce a different type of reflection. Simply by moving the lights further laterally, increasing the angle of incidence, the nasal tip appears more pointed, whereas an asymmetric positioning produces an asymmetric reflection on the tip, which could be mistaken for a real anatomical asymmetry. Even in a dedicated room for patient photography, with fixed light sources and a camera mounted on a fixed tripod, the variable of the patient position remains.

In discussing this topic, Jack Sheen stated that "There is no doubt that photographs can be manipulated. And lighting is probably the easiest, most effective way to manipulate an image" [10].

Meredith [6] includes positioning the patient too close to the background in his list of faulty techniques that are responsible for less-than-optimal results in facial photography. In his prescription, there should be at least 0.75 m between the back of the subject's head and the rear wall, to prevent shadows.

2.3.1 Point, Line, and Plane

Generally speaking, a photograph may be illegible due to underexposure (too much black) or overexposure (too much white). In clinical facial photography, the shadows (underexposed areas) may be divided into three subtypes: pointed, linear, and plane. Whereas the first two are positive because they underline some characteristics of the face (for instance, a depressed scar or a sulcus), the third is negative, as it hides other characteristics (for instance, the definition of the chin – neck angle).

In the same manner, the reflexes (overexposed areas) may also be divided into three subtypes: pointed, linear, and plane. Whereas the first two are positive because they highlight some characteristics of the face (for instance, a pointed nasal tip or a prominent zygomatic arch), the third is negative, as it cancels other characteristics.

The main aim of the lighting technique developed is to produce legible images, sometimes with points and lines.

2.3.2 A "Natural" Option

The sun is the main natural source of lighting, but for clinical purposes, it has a weak point: its distance from the subject, in spite of its great dimensions, makes it similar to a point light source, which, on a clear day, produces sharp shadows. Two symmetric lights of the same power, relatively far from the subject, produce unnatural lighting in which one corrects the shadow produced by the other's illumination. For clinical use, the best natural condition is a cloudy but bright day in which the light of one source, the sun, loses its contrast by the diffusion of the clouds, and the softened shadows on the subject show the main direction of the light itself. In this case, the observer easily perceives the natural modeling effect of the light on the surface of the face, whereas with two symmetric lights, only the reflection of the flash in the pupils of the eyes reveals the type of lighting used. In other words, if the observer is aware of the direction of the light, the reading of the images through its soft shadows is enhanced.

2.3.3 Problems with Two or More Lights

In my personal experience, the use of two or more flash units is counterproductive and unnecessary. The negative aspects of a multiple light system are:

- Increased cost (almost double).
- Occupies more space.
- More complex technique (increases the parameters that potentially require adjustments).
- The effects of any single-light source are difficult to assess due to the presence of other lights.

In a single flash system, the orientation of the light is easily adjusted from one view to another because the operator directly controls the shadows and the reflection on the face with the aid of the floodlighting. The reflecting panel, held by the patient, does not require any adjustment during the change from one view to another (keep the variables to a minimum!).

2.3.4 Avoid a False Asymmetric Face

The main views used to confirm or exclude the presence of facial asymmetry are frontal, extended, and basal. For that reason, any differences in side-to-side lighting during the shooting of these particular images may produce an erroneous conclusion. In any system, using two main lights, the power output of the two units, the type of soft boxes utilized, the orientation, the distance from the subject, the angles of incidence, and the height of the tripods must be identical. In other words, six different parameters set on the right unit must be reproduced exactly on the left. Any deviation from a perfect equilibrium produces a false asymmetric patient or changes the appreciation of a true asymmetry.

With my approach to lighting, symmetry is easily achievable in frontal, extended, and basal views, positioning the monolight directly in front of the subject at a higher level and asking the patient to hold the reflecting panel horizontally against her chest, just under the collarbone. In each case, the camera must be positioned perfectly frontal to the subject.

2.3.5 The Importance of Soft Box Size

The selection of the size of the soft box has repercussions on the quality and the ease of use. In particular, the large light banks (0.75 × 0.35 m) produce softer light and, because of their wide and homogeneous lighting, permit easy subject positioning. The small light banks (0.30 × 0.40 m), on the contrary, produce harder light and enhance the texture of the skin, and it is difficult to obtain the ideal position because the area covered with homogeneous light is smaller, and there is an increased likelihood of undesired shadows.

With the same emission power and distance from flash to subject, the smaller light bank also provides higher intensity and hence greater depth of field (the range within which objects are in focus).

2.3.6 Avoid Shadows on the Background Panel

Meredith's assertion that there is at least 0.75 m between the back of the subject's head and the rear wall to prevent shadows [6] is a misconception caused by poor lighting technique. If the light source is positioned too far from the subject, a sharp shadow is created on the background, even with a large soft box or umbrella to diffuse the light.

In summary, the keys to avoiding shadows are:

- Bring the flash near to the subject and the background.
- Diffuse the light with a 0.30 × 0.40 m or wider soft box.
- Use a reflecting panel under the face.

2.3.7 Advantages of Ceiling-Mounted Equipment

The advantages of ceiling-mounted equipment are sound. The floor is completely free of cables, tripod, stands, or other objects. The pantograph and rail system permit unrestricted horizontal and vertical movement of the monolight, while maintaining a relatively fixed distance from the subject and the background. Access to the area is easier for the patient, and at the end of the procedure, the equipment can be set aside to gain space for other activities in a few seconds.

2.4 The Seven Rules of Multiple Shots

1. Document every new patient with multiple shots whether or not she will be treated later.
2. Multiple shots of the same view ensure that if the patient blinks, you have plenty of non-blinking shots to choose from.
3. Multiple shots assure a better choice later.
4. After a rigorous capture of the standard view set, if you wish, perform multiple shots to document, in a personalized manner and without restrictions, the features of the face.
5. Use the skin marker to point out any particular deformity or lesion and perform multiple shots from different points of view to avoid shadows and reflections.
6. During capture of the full-face oblique view and full-face basal view, perform multiple shots in conjunction with small differences in head position.
7. Today, with digital cameras, the extra cost of multiple shots is small (one or 100 shots cost roughly the same). The methodology for better documentation must be cultivated daily, applying the seven rules of multiple shots, which also help to develop greater photographic skills. Clinical facial photography is, in a large part, a rigorous procedure, which requires a protocol to assure clarity and consistency, but, unfortunately, it is also, in a small part, an art.

References

1. Claman L, Paqtton D, Rashid R (1990) Standardized portrait photography for dental patients. Am J Orthod Dentofacial Orthop 98:197
2. Daniel RK, Hodgson J, Lambros VS (1990) Rhinoplasty: the light reflexes. Plast Reconstr Surg 85:859
3. DiBernardino BE, Adams RL, Krause J, Fiorillo MA, Gheradini G (1998) Photographic standards in plastic surgery. Plast Reconstr Surg 102:559
4. Ellenbogen R, Jankauskas S, Collini FJ (1990) Achieving standardized photographs in aesthetic surgery. Plast Reconstr Surg 86:955
5. Meneghini F (2001) Clinical facial photography in a small office: lighting equipment and technique. Aesthetic Plast Surg 25:299–306
6. Meredith G (1997) Facial photography for the orthodontic office. Am J Orthod Dentofacial Orthop 111:463
7. Morello DC, Converse JM, Allen D (1977) Making uniform photographic records in plastic surgery. Plast Reconstr Surg 59:366
8. Nelson GD, Krause JL (eds) (1988) Clinical photography in plastic surgery. Little, Brown and Company, Boston/Toronto
9. Sandler J, Murray A (1997) Clinical photography in orthodontics. J Clin Orthod 31:729
10. Sheen JH (1990) Discussion to: Daniel RK, Hodgson J, Lambros VS. Rhinoplasty: the light reflexes. Plast Reconstr Surg 85:867
11. Staffel JG (1997) Photo documentation in rhinoplasty. Facial Plast Surg 13:317
12. Tardy ME Jr, Thomas JR (1995) Facial aesthetic surgery, 1st edn, Year book. Mosby, St. Louis, pp 94–123
13. Tebbetts JB (1998) Photography and computer-assisted imaging in rhinoplasty – appendix B. In: Primary rhinoplasty. A new approach to the logic and the techniques. Mosby, St. Louis, p 581
14. Thomas JR, Tardy ME Jr, Prezekop H (1980) Uniform photographic documentation in facial plastic surgery. Otolaryngol Clin North Am 13:367
15. Zarem HA (1984) Standard of photography. Plast Reconstr Surg 74:137

Views of Clinical Facial Photography

3

Contents

The pictures in this chapter are taken from the scientific poster "Views of Clinical Facial Photography," conceived and realized by F. Meneghini in May 2003.

The photographic documentation of our patients must have the following important features: completeness, standardization, and quality. All physicians dealing with facial aesthetics need these documents for analysis, patient communication, planning, as an intraoperative tool, for early and late follow-up, for self-teaching and teaching objectives, and also for medicolegal purposes.

The previous chapter describes a personal technique used to obtain standardization and quality in lighting the face. This chapter illustrates how to position the patient's head and which views should be taken to obtain complete photographic documentation.

3.1 Natural Head Position

The natural head position (NHP) is a standardized and reproducible orientation of the head achieved when one is looking at a distant point in front of one, at eye level. The great majority of clinical photographs and direct clinical examination steps require the NHP; in addition, patient positioning for cephalometric analysis should be the NHP. The simplest way to obtain the NHP is to instruct the patient to look straight ahead at a point at eye level on the wall in front of him [4].

Sometimes, the orientation obtained seems unnatural to the examiner, but, on asking the

F. Meneghini, P. Biondi, *Clinical Facial Analysis*,
DOI 10.1007/978-3-642-27228-8_3, © Springer-Verlag Berlin Heidelberg 2012

patient to tilt the head upward and downward and then return to looking straight ahead to the point at eye level, we have noted that the final spatial orientation is very similar to the initial one.

The NHP is of paramount importance in facial analysis due to its reproducibility and, most importantly, because it is extremely simple to obtain. In contrast, the Frankfort horizontal and the other constructed planes utilized to orient the head and based on internal skeletal landmarks are "unnatural" and difficult to obtain clinically.

3.2 How to Obtain Life-Size Photographs

Frequently, the preoperative case study needs a soft-tissue cephalometric analysis on life-size photographs. As described by Bahman Guyuron [3], I place an opaque white ruler close to the subject while shooting the images, taking care that both are perfectly focused to ensure the accuracy of the enlargement. With conventional films, the printer must be as large as the subject in order to have a final 1:1 scale in the print. With a digital camera, I now use a quick and simple method:

- Transfer the image to the personal computer.
- With Adobe Photoshop software, adjust contrast and brightness.
- Save in JPEG format for storage.
- Import the image into a Microsoft Word document and enlarge or reduce it to obtain a life-size dimension.
- Insert the date, the name of the patient, and any useful clinical notes.
- Print on A4 paper (210×297 mm) format to obtain space around the image for all future handwritten notes.

3.3 The Poster "Views of Clinical Facial Photography"

The experience acquired documenting thousands of patients and teaching on the maxillofacial surgery postgraduate course at the University of Padua convinced me to produce a poster to inform my patients and instruct my young colleagues about clinical facial photography. Its actual dimensions are 0.70 m wide and 0.50 m high. A printable full-size electronic copy is available on Springer Extra Materials.[1]

The background consists of a drawing of a large open left hand. On the palm, the 11 basic views taken for all patients during the initial examination and any successive postoperative checkups are illustrated, independently of the type of treatment planned. On the thumb, we see the five views added to the previous basic series in the case of nasal feature documentation; on the index finger, the five views in the case of documenting dentofacial deformities and/or orthodontic problems are added; on the middle finger, the seven views in the case of documenting orbital and lid features, and on the ring finger, the three views in the case of documenting ear features. Thus, there are a total of 31 standard facial pictures illustrated in the poster, and only four of these are not in the NHP.

The small piece of 35-mm film, on the little finger, is a reminder of the necessity to take any other useful photographs required by a particular clinical case.

I recommend hanging the poster up in the examining room, near the blue background panel utilized for facial photography. The goals obtained using this visual tool are:

- First, strengthening the doctor's skills, as a communicator, during the first consultation
- Second, helping the patient to understand the necessity of complete facial documentation and to cooperate actively during the shoot
- Third, assisting the doctor in following a rigorous method and sequence in patient documentation so that no views are forgotten or technical errors made

[1] Section 1 on Springer Extra Materials (extras.springer.com)

3.4 The Shooting of a Complete Set of Clinical Facial Photographs (Step-by-Step Description)

3.4.1 Accompanying the Patient in the Photo Area

The ideal time, during the first consultation with a new patient, for a complete set of clinical photography is described in Chap. 1. Before asking the patient to sit on the rotating stool with rollers, I illustrate the basic and specific views utilizing the poster, underlining the fact that I will take two or three shots for each view to avoid the problem of blinking. When we are both sitting face to face, I instruct him on how to obtain the NHP and then start the set, taking the 11 basic views.

3.4.2 The Eleven Basic Views

This series of pictures is fundamental and should be taken for all patients. All the basic views presented in this book are taken at a fixed subject–camera distance of 1.5 m with a digital camera (Fujifilm digital camera FinePix S1 Pro) mounted with the 105 mm Micro-Nikkor lens. Care should be taken to maintain the camera at the same height as the subject [5].

The first two or three shots are the full face frontal view (Fig. 3.1). The patient is instructed to look at the lens of the camera, which is held perfectly frontal to the subject. I do not always continue with the next view, but I prefer to review these in the monitor of the digital camera to check the exposure, the shadows, the patient positioning, and the occurrence of blinking. Setting a good full face frontal view is essential because many of the parameters do not change during the rest of the procedure.

The next view is the full face basal view (Fig. 3.2). These photographs are taken with two or three small differences in the grade of head extension due to the difficulty in reproducing the same non-NHP orientation at the time of follow-up.

The more extended position (Fig. 3.2b) is ideal for the analysis of the nasal base and the shape and symmetry of the zygomatic arches and the inferior border of the mandible, but note that the dorsal profile of the nose is hidden completely by the nasal base compared with the less extended position (Fig. 3.2a).

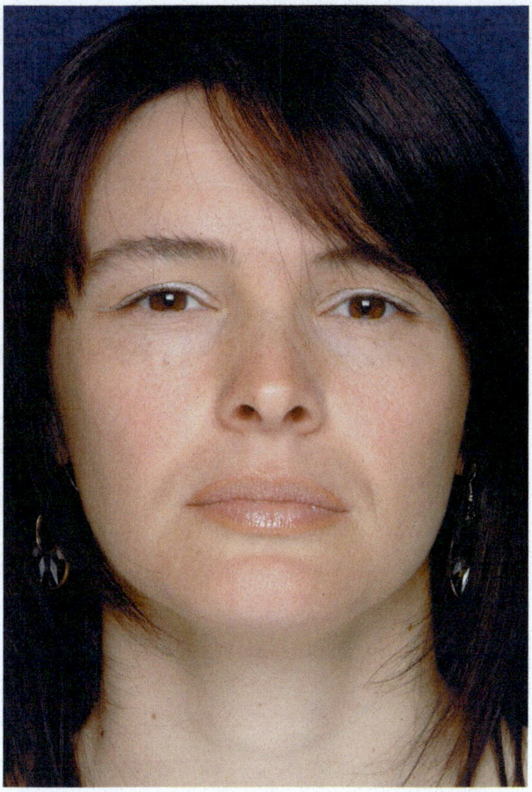

Fig. 3.1 Full face frontal view

For the next step, I ask the patient to return to the NHP and rotate the stool for the three full face oblique right views (Fig. 3.3). For a more precise head orientation, I find an object on the wall in front of the patient or a small part of it, at the same level as the patient's eyes, and I suggest that he looks at this point during shooting. Once the flash unit is oriented, I take these pictures, moving my camera from side to side to obtain three views with more or less rotation from the frontal view (to obtain these, I prefer to change the camera position instead of moving the patient's head).

These three oblique right views are taken to obtain more material for an in-depth analysis as well as to allow for the difficulty in reproducing the same head orientation in the future. Furthermore,

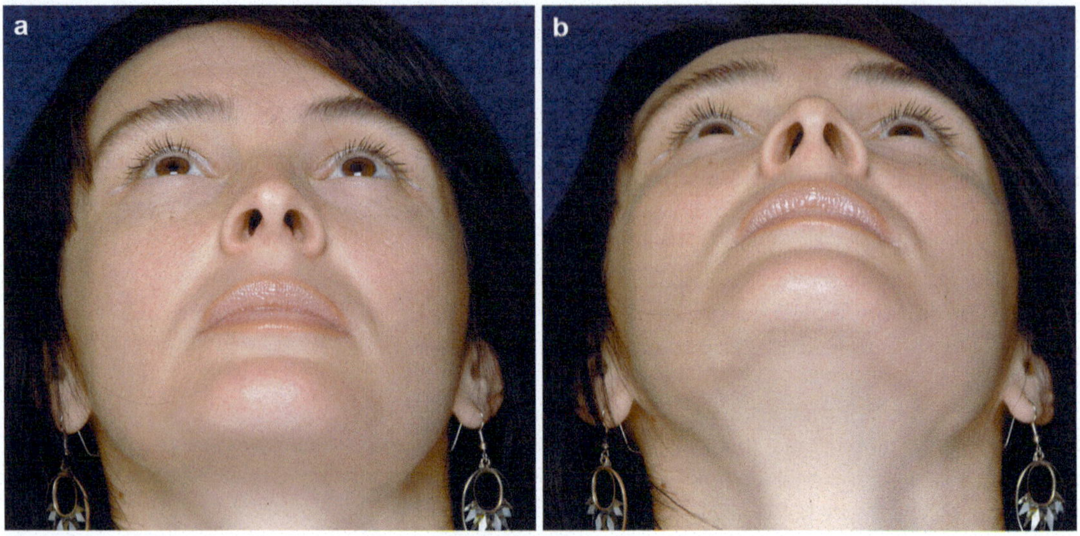

Fig. 3.2 Less extended (**a**) and more extended (**b**) full face basal views

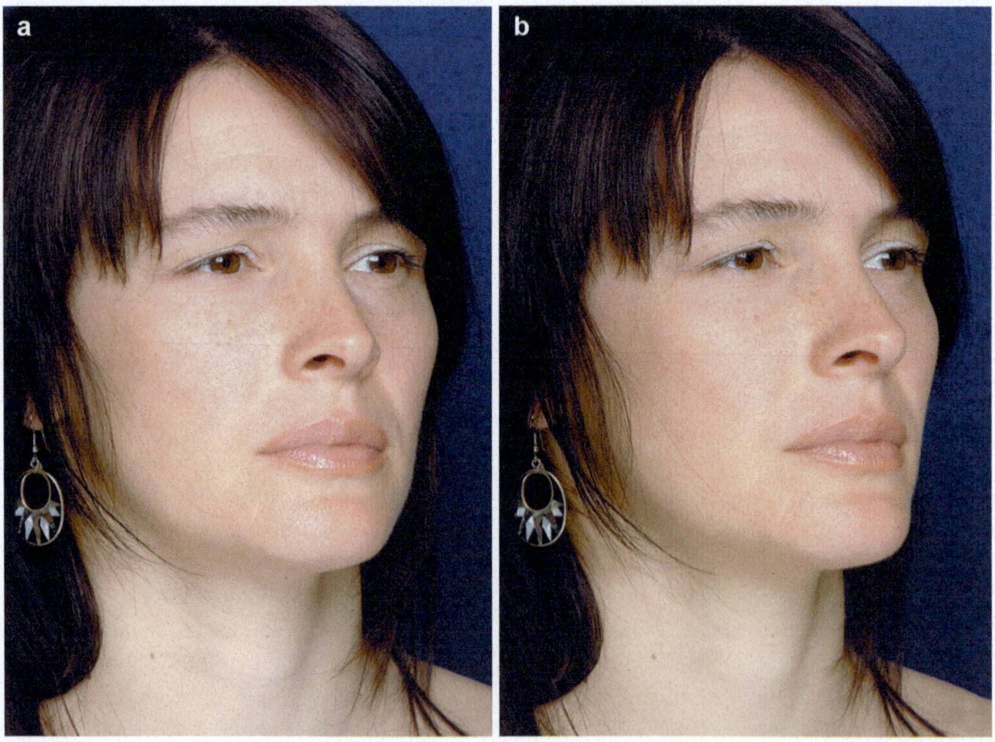

Fig. 3.3 Full face right oblique views (**a**–**c**)

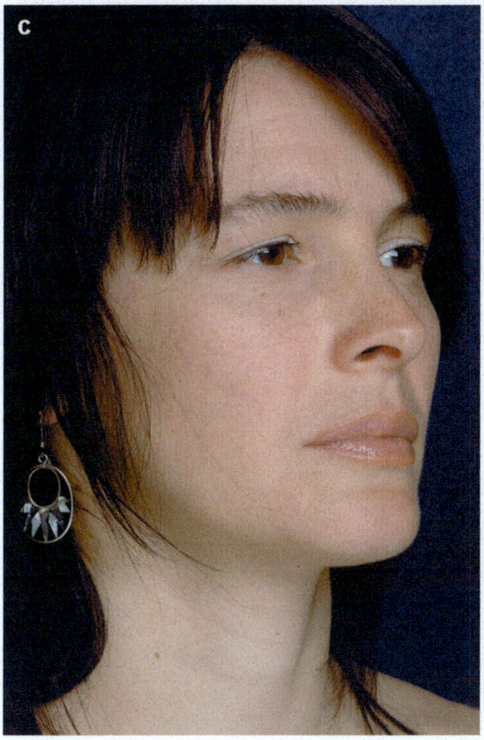

Fig. 3.3 (continued)

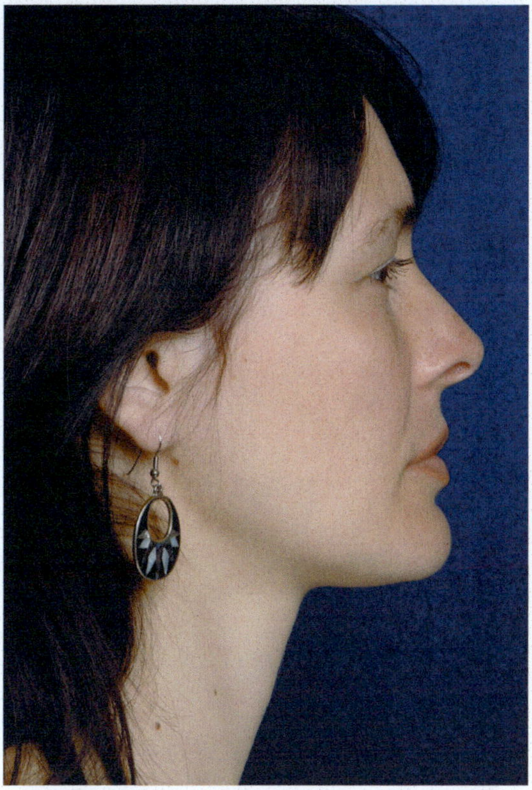

Fig. 3.4 Full face profile right view

each small difference in head rotation for the oblique views hides some facial details and highlights others; for example, the best oblique view to study the nasal outline is quite different from the best one to study the malar eminence.

The full face profile right view (Fig. 3.4) is taken next, taking care to orient the camera exactly perpendicular to the subject. In order to do that, during the framing, I move the camera slightly from side to side until the eyebrows are lined up.

After this, utilizing the same technique, the lighting system and the patient are oriented in the opposite positions for the full face oblique left views (Fig. 3.5) and the full face profile left view (Fig. 3.6).

3.4.3 The Five Nasal Views

If an in-depth study of nasal features is needed, as in the case of a rhinoplasty patient, the five nasal views are taken. With the patient sitting facing me, I ask him to tilt his face down and look at the reflecting panel; the perfect position for the facedown view (Fig. 3.7) is reached when the nasal dorsum is vertically oriented. This view is important clinically to check any asymmetry or external deformity of the nasal dorsum.

The next two nasal views are all close-up with a subject–camera distance less than 1.5 m and the presence inside the frame of a ruler, to permit a print at a 1:1 scale for successive analysis and precise surgical planning. The nasal base with ruler view (Fig. 3.8) is taken with the head in a more extended position, similar to that utilized for Fig. 3.2b, in which the dorsum is hidden completely by the nasal base. The right nasal profile with ruler view (Fig. 3.9) is taken in the NHP. The last two pictures, the depressor septi muscle action profile views, are useful for studying the effect of smiling on the tip of the nose caused by the activity of the depressor septi muscle. They are shot in rapid sequence and

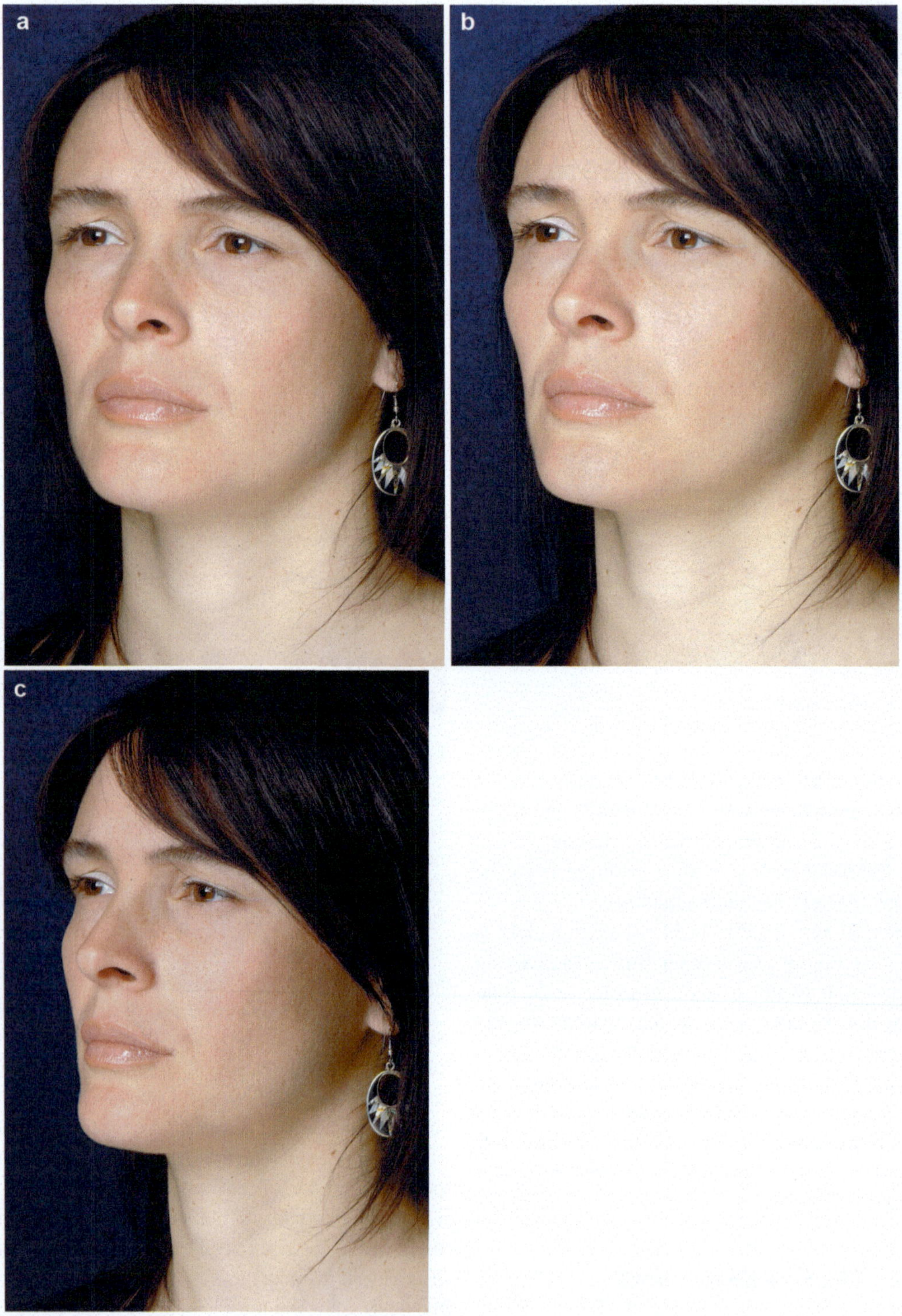

Fig. 3.5 Full face oblique views (**a**–**c**)

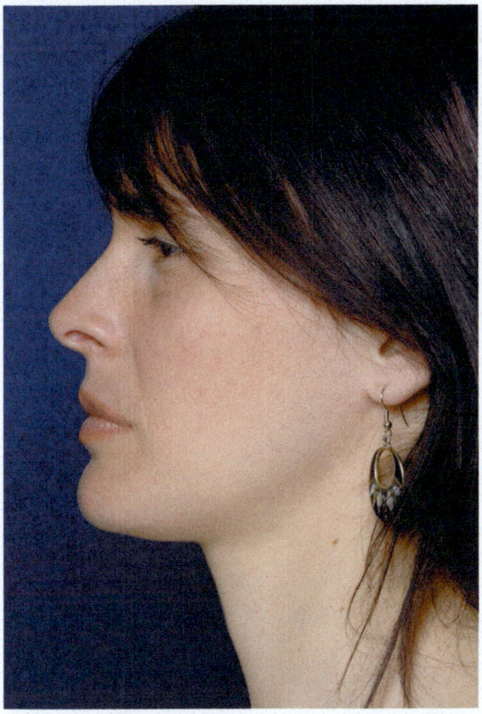

Fig. 3.6 Full face profile left view

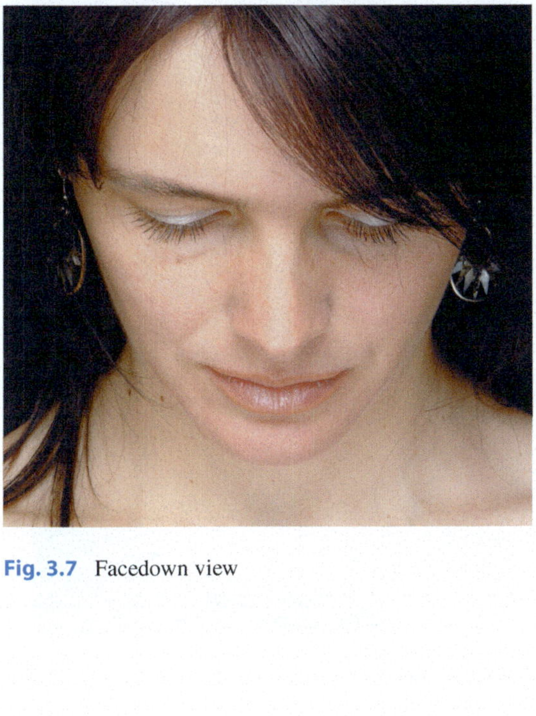

Fig. 3.7 Facedown view

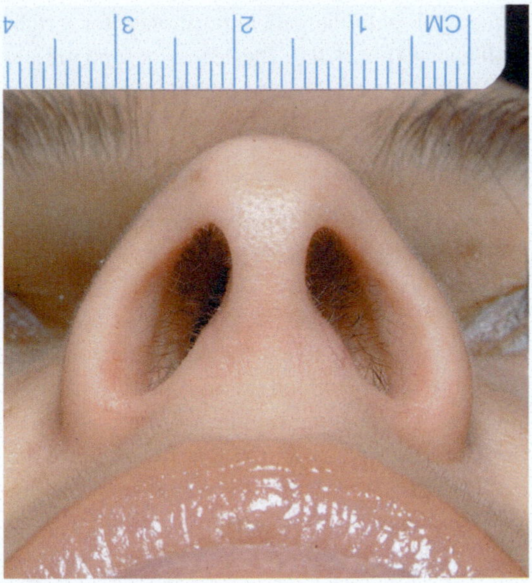

Fig. 3.8 Nasal base with ruler view

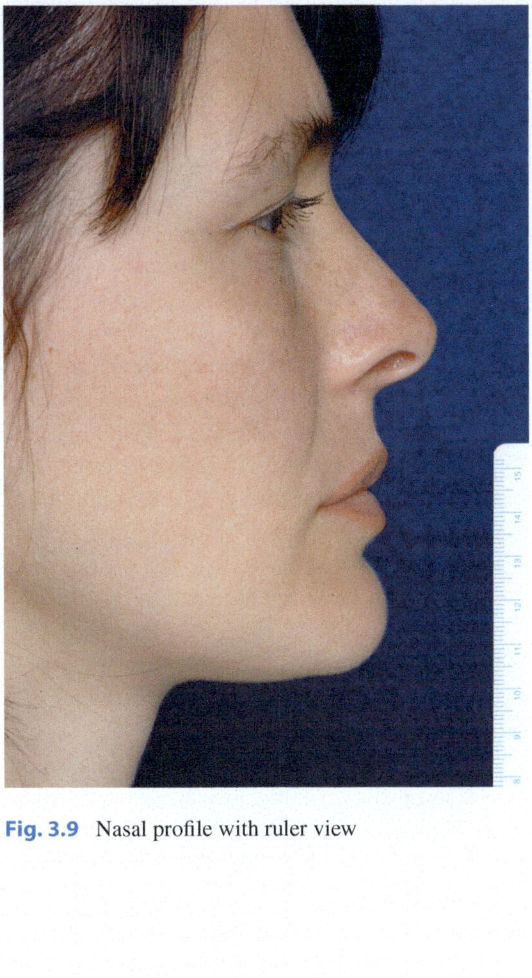

Fig. 3.9 Nasal profile with ruler view

in the NHP with the patient positioned for a right profile view (Fig. 3.10). The depressor septi muscle action profile views are also important for studying the range of movement of the upper lip.

3.4.4 The Five Orthognathic/Orthodontic Views

In the case of dentofacial deformities or dental malocclusions, the five orthognathic/orthodontic facial views are added to our documentation, along with three intraoral views (frontal, oblique right, and oblique left). All five facial views are in the NHP.

The first is the full face profile view during smiling, which permits the study of the relationship between the vertical and anterior–posterior position of the upper central incisors and the rest of the face (Fig. 3.11). Sometimes, in patients with maxillary deformities, the exposure of the upper incisors during smiling is impossible or severely reduced. In that case, I also favor the execution of a lateral cephalometric radiograph with the mandible in the rest position (not in centric occlusion) to study further the relationship between the upper lip and the upper incisors.

The second is the full face frontal view in posed smile (Fig. 3.12). The posed smile, also called the social smile, is voluntary, unstrained, and static; it is fairly reproducible. On the contrary, the unposed smile, also called the enjoyment smile, is involuntary and elicited by laughter or great pleasure (see Chap. 8 for more details on the posed smile) [1, 2].

The third picture is the full face frontal view with mouth retractors (Fig. 3.13). It is important to hold the two clear plastic mouth retractors horizontally and symmetrically. An interesting option is to mark, with a blue skin marker, some median facial points, such as the glabella, the tip of the nose, and the tip of the chin. The main goal of this particular view is to highlight facial and dental asymmetries together.

The final fourth and fifth pictures of this series, the close-up view of the lips at rest with ruler (Fig. 3.14), and the close-up view of the lips in posed smile with ruler (Fig. 3.15) are taken in rapid sequence with the patient positioned in frontal view. They are invaluable for smile analysis.

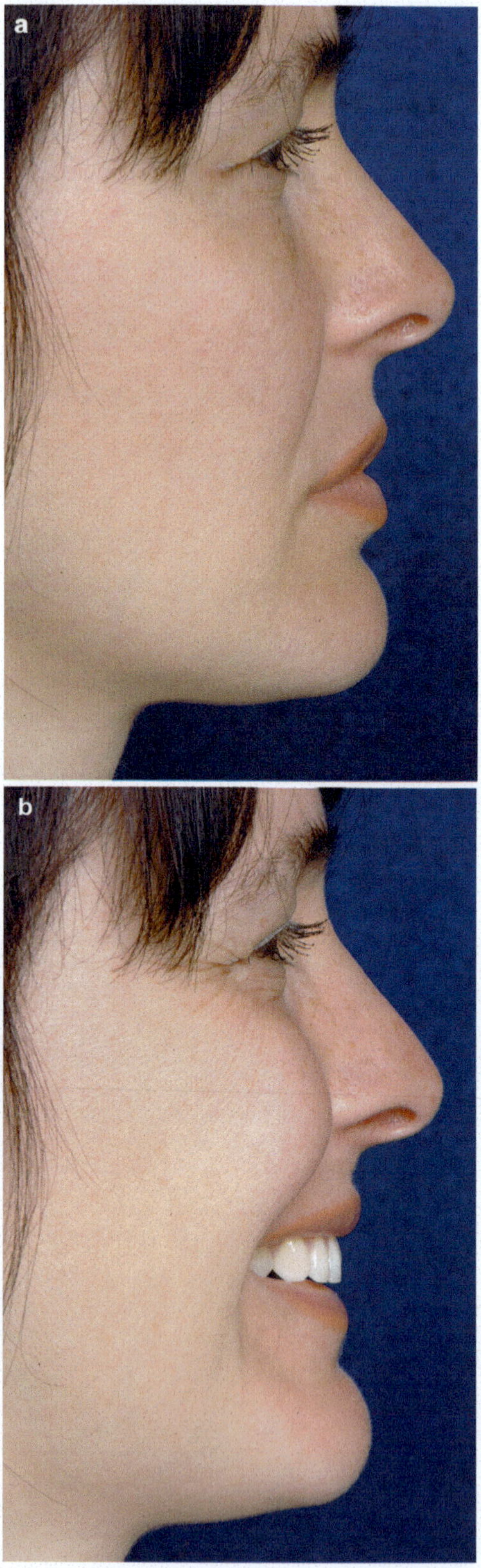

Fig. 3.10 Depressor septi muscle action profile views (**a**, **b**)

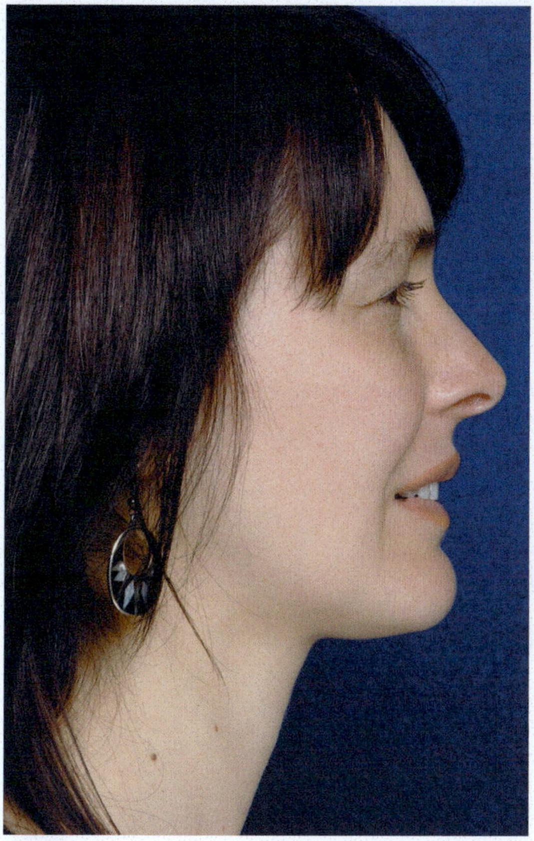

Fig. 3.11 (*Left*) Full face profile view during smiling

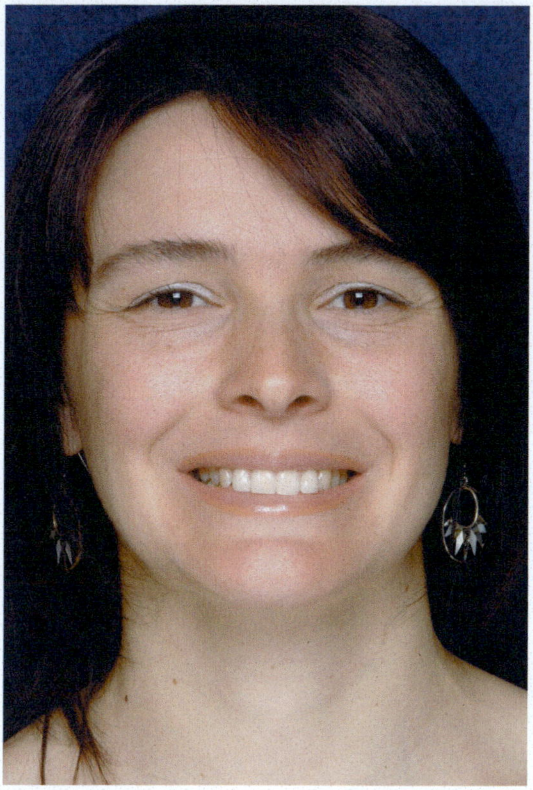

Fig. 3.12 (*Right*) Full face frontal view in posed smile

3.4.5 The Seven Eye Views

The seven eye views are necessary not only for the assessment of the globes and the eyelid but also for the eyebrows and the zygomatic, infraorbital, and paranasal regions. All are taken in the NHP and in close-up, five in frontal, one in oblique right, and one in oblique left view. The frontal ones are taken in rapid sequence, taking care that the patient does not move his head and maintaining the camera position fixed. The eye view looking straight ahead (Fig. 3.16) is taken first, then, maintaining the head position and the camera fixed, the patient is asked to turn his gaze upward, for the eye view looking up (Fig. 3.17) and downward, for the eye view looking down (Fig. 3.18).

Still in a frontal view, the next two shots are the unforced lid closure view (Fig. 3.19) and the forced lid closure view (Fig. 3.20), respectively.

The eye right oblique view (Fig. 3.21) and the eye left oblique view (Fig. 3.22) require changing both the patient and light source position and are taken last.

3.4.6 The Four Ear Views

The ear photographic documentation requires a precise and symmetric arrangement of the hair with two or three hairgrips. The frontal ear view (Fig. 3.23) and the rear ear view (Fig. 3.24) should be taken, maintaining the camera perpendicular to the subject in order to assess precisely the symmetry of the two ears. The successive pictures for the ears are the right ear close-up view (Fig. 3.25) and the opposite left ear close-up view taken maintaining the same subject– camera distance for comparison.

To document further the morphology and the actual dimensions of the ears, the rear ear view and the two ear close-up views can be taken positioning a ruler close to the subject.

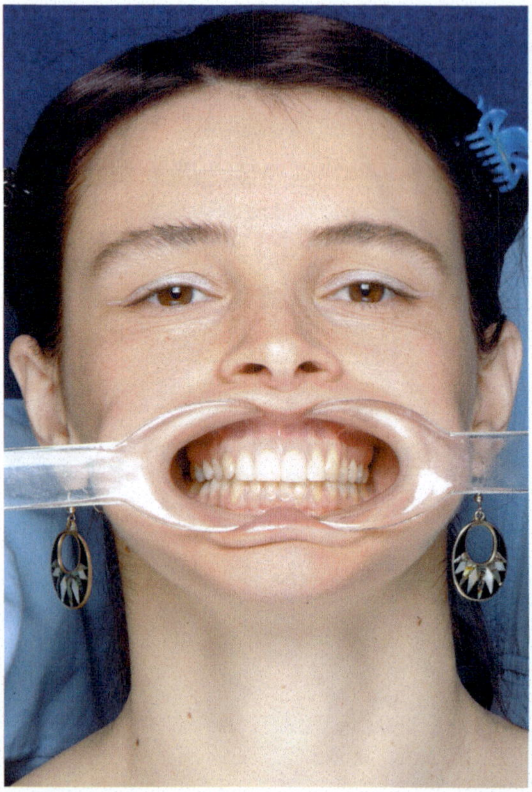

Fig. 3.13 (*Left*) Full face frontal view with mouth retractors

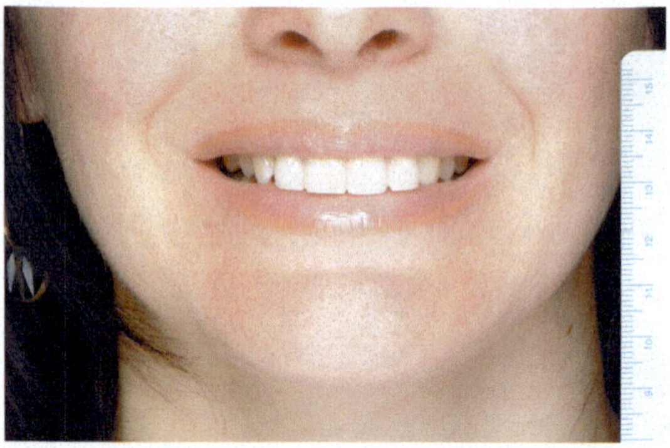

Fig. 3.15 Close-up view of the lips in posed smile with ruler

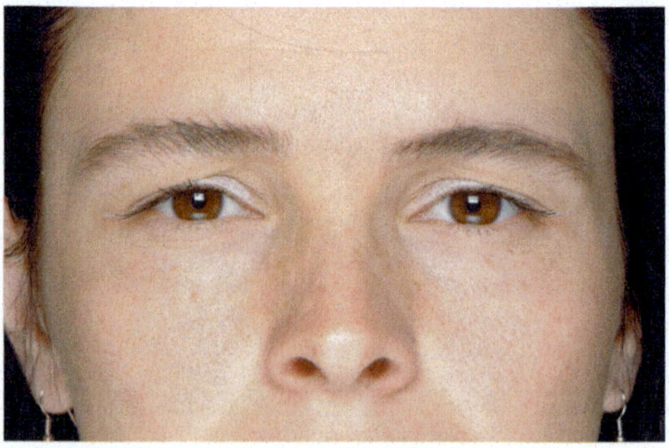

Fig. 3.16 Eye view looking straight ahead

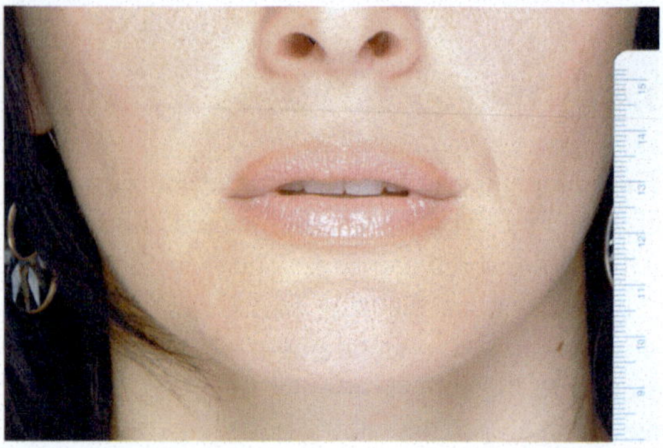

Fig. 3.14 Close-up view of the lips at rest with ruler

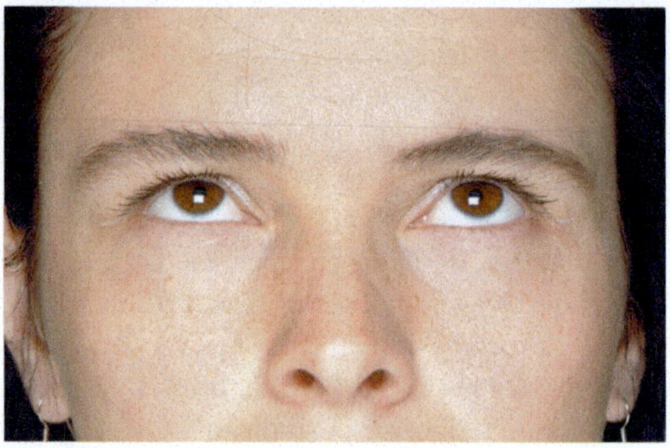

Fig. 3.17 Eye view looking up

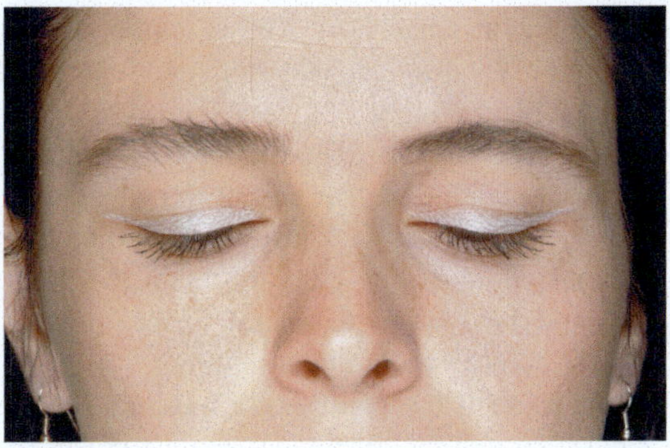

Fig. 3.18 Eye view looking down

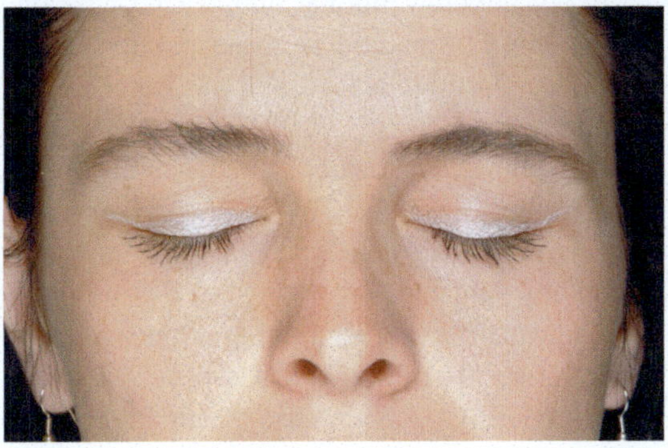

Fig. 3.19 Unforced lid closure view

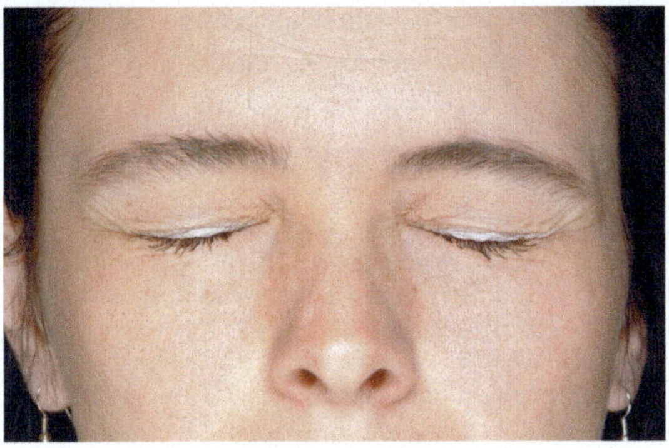

Fig. 3.20 Forced lid closure view

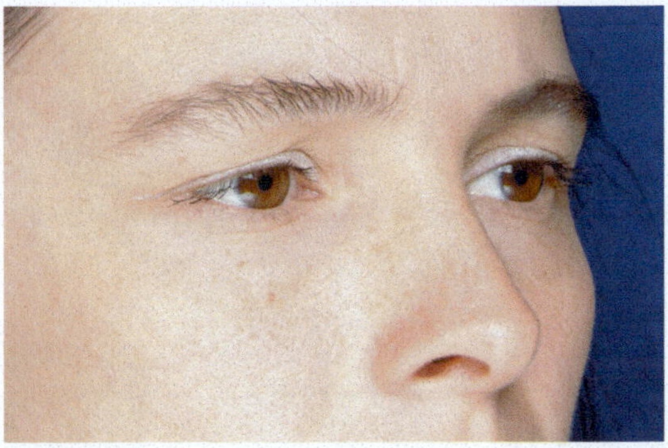

Fig. 3.21 (*Left*) Eye right oblique view

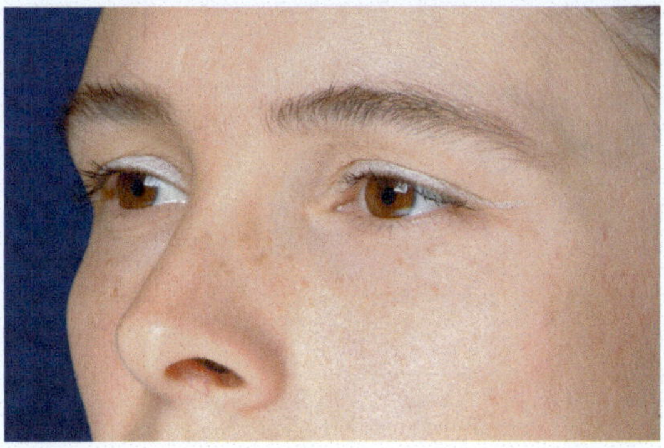

Fig. 3.22 (*Right*) Eye left oblique view

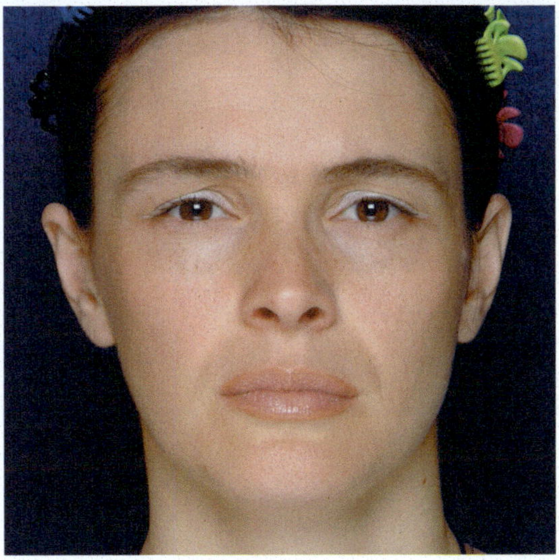

Fig. 3.23 Frontal ear view

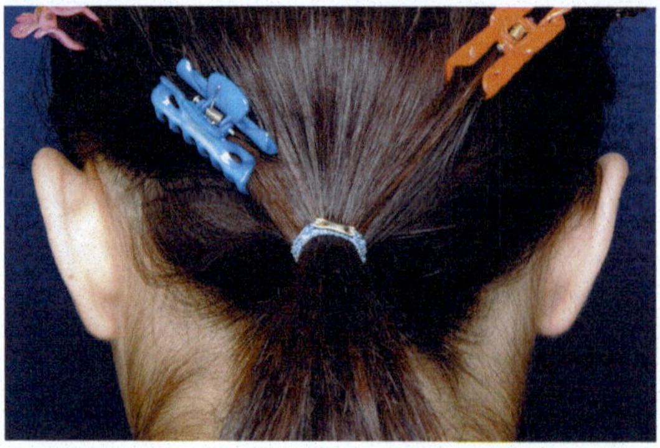

Fig. 3.24 Rear ear view

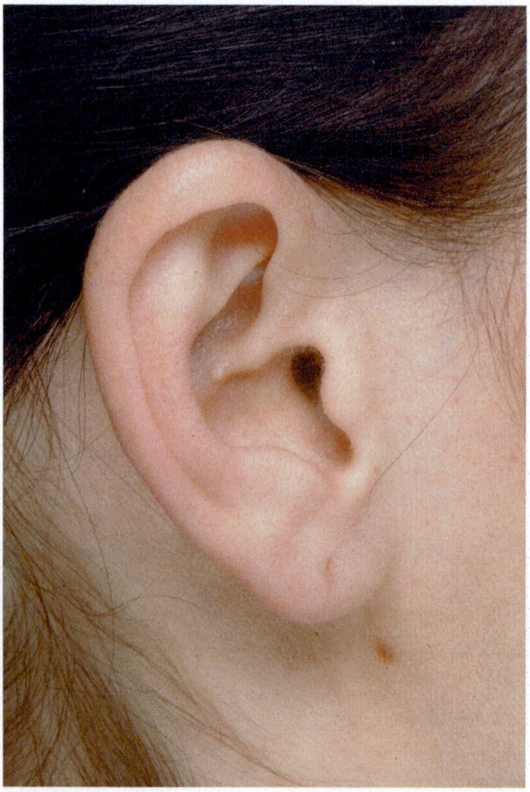

Fig. 3.25 Right ear close-up view

3.5 Final Remarks

The shooting of a complete set of quality clinical facial pictures is not an easy task. I strongly recommend that the reader practices taking pictures of a friend or colleague's face, utilizing the views discussed in this chapter as a template (see Exercise 2 in Chap. 14). The results obtained should be analyzed considering the following parameters separately:

- Patient positioning. This aspect is affected by the cooperation of your patient and your effective communication with him regarding the facial photography. How to obtain the NHP should be explained several times immediately before and during the sitting.
- Exposure. If the pictures are too light or too dark, correct the diaphragm and the power of lighting and standardize it for future sittings.
- Framing. The camera–subject distance depends on the focal length of the lens and the sensitive area of the conventional film or CCD. Again, you should standardize these parameters to obtain reproducible results in framing the subject.
- View points. The camera and the subject must be at the same level. When practicing, ask a third person to help you maintain the same camera–subject level.
- Shadows. The correct lighting of the subject is the most difficult technical aspect in clinical photography. Asymmetric shadowing "creates" an asymmetric face! The quality of the light is fundamental, and money spent on lighting equipment is more effective than money spent on high-tech cameras.

I have been struck how, after years spent documenting my patients with diligence and revising the collected material, my results are still improving.

References

1. Ackerman JL, Ackerman MB, Brensinger CM, Landis JR (1998) A morphometric analysis of the posed smile. Clin Ortho Res 1:2–11
2. Ackerman MB, Ackerman JL (2002) Smile analysis and design in the digital era. J Clin Orthod 36: 221–236
3. Guyuron B (1988) Precision rhinoplasty. 1. The role of life-size photographs and soft-tissue cephalometric analysis. Plast Reconstr Surg 81:489–499
4. Jacobson A (1995) Radiographic cephalometry. From basics to videoimaging. Quintessence Publishing, Chicago
5. Meneghini F (2001) Clinical facial photography in a small office: lighting equipment and technique. Aesthetic Plast Surg 25:299–306

The "Facial Points of Interest" 4

Contents

This chapter deals with references utilized for clinical facial analysis. I am convinced that judging the facial proportions and aesthetics utilizing internal and therefore "invisible" reference points, lines, and planes must be avoided. The inclination of the anterior cranial base, geometric center of the pituitary fossa, and other "invisible" references utilized in many cephalometric analyzes play a small role in the clinical decision-making process. So, more importance and emphasis is given to describing the points, lines, and regions of the external – visible – part of the face, together with the tissues that are under the skin and act as support structures.

The introductory topic is dedicated to how any observer, not necessarily a professional, identifies and studies the facial points.

4.1 Eye Movements and Visual Perception

Studies of eye movements during visual perception provide information concerning the nature of internal representations of an object in the memory [3].

Eye movements are necessary for a physiological reason: detailed visual information can be obtained only through the fovea, the small central area of the retina that has the highest concentration of photoreceptors. Therefore, the eyes must move in order to provide information about objects that are being inspected. When the retinal field is mapped onto the visual cortex, there is a considerable geometric magnification of the signals coming from the

F. Meneghini, P. Biondi, *Clinical Facial Analysis*,
DOI 10.1007/978-3-642-27228-8_4, © Springer-Verlag Berlin Heidelberg 2012

fovea and a consequent reduction of signals coming from the periphery. In about 1 s, we are able to fix two or three regions of interest (ROIs), which are also called significant points of fixation; a rapid eye movement, requiring a very short time period, connects one ROI to the next [3, 4].

We know this from the work of Albert Yarbus, a Russian psychologist active in the 1950s and 1960s. He developed the first apparatus that could track exactly where people centered their eyes as they looked at a photograph [1, 5].

The moments of eye fixation, made while viewing simple drawings, indicate that these ROIs correspond to the angles of the figure. Other studies added the points of maximum curvature and the so-called unusual details and unpredictable contours to the previous significant points of fixation [2–4].

Knowing these spontaneously selected ROIs facilitates clinical facial analysis, as it:

- Helps in distinguishing what is "captured" during our visual perception from what is not.
- Provides some facial points that can be considered more important than others.
- Permits the exclusion of some facial points, utilized in the previous analysis, as they are not detected as ROIs with direct examination and clinical photographs.
- Permits the construction of an exclusive, personalized, and unique approach to each clinical case utilizing the ROIs.
- Avoids treating a singular case by matching it with "normal templates" or "normal values."
- Helps the physician and the patient to discover and debate facial aesthetics with clinical photograph analysis. The ROIs are the same both for lay people and for the professional!
- Reduces the importance of abstract forms of analysis, such as cephalometric analysis, in planning the treatment and evaluating the results obtained.

4.2 From the Regions of Interest to the Facial Points of Interest

A human face is not a simple drawing like those utilized by Alfred Yarbus [5] for his study on eye movements, but, with different multiple views, it can be broken down into simple pictures. Chapter 3 is an example of that breakdown. Reviewing all the figures, we can note some points and lines that are evident in one view and completely hidden in another. This simple observation proves the limitation of the classic frontal and right profile views alone and the need for multiple views.

The reported experience gained studying eye movements during visual perception offers a new path for direct and photographic clinical analysis, helping us to identify something similar to Lawrence Stark's ROI in the face [3, 4]. There are three basic methods to identify a point utilizing the ROI principles:

- Search for an angle. The lip commissure, the lateral canthus, and the medial canthus are angular facial points of interest (Fig. 4.1).
- Identify the maximal curvature points on a curve. They are divided into two subgroups: maximal concavities and maximal convexities facial points of interest. In the profile view, the nasal radix and the labiomental sulcus are maximal concavities facial points of interest, whereas the nasal tip, the labrale superior and inferior are maximal convexities facial points of interest (Fig. 4.1).
- Search for an unpredictable curve or contour. A curve could be defined as unpredictable when it changes frequently and irregularly and so, from a visual point of view, has a large amount of information. A point of this type could be identified when a concavity turns into a convexity. The subnasal and the submental points are concavity/convexity facial points of interest (Fig. 4.1).

When two or more facial points of interest are spatially close to each other, as happens in the eye and perioral regions, the relative impact on the observer is high.

In the examples shown in Figs. 4.2, 4.3, 4.4, and 4.5, utilizing the frontal during smiling, profile, oblique, and nasal base views, some of the classical reference points are almost coincident with the facial points of interest; however, this is not always the case, especially when this search is performed in views other than the profile.

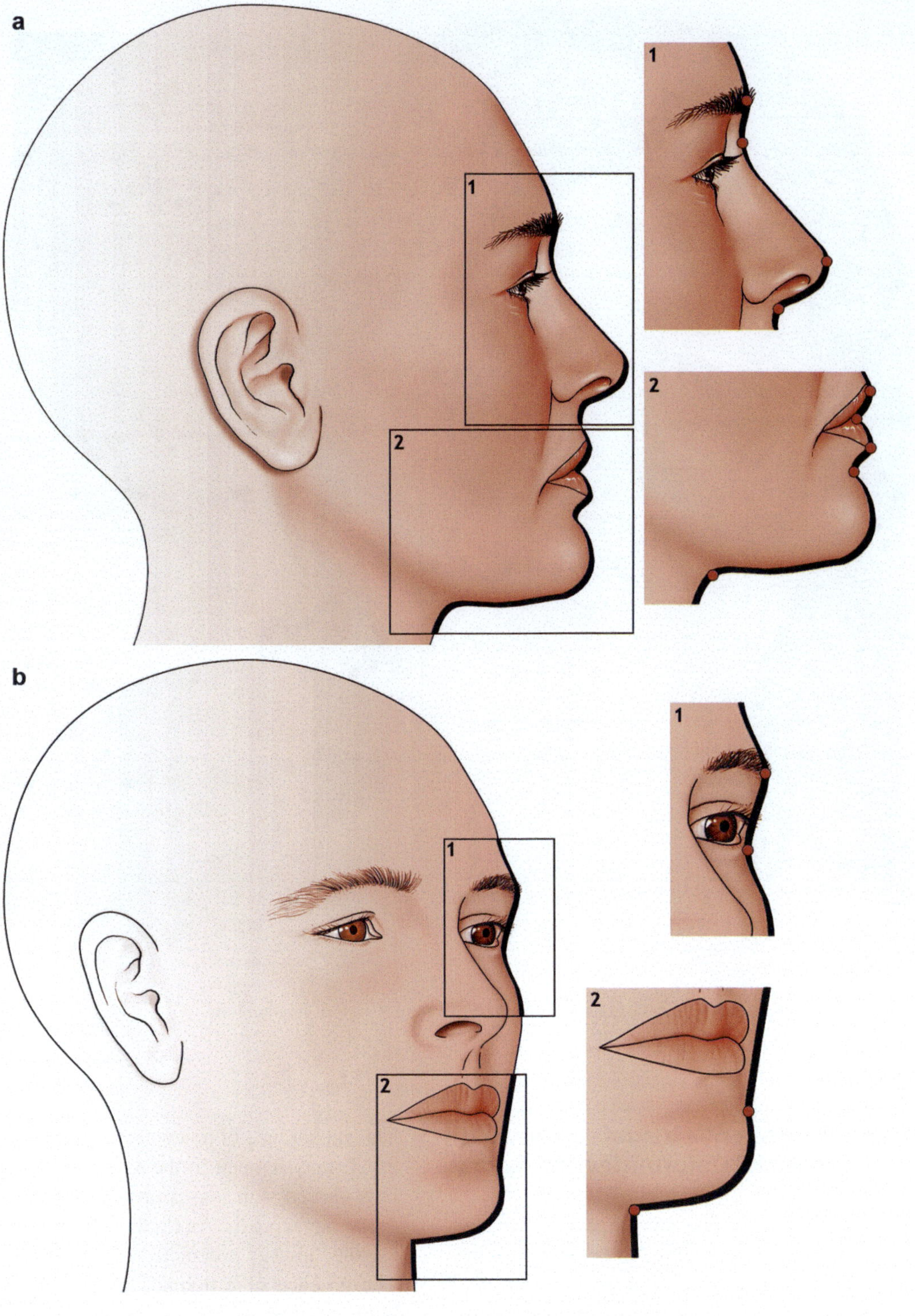

Fig. 4.1 Examples of angular facial points of interest, maximal concavities and maximal convexities facial points of interest, and concavity/convexity facial points of interest in profile (**a**) and oblique view (**b**)

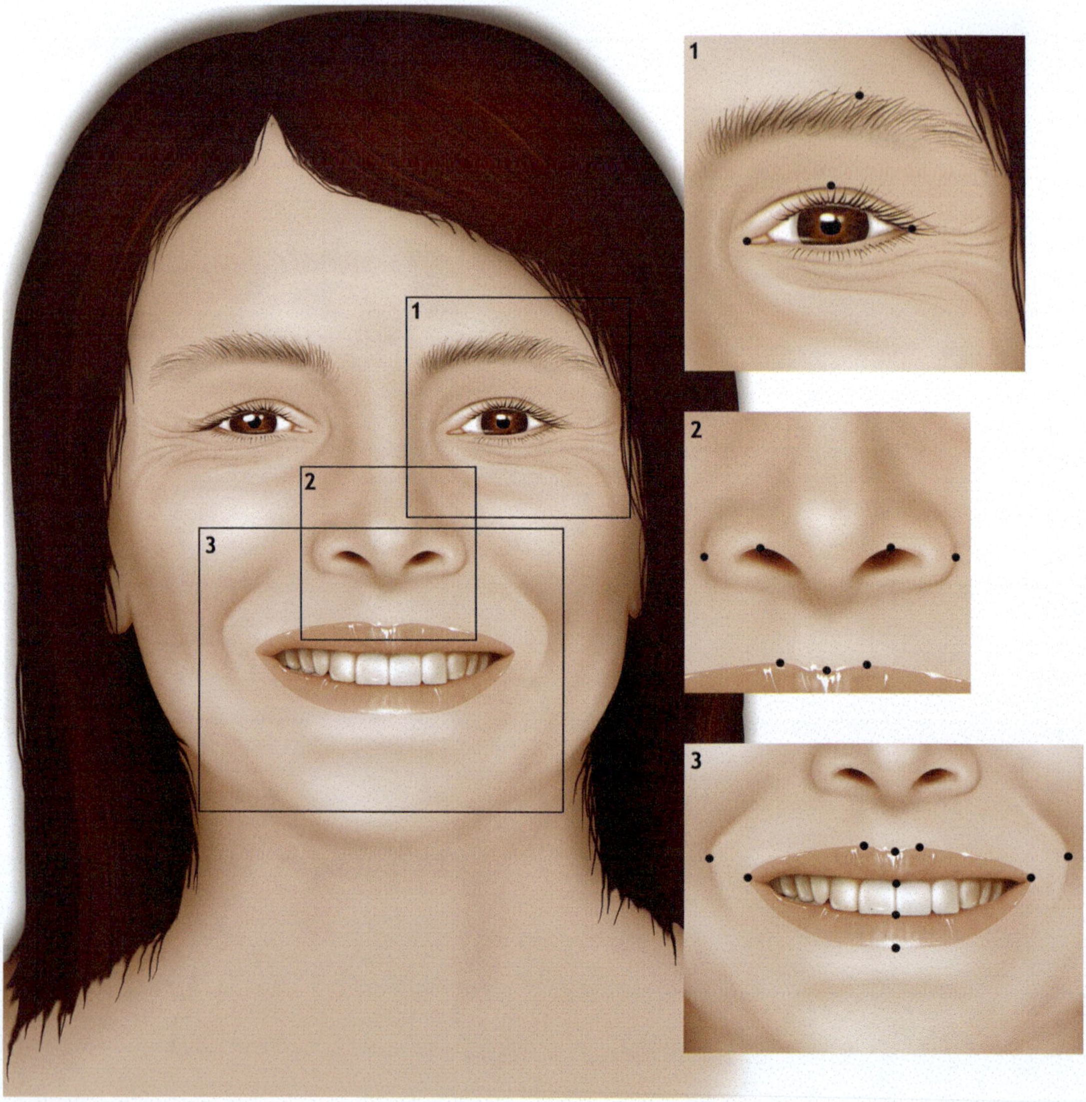

Fig. 4.2 Example of facial points of interest identified in a frontal view during smiling

4.3 A Different – Visual – Approach to Facial Deformities and Aging

What happens to our visual perception in cases of facial deformities or aging? I believe that the basic visual phenomena are these:

- The presence of one or more particular or distinctive facial points of interest. An example of this is the presence of a broken dorsal line in the case of a crooked nose (Fig. 4.6).
- The appearance of a new facial point of interest. It may happen in the aging face, when a new curved skin line is produced due to soft tissue facial ptosis. An example of this, regarding the "jowls," is depicted in Fig. 4.7.
- The absence of a normal and pleasant facial point of interest. An example of this is the absence of a distinguished nasal radix concavity, as in the so-called Greek nasal profile (Fig. 4.8).

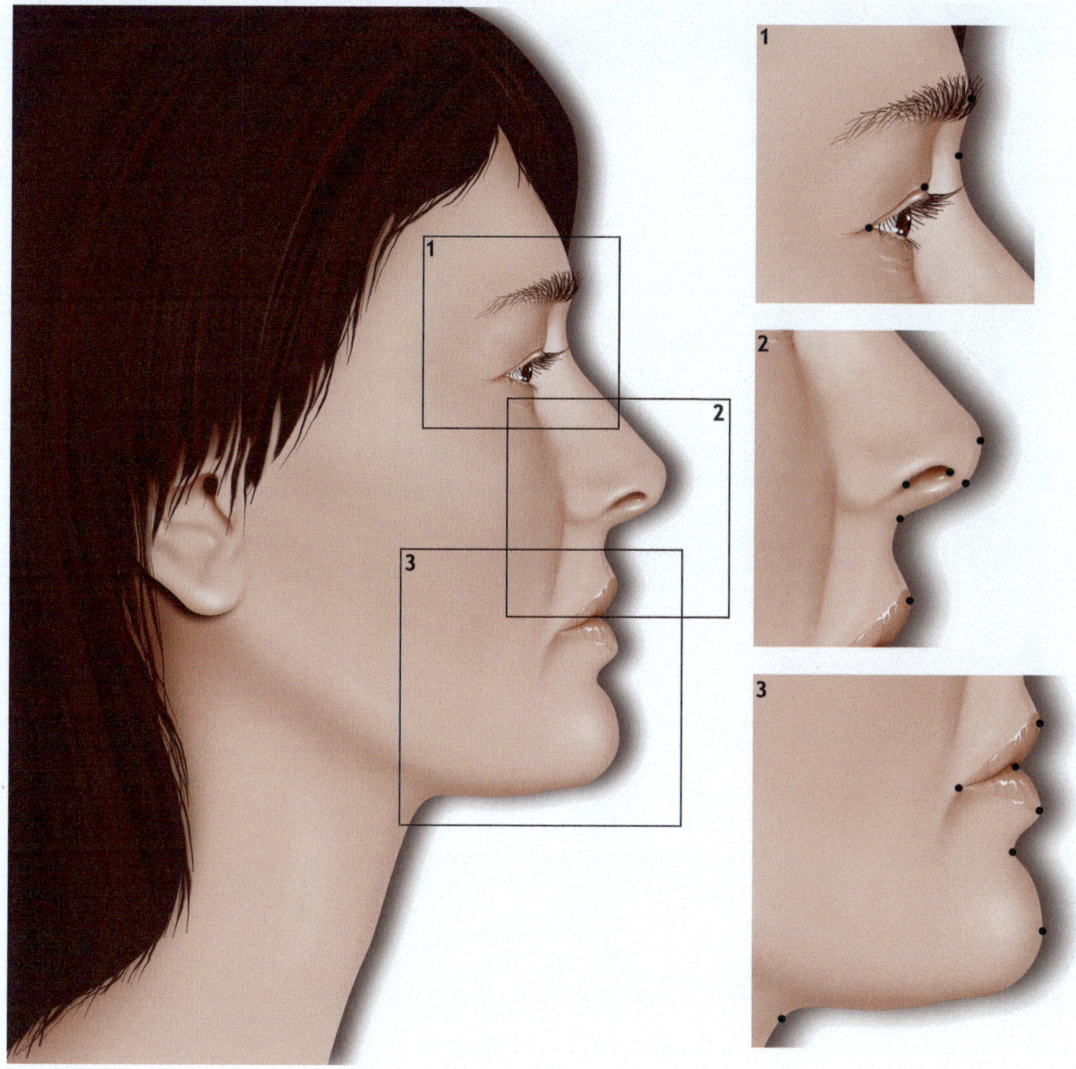

Fig. 4.3 Example of facial points of interest identified in profile view

- A change in the characteristics of a facial point of interest. An example of this is the transformation of a gentle curve into a deep sulcus, as happens to the chin–lip profile in the case of a deep bite dentofacial deformity or its flattening in the opposite case of an open bite class III skeletal pattern (Fig. 4.9).
- A change in the position of a facial point of interest. An example of this is the inferiorly positioned nasal radix, which makes the nose appear too short (Fig. 4.10).

Identifying and studying the facial points of interest can be very helpful in facial analysis and may be used to guide the treatment plan and to follow up the clinical case.

4.4 Adding Lines to the Facial Points of Interest

More frequently, the analytical value of some particular facial points of interest can be enhanced by adding a line. There are many ways of adding lines, such as:

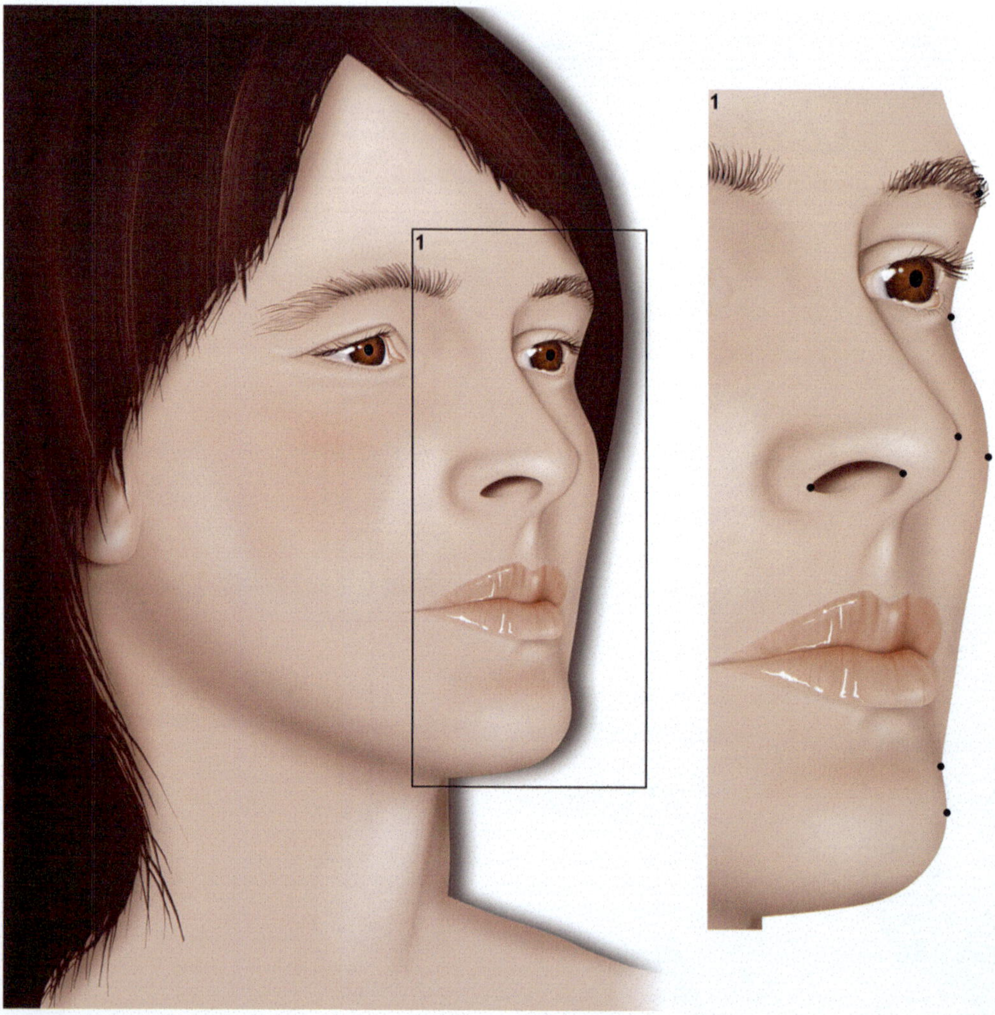

Fig. 4.4 Example of facial points of interest identified in an oblique view

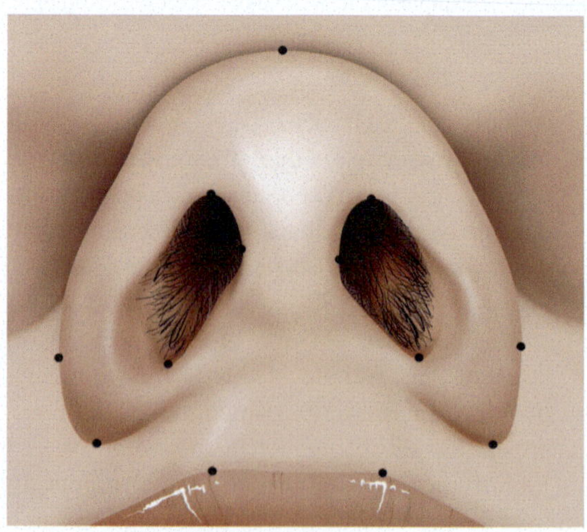

Fig. 4.5 Example of facial points of interest identified in a nasal base view

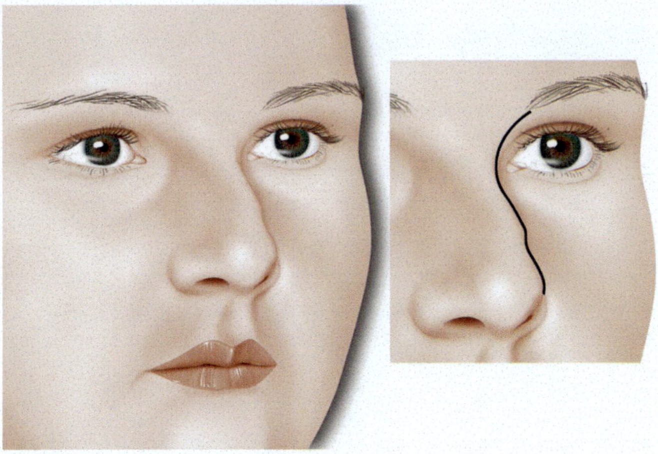

Fig. 4.6 Oblique view. Two facial points of interest related to a nasal deformity secondary to a trauma. The nasal dorsum outline is broken at the level of the deformity

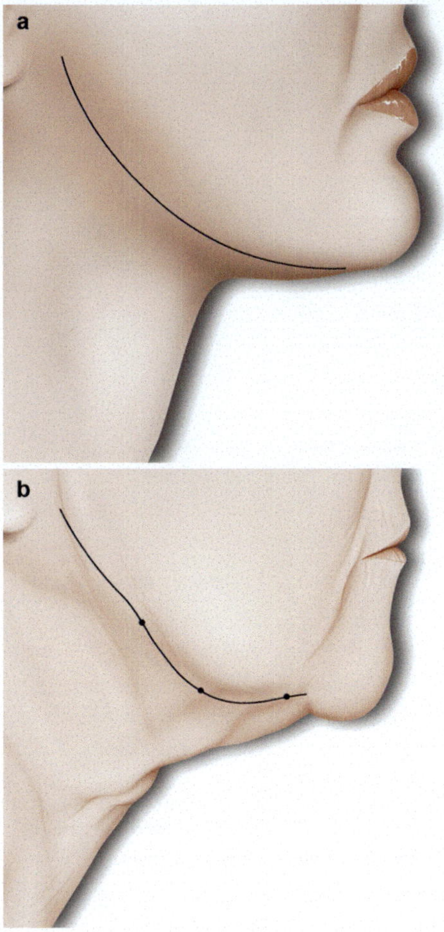

Fig. 4.7 Profile view. The appearance of new facial points of interest related to the aging process. The uninterrupted jaw line in a young girl (**a**) and the appearance of a convexity due to the ptosis of soft tissue in a 65-year-old woman (**b**)

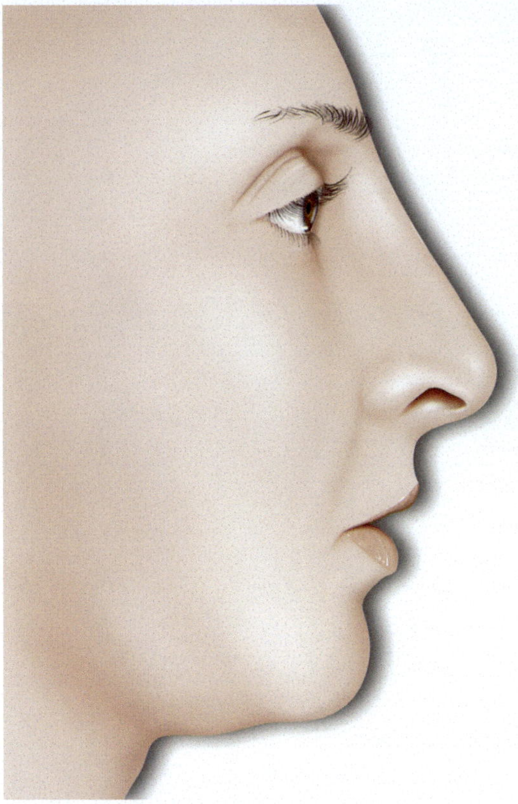

Fig. 4.8 Profile view. The absence of a facial point of interest from the nasal profile. The so-called Greek nasal profile in which the frontal and the nasal profiles are not separated by the concavity of the nasal radix

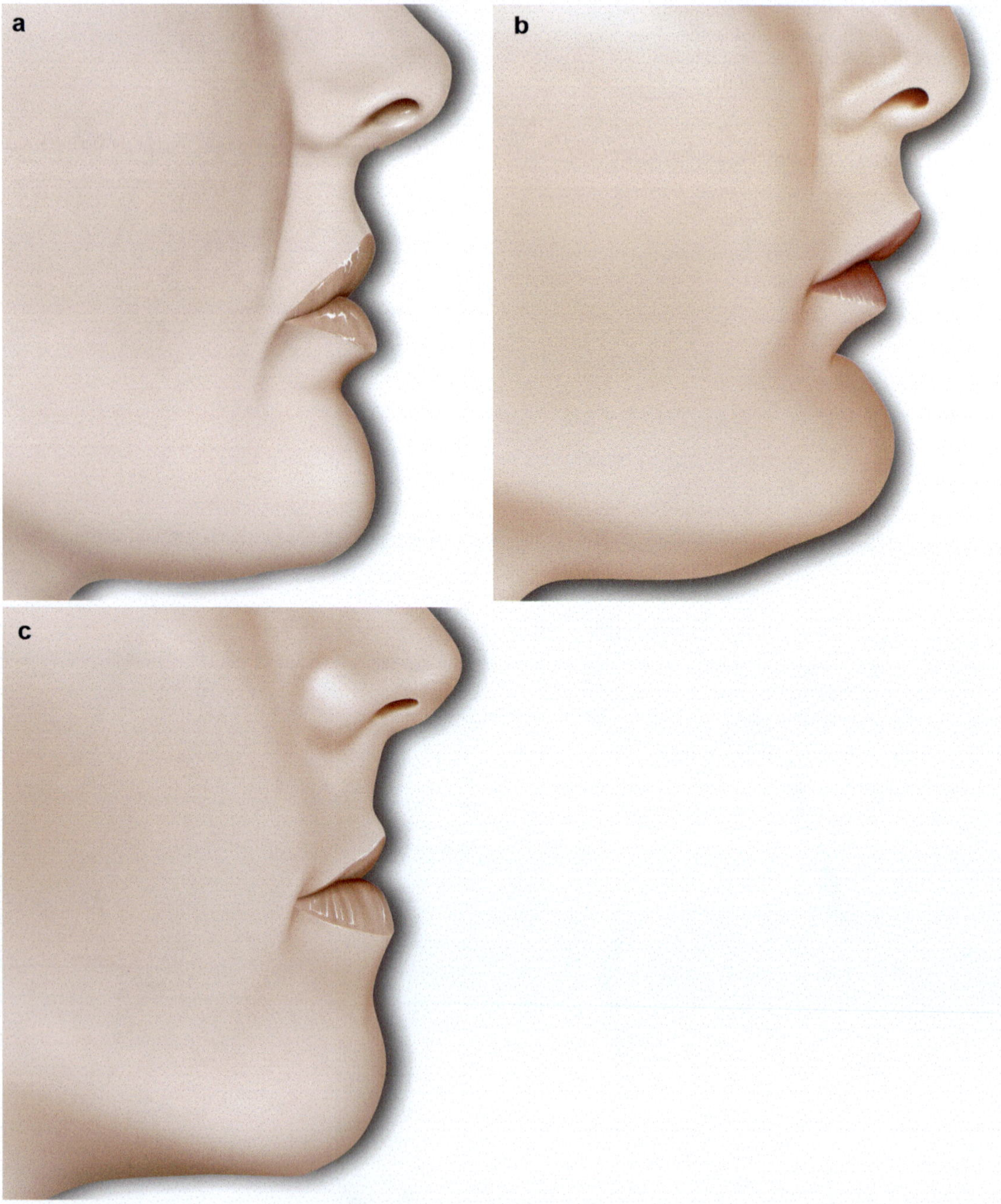

Fig. 4.9 Profile view. The change in shape of a facial point of interest. The pleasant gentle curve of the lower lip–chin profile in a balanced face (**a**), the deep sulcus in a deep bite dentofacial deformity (**b**), and the flat sulcus in an open bite case (**c**)

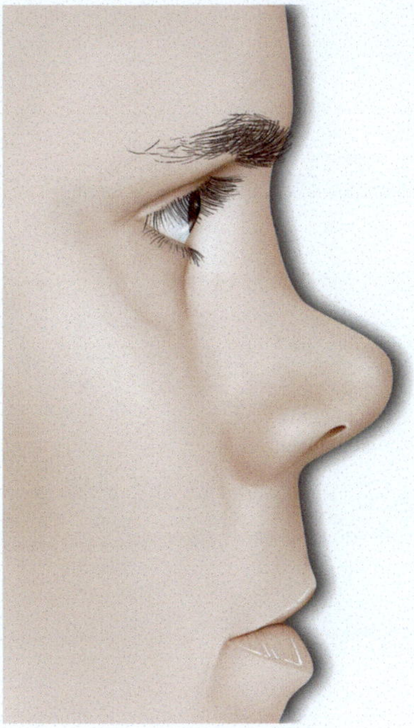

Fig. 4.10 Profile view. The change in position of a facial point of interest. The inferiorly positioned nasal radix makes the nose appear too short

- In pictures taken in the natural head position, we can utilize perpendicular or horizontal lines passing through a facial point of interest. An example of this is shown in Fig. 4.11a, in which a horizontally and a vertically oriented line passing through the subnasale helps in judging the columella–upper lip profile.
- In frontal and basal views, a line passing through two opposite side points helps to detect the symmetry of a facial region (Fig. 4.11b).
- In all cases, drawing a line that passes through two facial points of interest can underline a particular facial feature or deformity (Fig. 4.11c).

4.5 Illusion in Clinical Facial Analysis

Some fixed distances between points or regions can be perceived as long or short by the observer, depending on the shape and volume of other facial features. Typically, in the frontal view, the measurable distance between the medial canthus is not influenced by lowering or augmenting the nasal profile with a rhinoplasty procedure, but the visual effect obtained clearly modifies how the observer judges this distance. Again, in profile view, the anterior or posterior surgical repositioning of the chin greatly influences how one perceives the nasal tip projection.

Sometimes, in the analysis of a clinical case, the mean distance in millimeters between two points or the mean angular value in degrees between two lines should be reconsidered after studying the effects of visual illusion sustained by the other parts of the face.

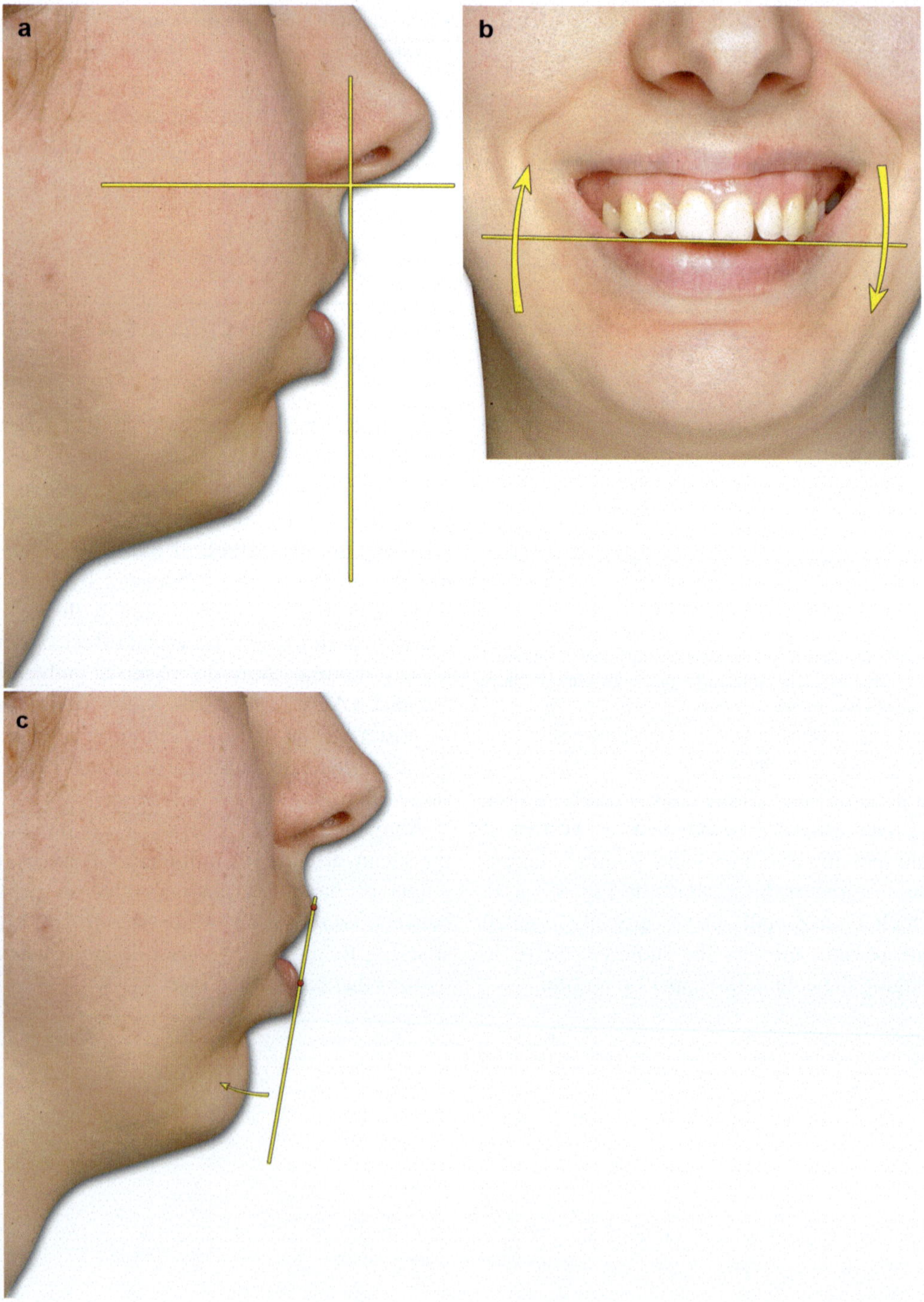

Fig. 4.11 A *horizontal* and a *vertical line* passing through the subnasale, in profile view taken in the natural head position, helps to distinguish the relative inclination of the upper lip and the columella (**a**). A *line* connecting the two upper cuspid margins, in a frontal view while smiling, gives an idea about the tilt of the upper dental arch (**b**). Connecting the upper and lower lip facial points of interest with a line assists in assessment of the projection of the chin (**c**)

References

1. Brooks RA (2003) Robot. The future of flesh and machines. Penguin, London
2. Macworth NH, Morandi AJ (1967) The gaze selects information details within pictures. Percept Psychophys 2:547–551
3. Noton D, Stark L (1971) Eye movements and visual perception. Sci Am 224:34–43
4. Stark LW, Privitera CM, Yang H, Azzariti M, Fai Ho Y, Balckmon T, Chernyak D (2001) Representation of human vision in the brain: how does human perception recognize images? J Electron Imaging 10:123–151
5. Yarbus AL (1967) Eye movements and vision. Plenum, New York

Basic Facial Analysis

5

Contents

During the first session with a new patient, the analysis and discussion are often focused on a particular facial feature, such as "the nasal hump," "the crowded upper anterior teeth," or "the periorbital wrinkles." This is related to a common idea among patients that there is only one single major problem, which needs treatment, and many minor or "not-detected" details, which are entirely acceptable. I favor this initial approach in every case, writing an itemized list of the patient's concerns to reassure her about my understanding of her wishes.

Even if I confirm the patient's concerns, a basic analysis of the entire face must be done next in order to separate the problem into its absolute and relative values.

For example, in the case of a large nose, what is the role of the nose itself and what is the role of a deficient paranasal region, a total hypoplasic maxilla, or a flat lower-lip-chin profile?

5.1 Regions of the Face and Neck

The surface of the face and neck can be divided into basic regions or frames as follows [6]:

1. Forehead region
2. Temporal region
3. Zygomatic arch
4. Malar region
5. Orbital region

F. Meneghini, P. Biondi, *Clinical Facial Analysis*,
DOI 10.1007/978-3-642-27228-8_5,

6. Infraorbital region
7. Nasal region
8. External ear
9. Parotid-masseteric region
10. Buccal region
11. Oral region
12. Chin region
13. Mandibular border region
14. Mandibular angle region
15. Suprahyoid region
16. Submandibular triangle
17. Carotid triangle
18. Retromandibular fossa
19. Median cervical region
20. Sternocleidomastoid region

The landmarks of these anatomical regions are not always obvious, as depicted in Fig. 5.1.

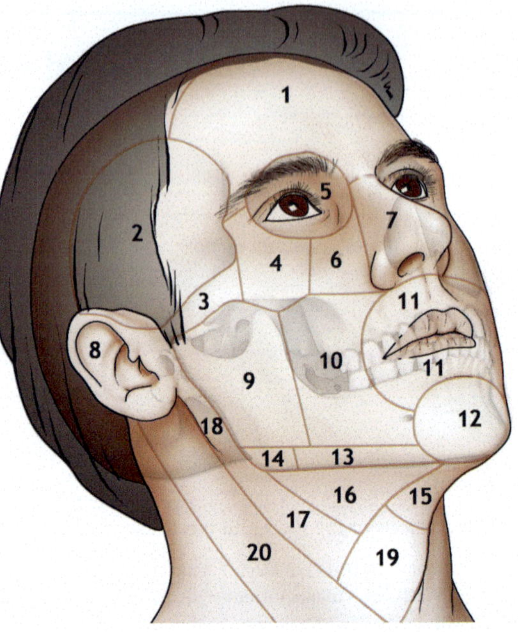

Fig. 5.1 Regions of the face and neck: *1* forehead region, *2* temporal region, *3* zygomatic arch, *4* malar region, *5* orbital region, *6* infraorbital region, *7* nasal region, *8* external ear, *9* parotid–masseteric region, *10* buccal region, *11* oral region, *12* chin region, *13* mandibular border region, *14* mandibular angle region, *15* suprahyoid region, *16* submandibular triangle, *17* carotid triangle, *18* retromandibular fossa, *19* median cervical region, *20* sternocleidomastoid region

5.2 Basic Qualitative Facial Analysis (Without Measurements)

The preliminary analysis – the most important – of a clinical case first requires exploring some basic facial features without taking any metric or angular measurements. These quantitative measurements are frequently at variance with each other: the same nasal tip can be 2 mm under-projected utilizing the norms proposed by Doctor JX, 1 mm under-projected utilizing the parameters of Doctor JJ, or normal utilizing the data of Doctor JK! Furthermore, are the subject's sex, age, height, weight, race, hormonal balance, head positioning, and many other variables all taken into account in these normative data? I think not.

So, a general assessment must be created without comparing it to normative values or a given template but using only adjectives and referring them to the whole face and to the main facial subunits, lines, and points. Some of the most utilized adjectives are normal, symmetric–asymmetric, present–absent, long–short, large–small, wide–narrow, deep–shallow, convex–concave, full–hollow, open–closed, acute–obtuse, straight–curved, projected–depressed, balanced–unbalanced, and deviated–centered.

A particular effort is made to recognize which areas are in an ideal position and/or have a normal shape and volume, as they will be used in evaluating and comparing the other regions.

5.2.1 Frontal View Analysis

Frontal analysis starts by assessing the transverse and vertical facial dimensions and general symmetry. The relationship between the bitemporal, bizygomatic, bigonial, and mental widths, also in comparison with facial heights, determines the facial form, which varies from wide to narrow, from long to short, and from square to triangular (Fig. 5.2). The grade of angularity and skeletonization of the facial form should also be noted.

Symmetry is always checked. Many patients are unaware of minor facial asymmetries, and if they

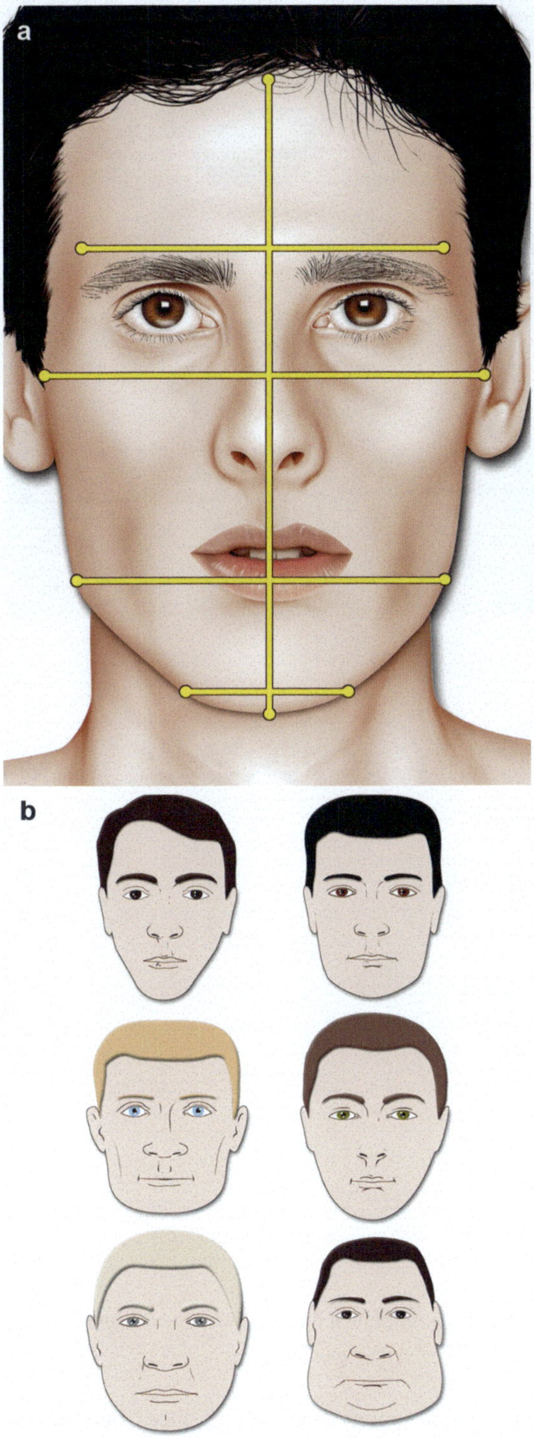

Fig. 5.2 The bitemporal, bizygomatic, bigonial and mental widths, and the total facial height (**a**). Examples of differences in facial form obtained by varying the width of the face at different levels (**b**)

discover these in the postoperative period, it will lead to patient dissatisfaction and misunderstanding. My preferred way to document and show all the facial asymmetries to the patient requires the marking of the midline skin points, using a fine-tip surgical skin marker and taking the frontal, basal, and facedown views again (Fig. 5.3). If the facial asymmetry is located in a lateral structure and not in the midline, as in the case of unilateral upper lid ptosis, a simple picture taken in frontal view is the best way to communicate this to the patient.

My attention is almost always focused on the central oval of the face. This extended facial region, described by Oscar Ramirez in his articles on facial rejuvenation, is also of interest in every basic facial analysis [7]. The central oval of the face comprises the eyes, the eyebrows, the zygoma, the nose, the mouth, and the chin, as depicted in Fig. 5.4.

5.2.2 Basal View Analysis

The basal views offer an additional check in the evaluation of general facial symmetry. The shape of the nasal base, the projection of the nasal tip and eye globes, and the shape of the zygomatic arches and chin are all evaluated and judged utilizing the basal view (Fig. 5.5).

5.2.3 Oblique Views Analysis

There are multiple oblique views because, from the pure frontal to the pure profile views, we can find 89 different head positions to the right and 89 different head positions to the left by making small intermediate rotations of 1°. When we try to document a nose with a dorsal deformity, the best oblique view is quite different with the oblique view we need to judge the spatial position of the malar eminence, as depicted in Fig. 5.6.

As recommended in Chap. 3, in every clinical case, I prefer to take at least three different right and left oblique views, changing the camera position and maintaining the position of the subject, with the lighting system fixed.

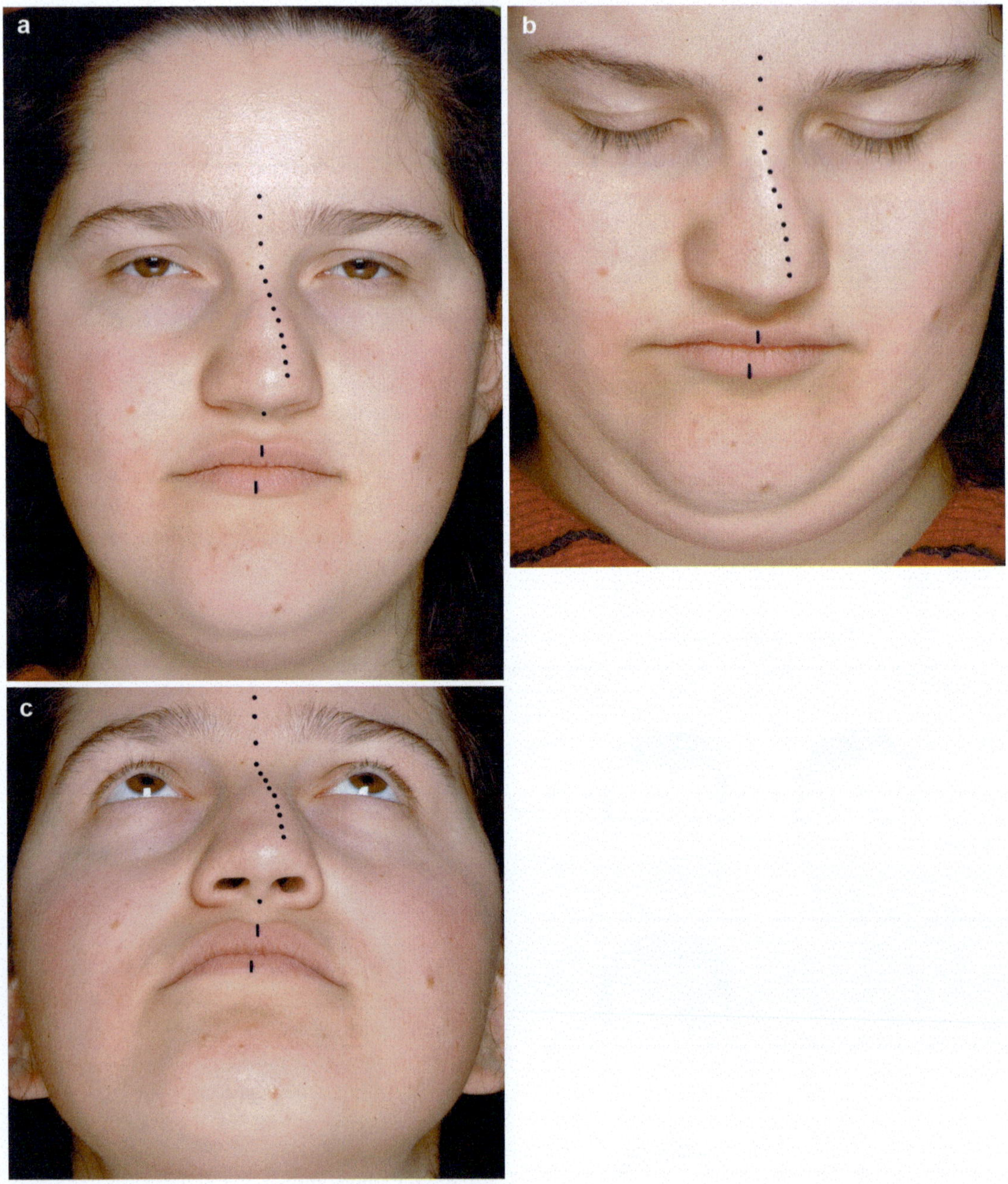

Fig. 5.3 Frontal (**a**), facedown (**b**), and basal (**c**) views with midline facial points, marked with *blue ink*, in a clinical case of posttraumatic nasal asymmetry

Ideally, an oblique view should be considered as being composed of two distinct components, which need to be analyzed separately.

The first one (Fig. 5.7) is the half of the face that is facing the camera (or the eyes of the observer) and is a great aid in the evaluation of the lateral components of the face such as the temporal, zygomatic, orbital, cheek, paranasal, preauricular, and mandibular angle. This component is usually familiar to the patient, as is the frontal view, so it is utilized extensively during communication with her.

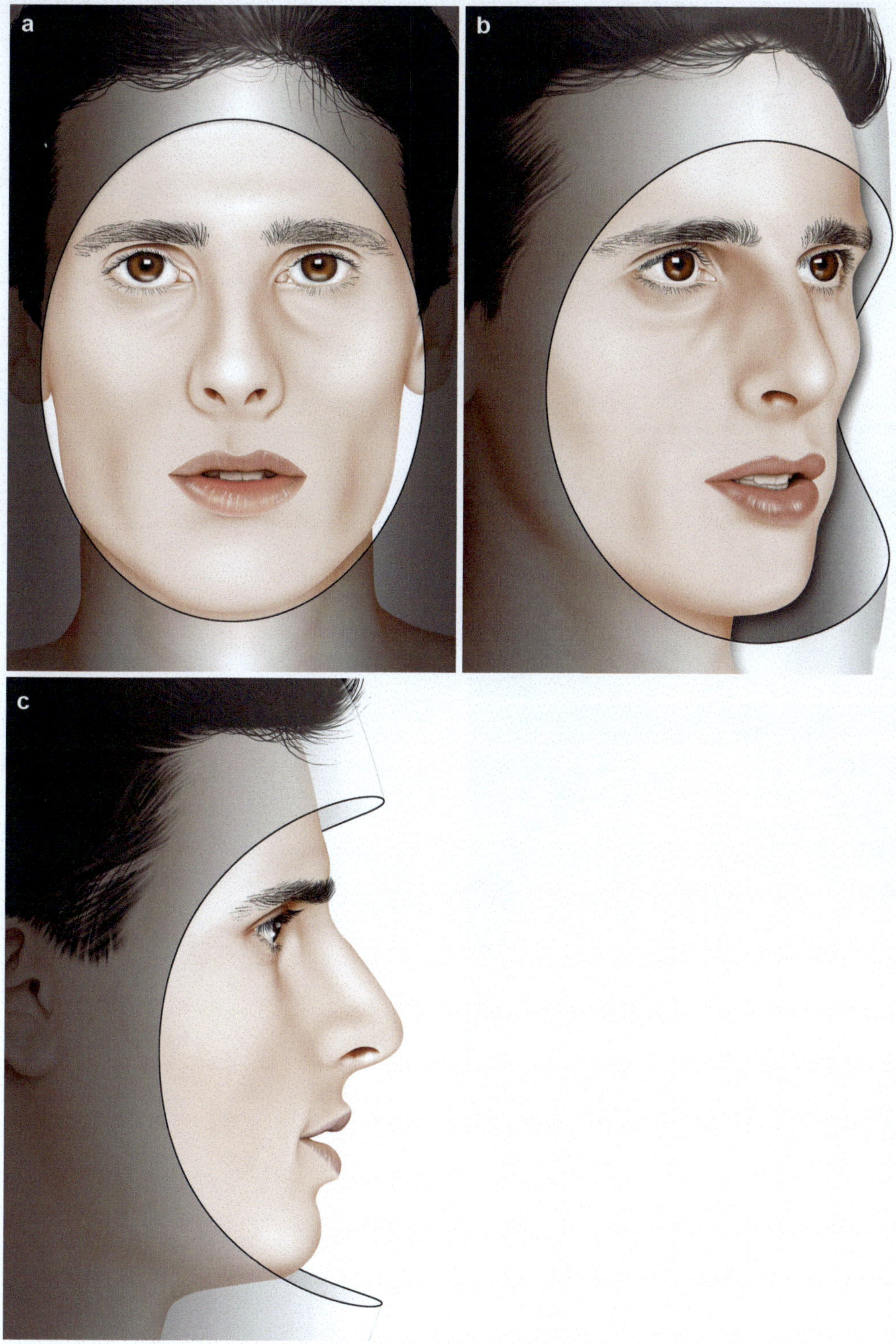

Fig. 5.4 The central oval of the face in frontal (**a**), oblique (**b**), and profile views (**c**)

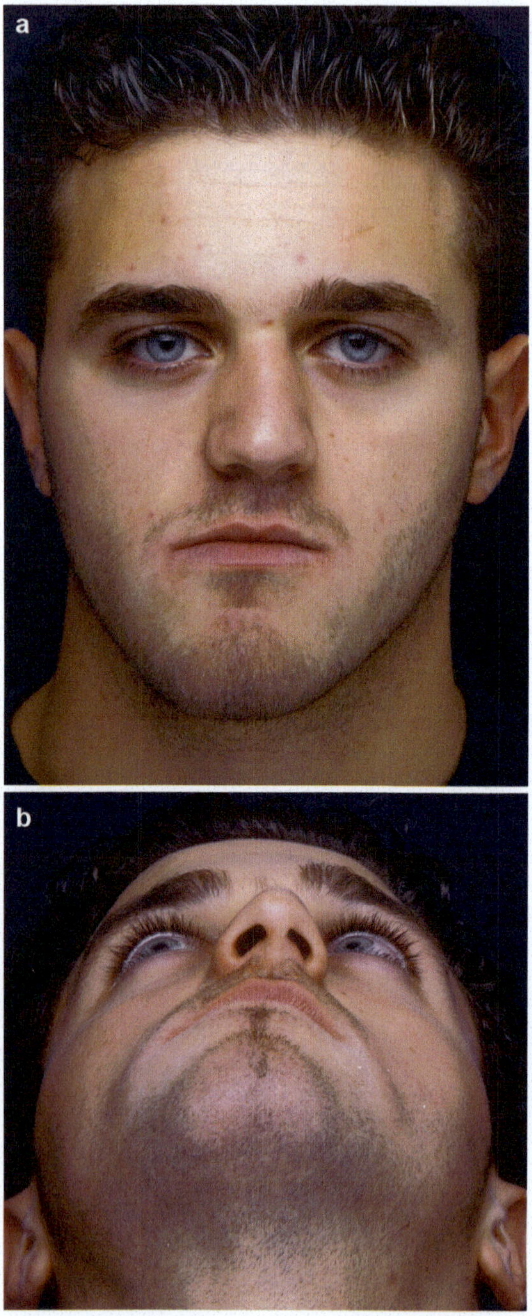

Fig. 5.5 Frontal (**a**) and basal (**b**) views in a clinical case of facial asymmetry

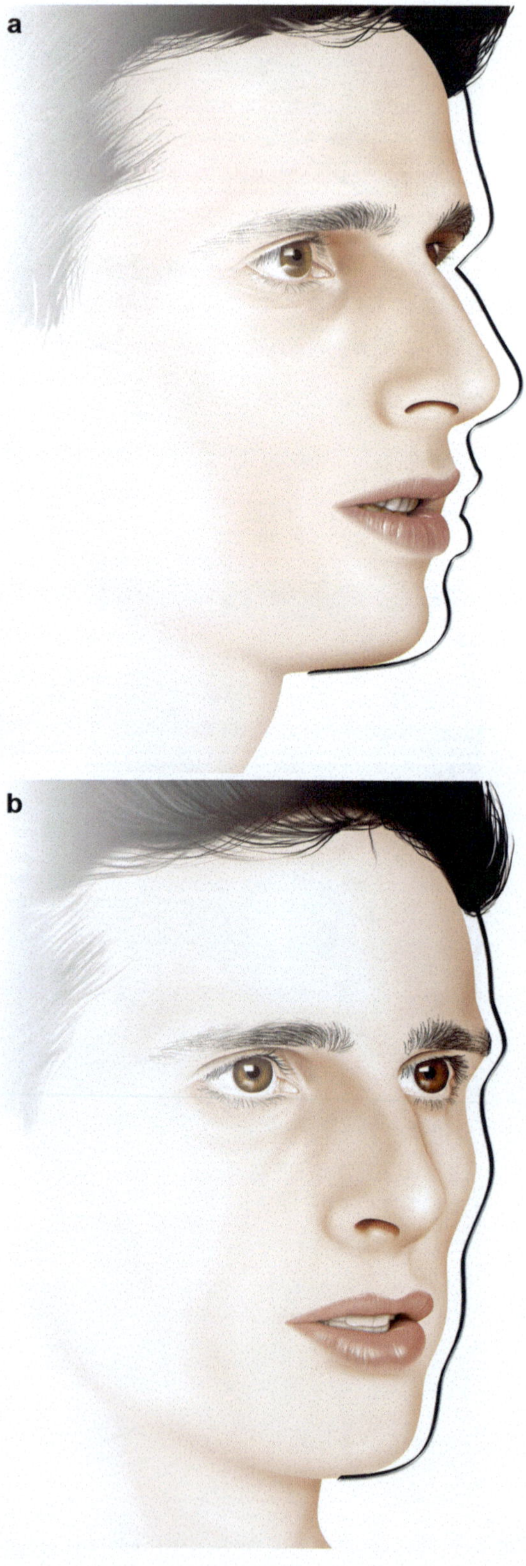

Fig. 5.6 A more rotated oblique view is preferred to document the nasal pyramid (**a**), whereas a less rotated oblique view is necessary to document the shape of the orbito-zygomatic region (**b**)

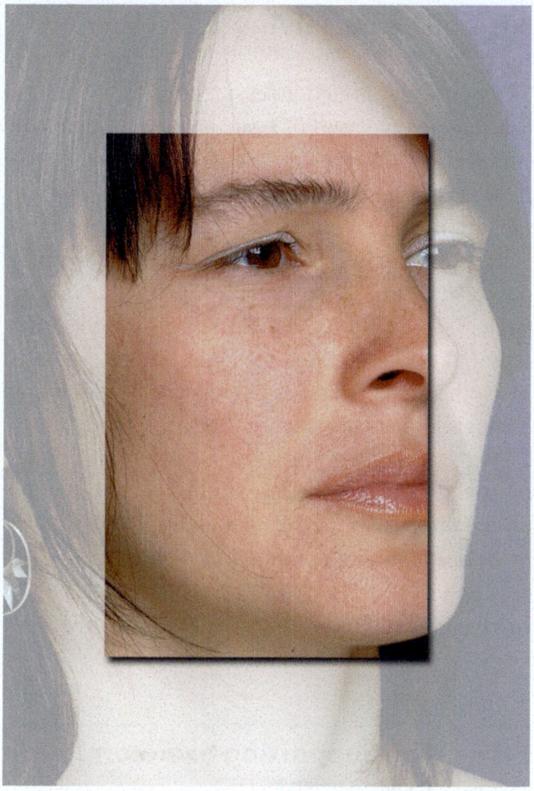

Fig. 5.7 The first component of the oblique views is facing the camera or the observer's eyes. It is a great aid in the evaluation of the lateral regions of the face such as the temporal, zygomatic, orbital, cheek, preauricular, and mandibular angle

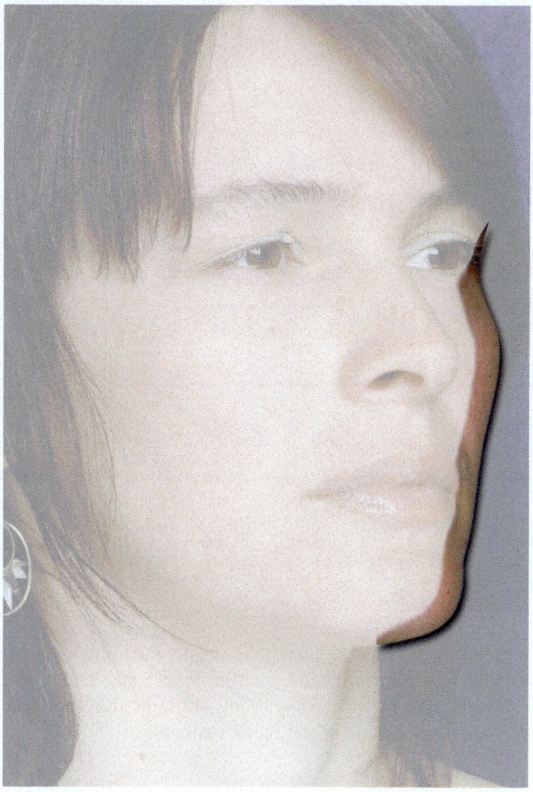

Fig. 5.8 The second component of the oblique views is the opposite profile of the face that emerges on the background panel. In a youthful subject, it is composed of a series of gentle curves, which resembles the outline of an ogee

The second component (Fig. 5.8) is the profile of the opposite side of the face that emerges on the background panel. In a youthful subject, it is composed of a series of gentle curves, which resembles the outline of an ogee. Here is how J. William Little describes these curves: "the youthful facial ogee typically arises from a high, subtle lid–cheek interface and rises gradually and gracefully to a broad, uniform convexity that peaks near or above the nasal tip. It then continues as a descending convex curve to the level of the upper lip, where it rapidly reverses itself through the occlusal plane, entering a limited concavity that rises slightly at the mandibular border before curving acutely around that structure into the neck" [4].

5.2.4 Profile View Analysis

The profile view is both the most utilized by the doctor and the least known by the patient herself. Without a couple of mirrors specifically oriented or a photographic camera, nobody can observe her own profile. How many pictures, captured in profile view, do you have in your personal album? And how many times have you looked at your profile, using two mirrors, in the last year? For that reason, even if the profile view analysis is fundamental for planning and visualizing the treatment goals, it must not be overemphasized to the patient, stating that it is only in the eyes of the beholder. In all cases, the profile view is essential to judge some basic facial parameters, such as:

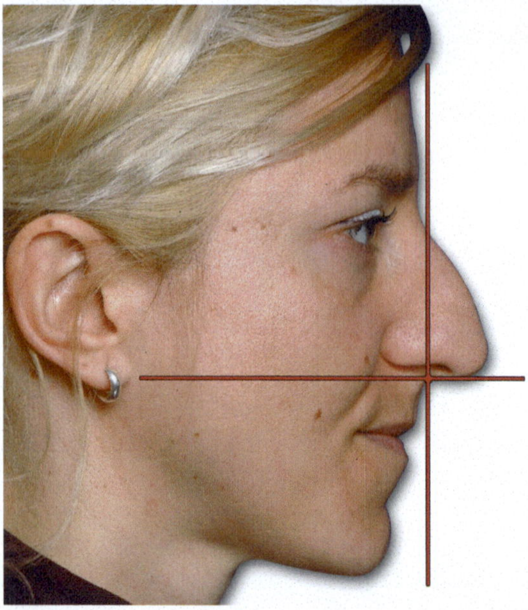

Fig. 5.9 In this photograph, taken in profile view with the subject in the natural head position, *horizontal* and *vertical reference lines*, both passing through the subnasal point, aid evaluation of the facial features

- The total face height; the heights of the upper, middle, and lower facial thirds separately; as well the heights of the basic regions of the face (forehead, orbit, nose, upper lip, lower lip, and chin)
- The sagittal (posteroanterior) projection of the orbital ridges, zygoma, nasal radix and tip, lips, and chin
- The slope of forehead, nasal, infraorbital, columellar, upper and lower lips, submental, mandibular border, and neck outlines
- The general shape of the facial profile itself in terms of concavity–convexity

For a better evaluation of the profile view, I suggest adding two reference lines, one horizontal and one vertical, both passing through the subnasal point, as depicted in Fig. 5.9.[1] With this approach, the vertical and sagittal position of many points, as well as the incline of some facial outlines, can be studied and recorded.

5.3 The Facial Angles

The construction and assessment of facial angles is a fundamental part of basic analysis. Again, the comparison of a clinical case with an average template or normative data is seldom necessary. The most utilized photographic and radiographic view is the profile view, but all of the clinical views proposed in Chap. 3 are suitable for an analysis by angles. In many cases, the two straight lines required to construct an angle are drawn connecting some facial points of interest and/or extending a facial outline, as shown in Figs. 5.10 and 5.11.[2]

For the angles constructed utilizing views taken in the natural head position, I favor breaking up the angle into its two elementary components by dividing it with a horizontal or vertical line, as depicted in Fig. 5.12. In this manner, each incline can be assessed independently from the others.

5.4 The Supporting Skeleton Assessment

Figure 5.13 illustrates the three main supporting structures of the facial soft tissue envelope: the bony, the cartilaginous, and the dental structures. It can be noted that the major determinant of facial support and shape is a relatively small portion of these three components (Fig. 5.13b, c). The eye globe, with its fixed spatial position, may be assumed to be a skeletal supporting structure for the lids.

5.5 Facial Soft Tissue Envelope Assessment

The assessment of skin and soft tissue needs visual and manual inspection. Skin tone, elasticity, ptosis, pigmentation, dynamics, and scars should be shown to and discussed with the patient. Any pigmented lesion or scar must also be documented with multiple photographs (taken at

[1] The complete clinical facial photographic documentation of this clinical case is available in Sect. 4 on Springer Extra Materials (extras.springer.com) (clinical case no. 1).

[2] The complete clinical facial photographic documentation of the clinical case of Fig. 5.11b is available in Sect. 4 on Springer Extra Materials (extras.springer.com) (clinical case, *a* and *b*, no. 2).

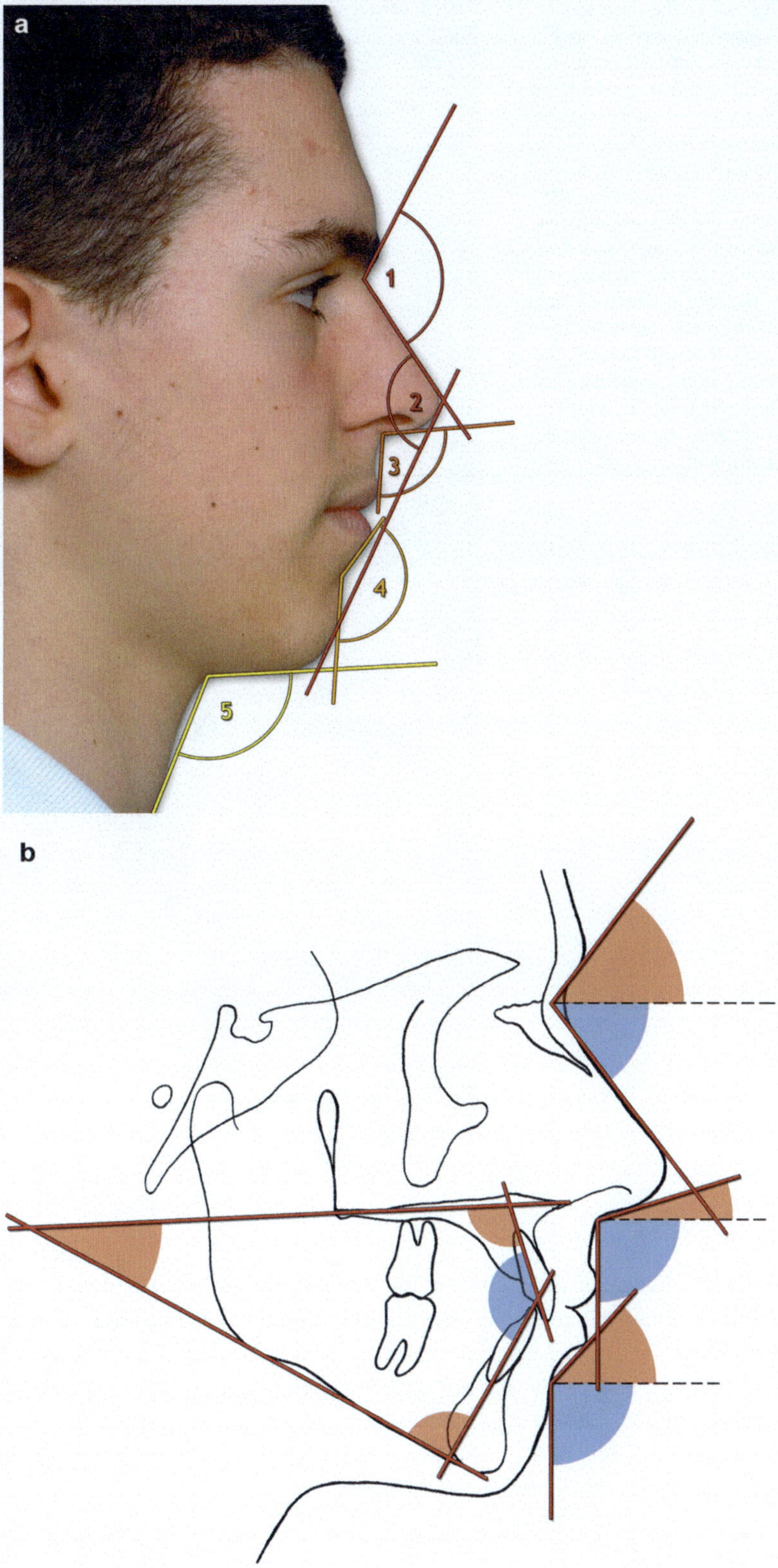

Fig. 5.10 Angles constructed over a photographic (**a**) and cephalometric tracing (**b**) profile view of the same patient

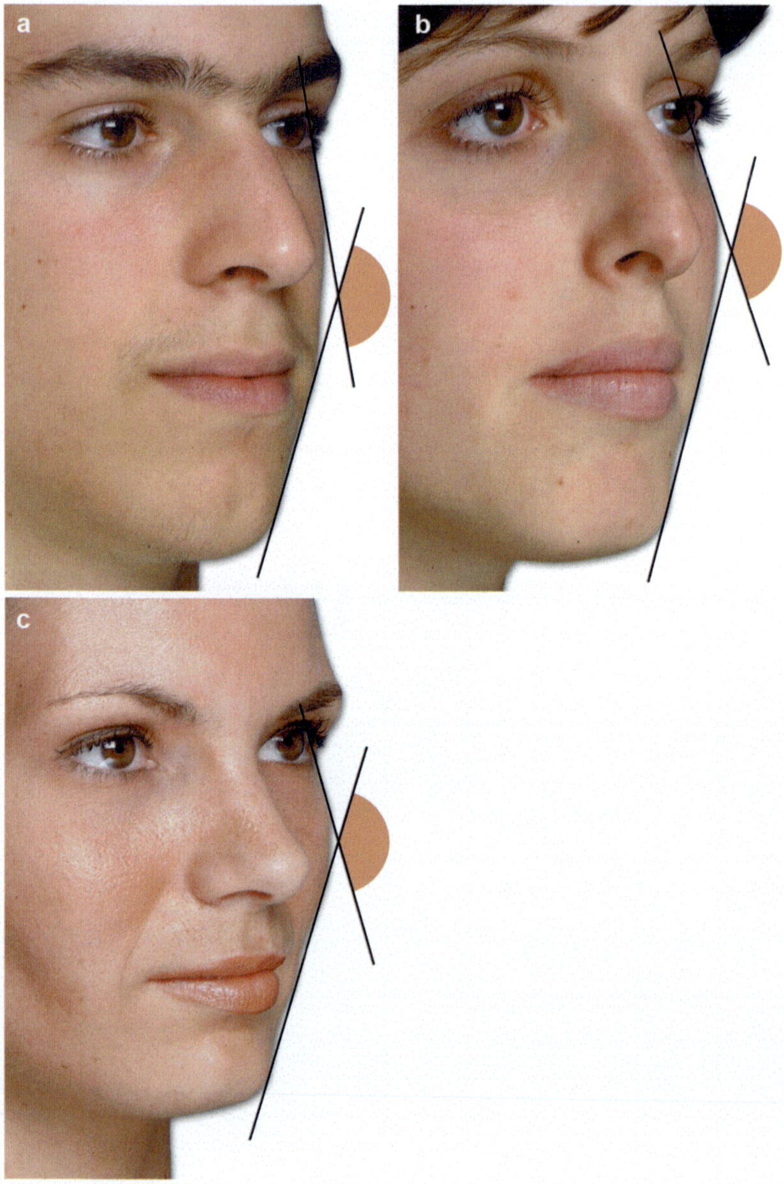

Fig. 5.11 The same angle constructed over the ogee curve of three different young subjects in which the projection of malar eminence increases from (**a**–**c**). There are three parameters to consider: the degree of the angle, the background area between the angle and skin profile, and the vertical level of the face at which the angle is positioned. In these three cases, from *left* to *right*, the degree of the angle decreases, the background area also decreases, and the vertical position of the angle is higher

different distances and varying the light incidence), utilizing a ruler, to assess its evolution with time.

To further document and register the characteristics of the facial soft tissue, I suggest the utilization of the fixed, step-by-step method reported in the facial soft tissue analysis checklist, in which each parameter considered must be assessed utilizing a progressive scale.

The first parameter considered is the phototype, utilizing the Fitzpatrick classification, which divides the skin type based on its color and its reaction to the first summer exposure (Table 5.1) [5].

The second parameter considered is the structure of the rhytids with and without expression, utilizing the Glogau classification (Table 5.2) [1, 2].

The third parameter considered is the general grade of skeletonization–fullness of the face. The scale ranges from grade I, in the case of extreme (pathological) thin facial soft tissue envelope

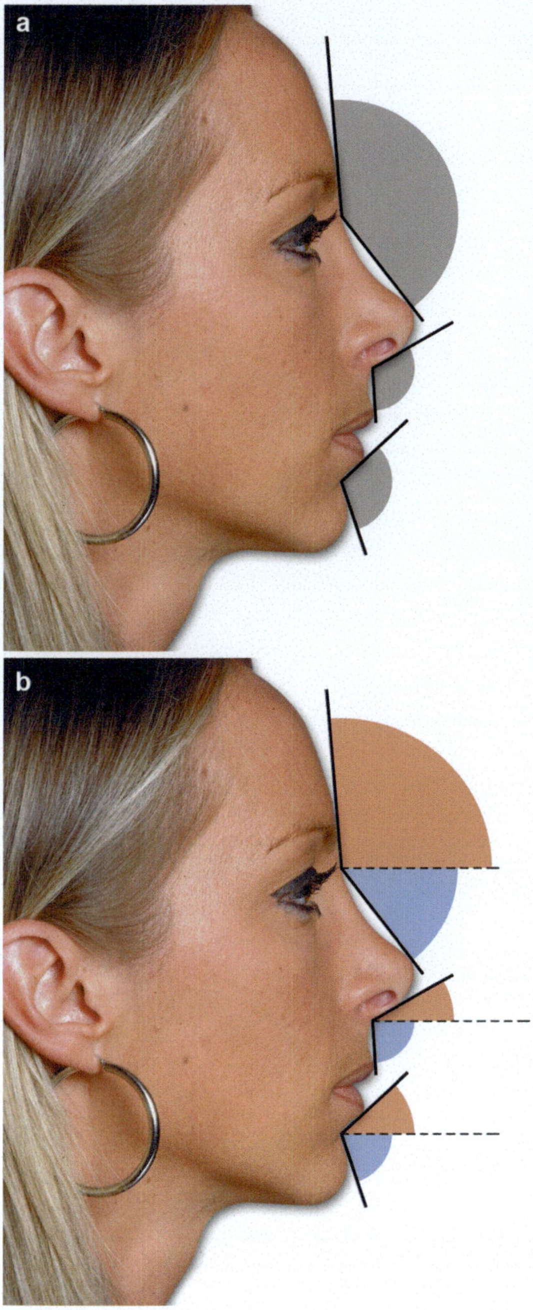

Fig. 5.12 The absolute value of some facial angles (**a**) can be broken up into their two elementary components by a *horizontal* or *vertical line* (**b**). For example, the too wide subnasal angle of this clinical case is due more to an upward rotated columella and less to a clockwise rotated upper lip

with greatly accentuated bony rims, eye globe, masseter muscle, and sternocleidomastoid muscle, to grade V, in which the fat accumulation significantly obscures the underlying skeletal shape. It is important to exclude some regions, like the nasal one, which may have a different grade of skeletonization compared to the rest of the face (Table 5.3).

The fourth parameter considered is the soft tissue laxity grade or the range of passive mobility of the skin over the skeletal and muscular underlying structures and is correlated to the grade of ptosis displayed. The scale ranges from grade I, in the case of an ideal and youthful subject with absence of laxity, to grade V, in which the ptosis is extreme and easy to mobilize with digital traction. Once again, some areas of the face, such as the medial canthus, should not be included in this general evaluation (Table 5.4).

The fifth parameter considered is the active spontaneous mobility grade, due to facial muscular contraction, that is exhibited during a conversation by the patient. The scale ranges from grade I, in the case of very low muscular activity, to grade V, characterized by an excessive mimetic activity. This evaluation is of special importance in the orbital and perioral region due to the functional and aesthetic role played by these muscles (Table 5.5).

This systematic assessment of the basic soft tissue envelope can reveal many previously undetected problems that may lead to a less than ideal final aesthetic outcome of our treatment.

5.6 Facial Soft Tissue Analysis Checklist[3]

- Fitzpatrick phototype classification:
  - □ I Very white or freckled
  - □ II White
  - □ III White to olive
  - □ IV Brown
  - □ V Dark brown
  - □ VI Black
- Glogau wrinkles classification:
  - □ I No wrinkles
  - □ II Wrinkles in motion
  - □ III Wrinkles at rest
  - □ IV Only wrinkles

[3]Section 2 on Springer Extra Materials (extras.springer.com).

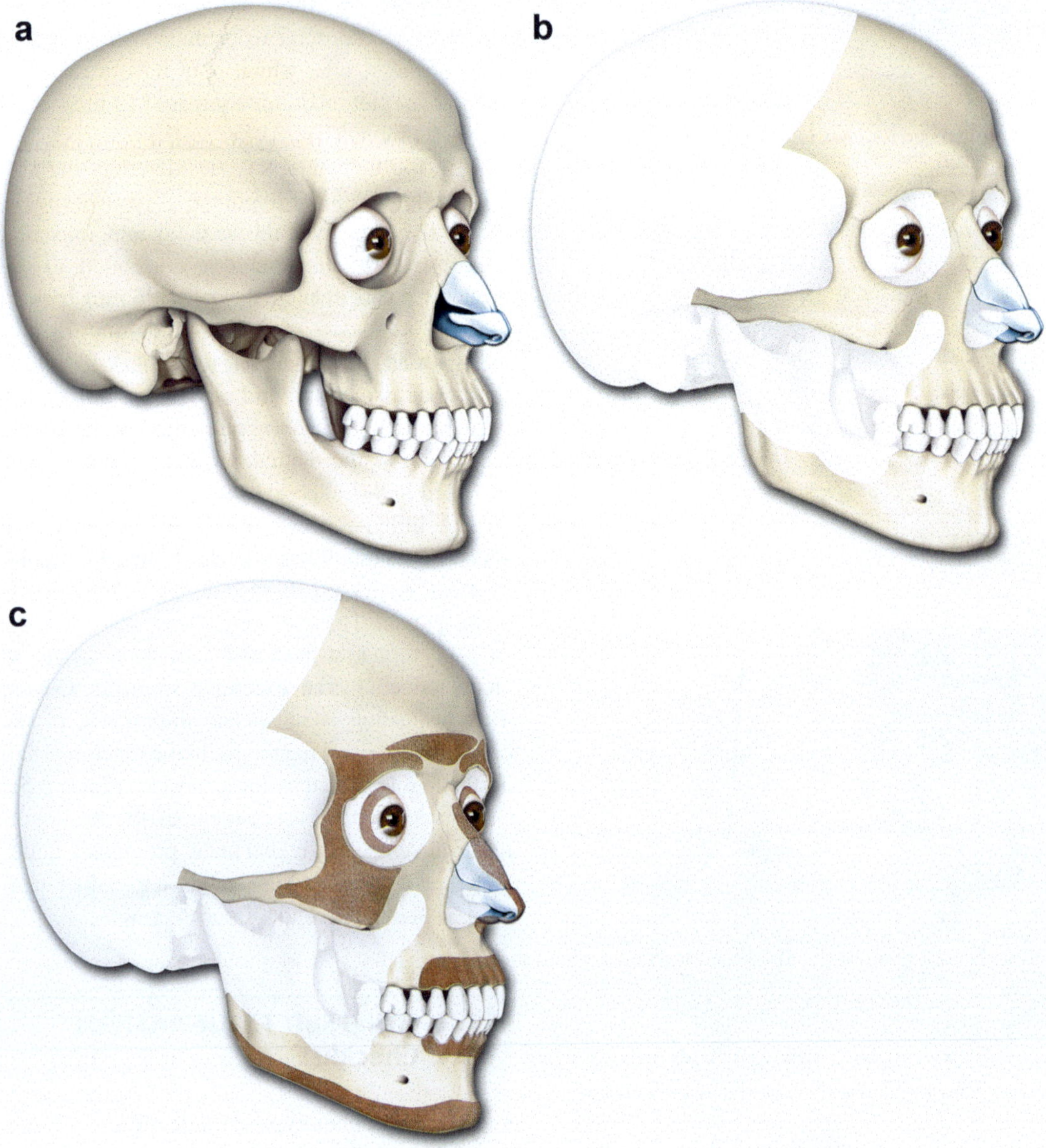

Fig. 5.13 The portions of the bony skeleton (*pale yellow*), the teeth (*white*), and the nasal cartilage (*pale blue*) as well the eye globe responsible for the "aesthetic" support of the facial soft tissue envelope are illustrated (**a**). In (**b**, **c**), the main structures of support are *highlighted*

- Facial skeletonization–fullness classification:
  - □ I Extremely thin (pathological)
  - □ II Thin
  - □ III Slightly thin
  - □ IV Ideal thickness for age and sex
  - □ V Slightly thick
  - □ VI Thick
  - □ VII Extremely thick (extremely obese patients)
- Facial soft tissue laxity classification:
  - □ I Ideal for sex and age (no evidence of laxity)
  - □ II Initial and localized laxity
  - □ III Moderate laxity

Table 5.1 The Fitzpatrick classification of sun-reactive skin types

Skin type	Color	Reaction to sun
I	Very white or freckled	Always burns
II	White	Usually burns
III	White to olive	Sometimes burns
IV	Brown	Rarely burns
V	Dark brown	Very rarely burns
VI	Black	Never burns

From [5]

Table 5.2 The Glogau wrinkles classification51

Progressive degrees of photodamage	Typical attributes
Type I: No wrinkles	Typical age 20s–30s
Early photoaging	
Mild pigmentary changes	
No keratoses (skin overgrowths)	
No or minimal wrinkles	
Type II: Wrinkles in motion	Typical age 30s–40s
Early to moderate photoaging	
Early senile lentigines	
Palpable but not visible keratoses	
Parallel smile lines beginning to appear lateral to mouth	
Type III: Wrinkles at rest	Typical age 50 or older
Advanced photoaging	
Obvious dyschromias, telangiectasias	
Visible keratoses	
Parallel smile lines beginning to appear lateral to mouth	
Type IV: Only wrinkles	Typical age 60 or above
Severe photoaging	
Yellow–gray skin	
Prior skin malignancies	
No normal skin	

Adapted from [5] and [1]

- □ IV Advanced laxity
- □ V Extreme laxity
- Facial soft tissue active mobility range:
  - □ I Limited
  - □ II Slightly limited

Table 5.3 The facial skeletonization–fullness classification

Degrees of skeletonization	Clinical attributes
I Extremely thin	Pathologically skinny subjects
II Thin	Skinny subjects Underlying bony and muscular structures easy to recognize
III Slightly thin	Acceptable thin soft tissue envelope Slight underweight may be associated
IV Ideal thickness	Ideal soft tissue thickness for age and sex
V Slightly thick	Acceptable thick soft tissue envelope Slight overweight may be associated
VI Thick	Overweight subjects Underlying bony and muscular structures difficult to recognize
VII Extremely thick	Extremely obese patients (pathological)

  - □ III Ideal
  - □ IV Slightly excessive
  - □ V Excessive
- Facial soft tissue active mobility symmetry:
  - □ Symmetric
  - □ Asymmetric (describe the asymmetry)

5.7 The Overweight Patient, Facial Analysis, and Surgical Treatment

Some facial areas, such as the cheeks, the preauricular area, the neck, and the submandibular and submental areas, are more prone to fat accumulation. Others, such as the nasal dorsum and the forehead, are less influenced by fat variations. In some overweight patients, the excess of facial fat can negate the aesthetic results of surgery, and as for some body surgical treatments, decisions about treatment should be deferred until appropriate weight reduction is realized and stabilized.

Table 5.4 The facial soft tissue degree of laxity scale (the ptosis scale)

Degrees of laxity	Clinical attributes
I Ideal	No sign of laxity
	Typical age up to 20s
II Initial and localized	Difficult to detect by layperson
	Typical age 20s–30s
	Localized in small facial areas such as upper lids or around lip commissures
III Moderate	Detectable by laypersons
	Typical age 30s–40s
	Localized mainly in some facial areas
IV Advanced	Diffuse laxity
	Skin easy to redrape in its original position with digital traction (passive repositioning)
V Extreme	Diffuse facial skin ptosis
	Ptosis sometimes extended to nasal tip
	Functional impairment due to ptosis (e.g., visual field reduction secondary to upper lid ptosis)

Table 5.5 The spontaneous facial musculature activity classification

Degrees of muscular activity	Clinical attributes
I Limited	Reduced ability in producing specific facial expressions
	Sometimes correlated to obesity or aging
	May be pathological
II Slightly limited	The range of movement is limited, but the ability to communicate emotions is maintained
	Some asymmetric muscular contraction may be possible
III Ideal	The range of movement is appropriate when the subject tries to communicate emotions to others
	Some minor asymmetric muscular contraction may be possible
IV Slightly excessive	The range of movement is enhanced, but the ability to communicate emotions is maintained Some asymmetric muscular contraction may be possible
V Excessive	The excessive facial muscular contraction reduces the ability of the subject to produce a specific facial expression
	May be pathological

5.8 From Specific to General: A Reversed Approach to Basic Analysis

This chapter is dedicated to basic facial analysis, which is mainly conducted observing the entire face. But often, we need the input offered by a small particular to find out or confirm a general feature of the whole face. In other words, we should combine two key clinical approaches: "from general to specific" and, its reverse, "from specific to general."

An example of the latter is given by the presence of the inferior scleral show. This is the presence of a small portion of white sclera between the iris and the lower lid margin in a subject examined in the natural head position and straight gaze. Tilting the head down or orienting the gaze upwards can produce a false scleral show (Fig. 5.14).

A true scleral show can be a sign of regional problems, such as a retracted lower lid or

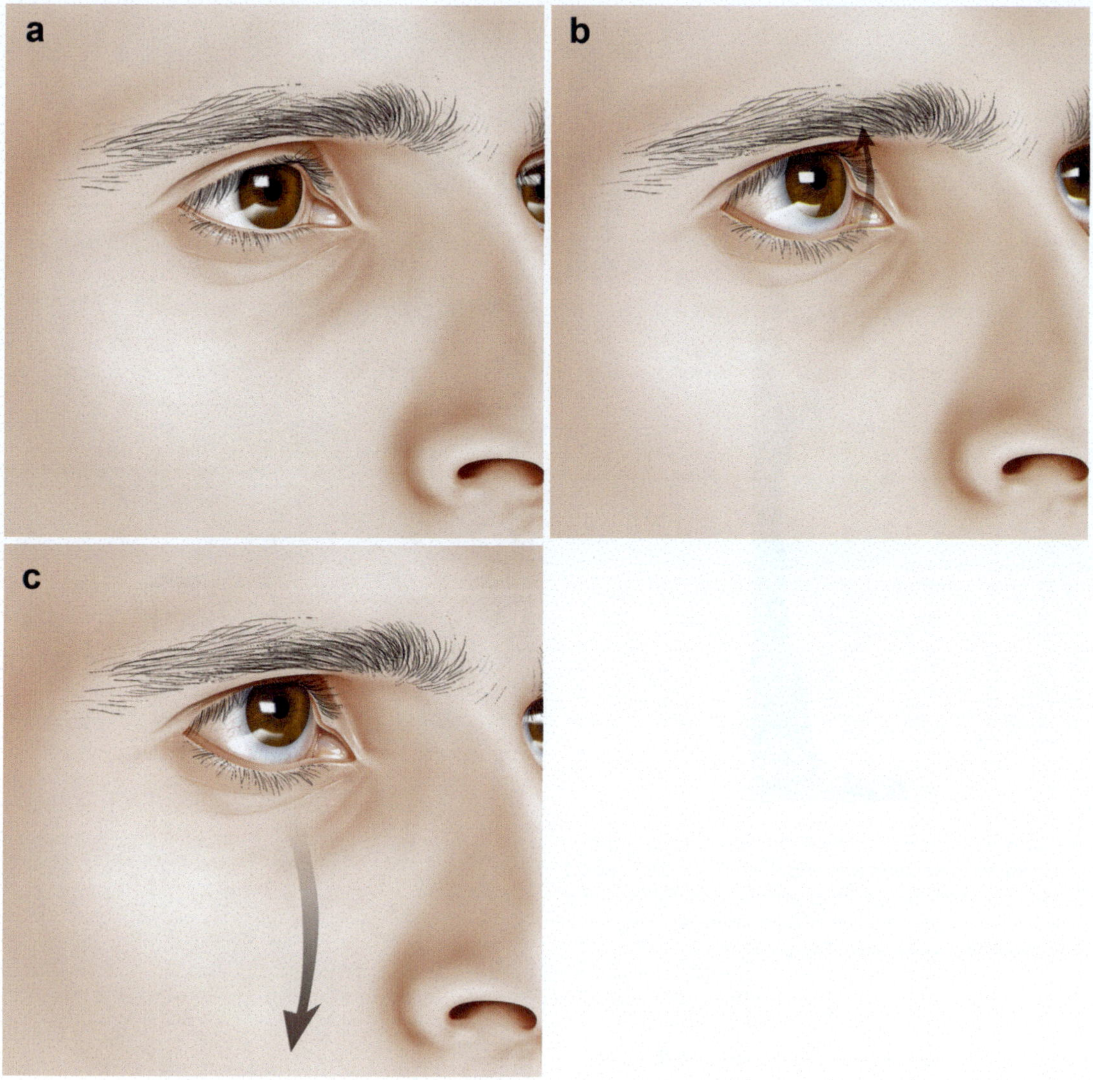

Fig. 5.14 Errors in detecting the inferior scleral show. Oblique close-up view taken in the natural head position and straight gaze with no evidence of scleral show (**a**). The same subject in upward-oriented gaze (**b**) and in head-tilted-down position (**c**) with the appearance of false scleral show

exophthalmia, but also of a whole facial problem such as a hypoplasia of the middle third of the face (Fig. 5.15).

Another specific key point to observe is the sharpness and the incline of the mandibular border outline in profile and oblique views. Its definition is related to the soft tissue thickness and ptosis (Fig. 5.16), whereas the degree of rotation is clearly connected with the vertical feature of the lower third of the face, the chin projection, and contour (Fig. 5.17).

5.9 Basic Analysis: Preferred Terms[4]

In this and the subsequent chapters, the reader will find one or more sections, presented as an alphabetically ordered glossary, that gives the related terminology used in the text, along with short

[4]Section 3 on Springer Extra Materials (extras.springer.com).

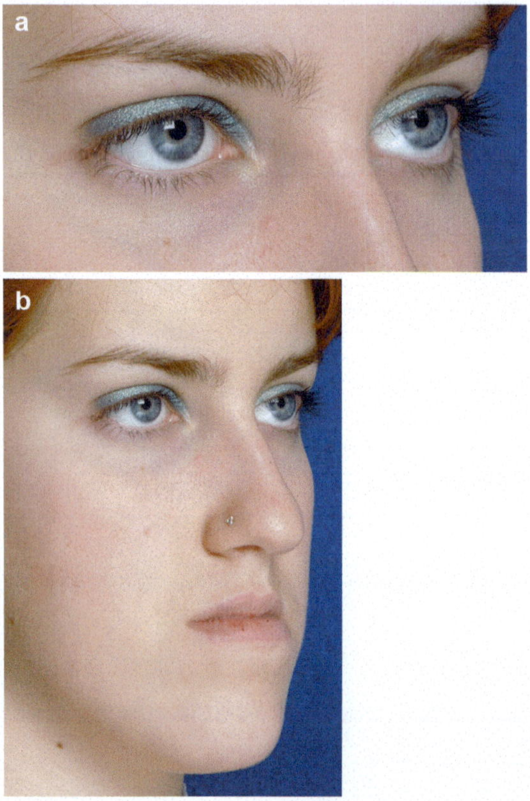

Fig. 5.15 A clinical case in which the scleral show (**a**) is a sign of marked maxillary hypoplasia (**b**). The scleral show is the presence of a small portion of the white sclera between the iris and the lower lid margin in a subject in the natural head position and straight gaze

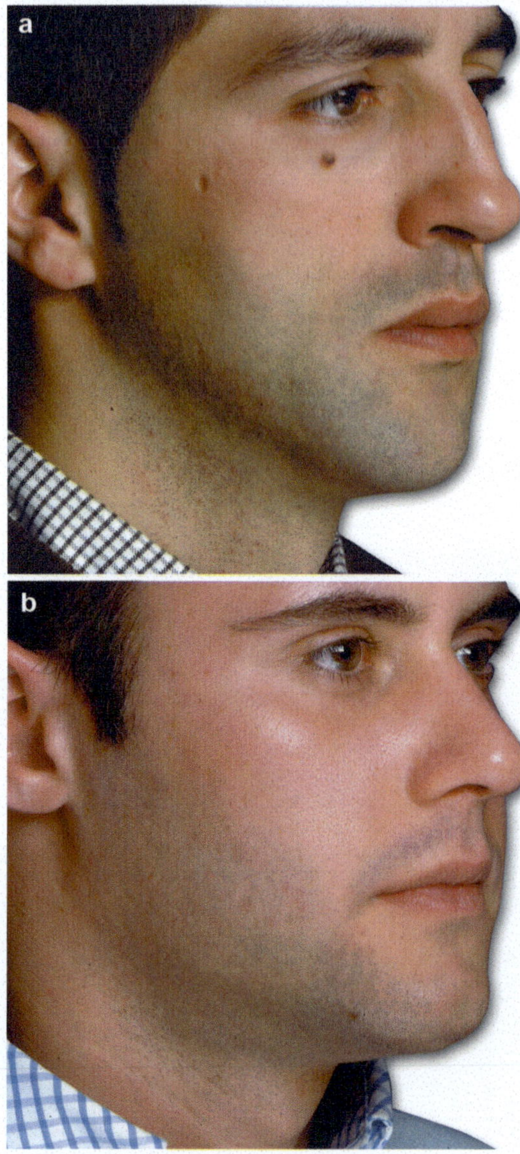

Fig. 5.16 Facial soft tissue thickness can be appreciated by judging the mandibular border outline and shadowing in oblique and profile views. Two oblique views of young male subjects with moderately thin (**a**) and moderately thick (**b**) soft tissue envelope revealed utilizing the mandibular border outline

definitions. The following list explains the essential terminology utilized for basic facial analysis:

- *Bigonial width* – The width of the face, measured between the skin outline at the level of the mandibular angles, in frontal view.
- *Bimental width* – The width of the face, measured between the skin outline at the level of the chin, in frontal view.
- *Bitemporal width* – The width of the face, measured between the skin outline at the level of the temporal region, in frontal view.
- *Bizygomatic width* – The width of the face, measured between the two zygomatic arches at their maximal distance, in frontal view.
- *Central oval of the face* – The extended central region of the face. It is comprised of the eyes, the eyebrows, the zygoma, the nose, the mouth, and the chin [7].
- *Concave–convex profile* – The anterior–posterior relationship of the whole facial profile. It varies from concave, due to a relative posteriorly positioned middle third, to convex, due to a relative anteriorly positioned middle third. This classification does not define which third of the face is responsible for the deformity.

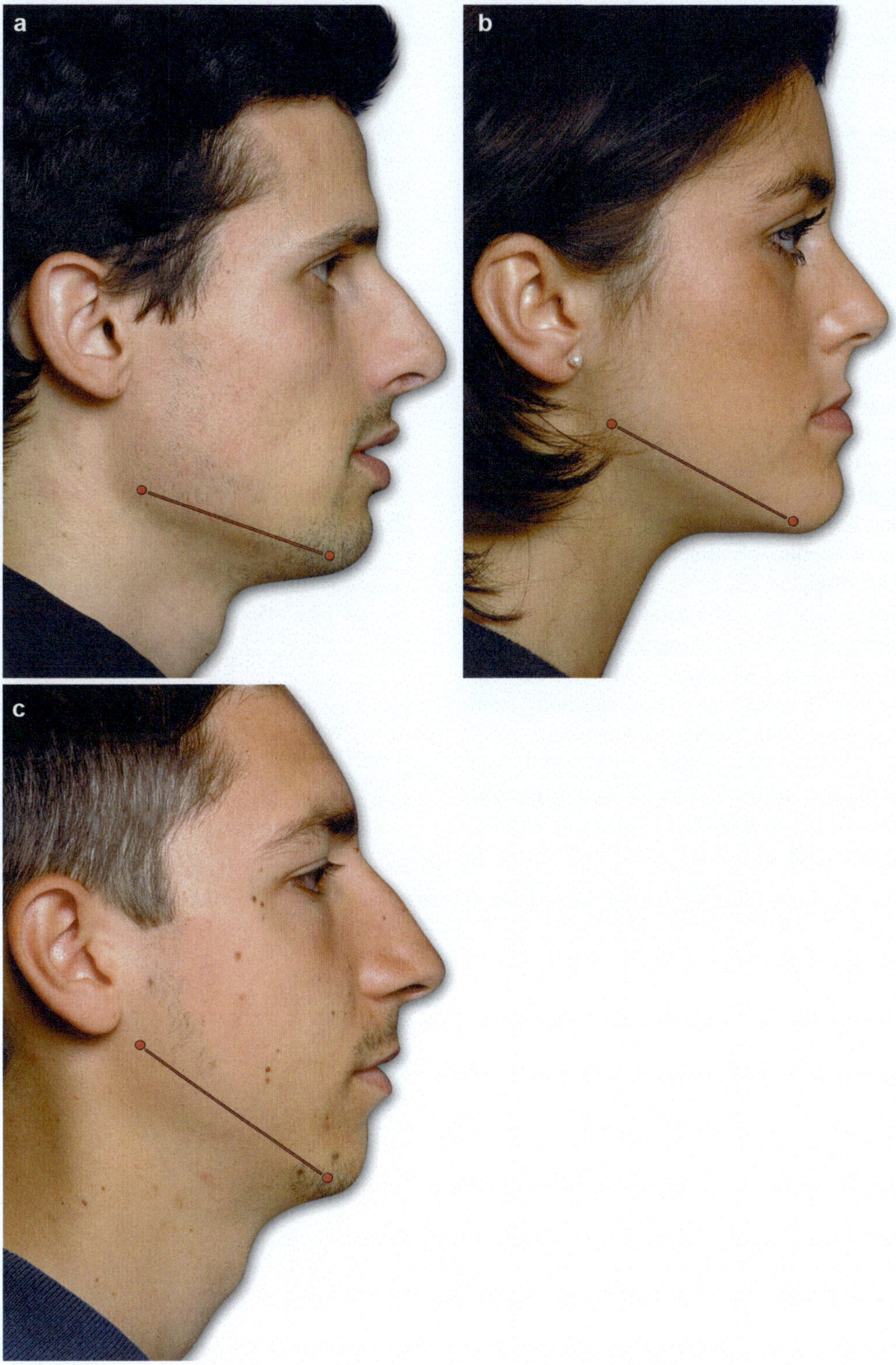

Fig. 5.17 Different degrees of mandibular border rotation in profile view. Counterclockwise rotation associated with reduction of the facial lower third height and well-shaped chin outline (**a**). Normal incline of the mandibular border in a subject with thin soft tissue thickness and maintenance of good chin contour (**b**). Clockwise rotation of the mandibular border associated with loss of chin projection, increased facial lower third, and poor profile aesthetics (**c**)

- *Facial height* (*total facial height*) – The distance between the trichion and soft tissue menton.
- *Hairline* – The edge of hair round the face.
- *Wide–narrow face* – The predominance and the reduction, respectively, of the four widths of the face over the total facial height.
- *Long–short face* – The predominance and the reduction, respectively, of the total facial height over the four widths of the face.
- *Menton* (*soft tissue menton*) – Lowest point on the contour of the soft tissue chin. In cephalometric analysis, it is found by dropping a perpendicular from the horizontal plane through the skeletal menton [3].
- *Subnasal* – The point at which the columella merges with the upper lip in the midsagittal plane [3]. It varies widely in relation to the caudal septum prominence and nasal spine morphology.
- *Malar eminence* – The point of maximal outer projection of the malar region.
- *Mandibular border outline* – The skin contour line that separates the mandibular body from the submental and submandibular ones.
- *Ogee curve* – The outline of the middle and the lower third of the face viewed in oblique view. This term was introduced by J. William Little and is correlated to the characteristics of the youthful face [4].
- *Triangular–square face* – The classification of the whole face in frontal view based on the relationship between the upper widths (bitemporal and bizygomatic) and the lower ones (bigonial and bimental).
- *Trichion* – The hairline midpoint.

References

1. Bauman L (2002) Photoaging. In: Bauman L (ed) Cosmetic dermatology: principle and practice. McGraw-Hill, New York
2. Glogau RG (1994) Chemical peeling and aging skin. J Geriatr Dermatol 12:31
3. Jacobson A, Vlachos C (1995) Soft tissue evaluation. In: Jacobson A (ed) Radiographic cephalometry: from basics to videoimaging. Quintessence, Chicago
4. Little JW (2000) Volumetric perceptions in midfacial aging with altered priorities for rejuvenation. Plast Reconstr Surg 105:252–266
5. Monheit GD (2002) Combination chemical peelings. In: Lowe NJ (ed) Textbook of facial rejuvenation. The art of minimally invasive combination therapy. Martin Dunitz, London
6. Platzer W (1985) Atlas of topographical anatomy. Georg Thieme Verlag, Stuttgart
7. Ramirez O (2000) The central oval of the face: tridimensional endoscopic rejuvenation. Facial Plast Surg Clin North Am 16:283–298

Forehead, Eyebrows, and Eyes

6

Contents

Looking at the upper third of the face, we can note its role in facial expression. The acts of blinking, raising or lowering the eyebrows, frowning the glabella, elevating the upper lids, closing the eyes, and rotating the eye globes up or down are essential in communicating approval or disapproval, attention, surprise, indifference, and many other emotions. In the long term, the aging process progressively changes the external aspect of the upper third, as well as its dynamics.

For these reasons, the analysis of the upper third of the face is not limited to a simple three-dimensional assessment of symmetry, proportion, and shape of the region, but must include the fourth dimension of dynamics and the fifth dimension represented by the effects of the aging process.

6.1 Forehead Analysis

The forehead occupies the upper third of the face entirely, and its bony shape and muscle activity are intimately associated with the aesthetics and functions of the orbital and nasal units; its width is about twice its height.

Two skeletal subunits can be considered: the supraorbital bar and the upper forehead [5]. The supraorbital bar, corresponding to the supraorbital rim and glabellar area, greatly influences the aesthetics of the brow, the upper lid, and the nasal radix, due to its direct structural support. Its shape varies widely with the development of the frontal sinus, with more angularity and anterior prominence in male subjects than in female ones.

F. Meneghini, P. Biondi, *Clinical Facial Analysis*,
DOI 10.1007/978-3-642-27228-8_6, © Springer-Verlag Berlin Heidelberg 2012

The upper forehead, located above the supraorbital bar, consists of a slight vertical and transversal convexity. The palpable and often visible rim of the temporal fossa, also called the temporal ridge, is the lateral boundary of the forehead. The hairline, which defines the forehead upper boundary, is quite different between the sexes and, especially in relationship with men's anterior balding, can change with age.

When analyzing the bony forehead, three important aesthetic characteristics should be considered: the general shape, the slope, and the morphology of the supraorbital bar. The outline, in profile and oblique views, varies from round to flat with, sometimes, an inferior concavity defining the supraorbital ridge. The basal view is useful in defining the symmetry and the grade of transversal convexity.

The soft tissue analysis of the forehead should recognize the glabellar frown lines and the transverse forehead wrinkles or furrows along with the evaluation of the regional muscle dynamics.

Even if the forehead can be reshaped surgically with specific procedures, in the vast majority of cases, it should be considered as a stable and highly visible skeletal structure that can be utilized as a reference in the process of analysis of the shape, volume, and spatial orientation of other structures such as the nose, the midface, the anterior teeth, and the chin.

The temporal region, which is bounded inferiorly by the zygomatic arch, anteriorly by the posterior rim of the frontal process of the malar bone and the zygomatic process of the frontal bone, and superiorly by the rim of the temporal fossa, can vary from slightly concave to slightly convex depending on the volume of temporal muscle and subcutaneous fat. The shape and location of the temporal hairline have an important role as a boundary in the aesthetics of the upper third of the face.

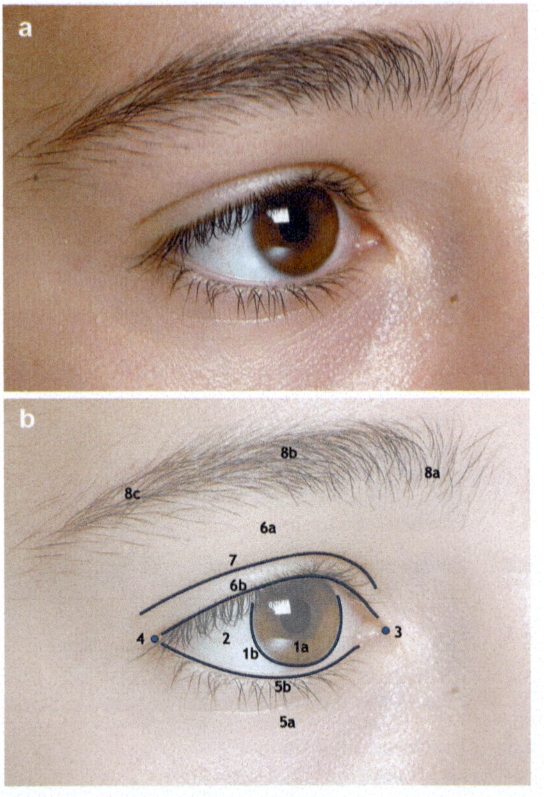

Fig. 6.1 Close-up oblique view of orbital region in a young subject (**a**). Basic elements of normal surface anatomy of the orbital region (**b**): *1a* iris, *1b* limbus (the circular line separating the iris from the white sclera), *2* white sclera, *3* medial canthus, *4* lateral canthus, *5a* lower lid, *5b* lower lid free margin, *6a* upper lid, *6b* upper lid free margin, *7* upper lid crease, *8a* medial third of the eyebrow (head), *8b* central third of the eyebrow (body), and *8c* lateral third of the eyebrow (tail)

6.2 Eyebrow, Eye, and Lids Analysis

From the aesthetic and functional point of view, there is no sense in evaluating the eyebrow separately from the upper lid or any other component of the orbital region. Figure 6.1 shows the surface anatomy of the orbital region along with the related basic terminology.

The assessment of the skeletal support sustained by the orbital ridges and the globe to soft tissue requires the visualization in profile view of three different vertical reference lines, which, in the frontal view, pass through the center of the iris (Fig. 6.2a):

- The corneal line. This is the reference line and requires that the eye globe be in a normal sagittal position.
- The upper orbital rim line. This is 8–10 mm anterior to the corneal plane line depending on the pneumatization of the frontal sinus and the morphology of the supraorbital bar [6].

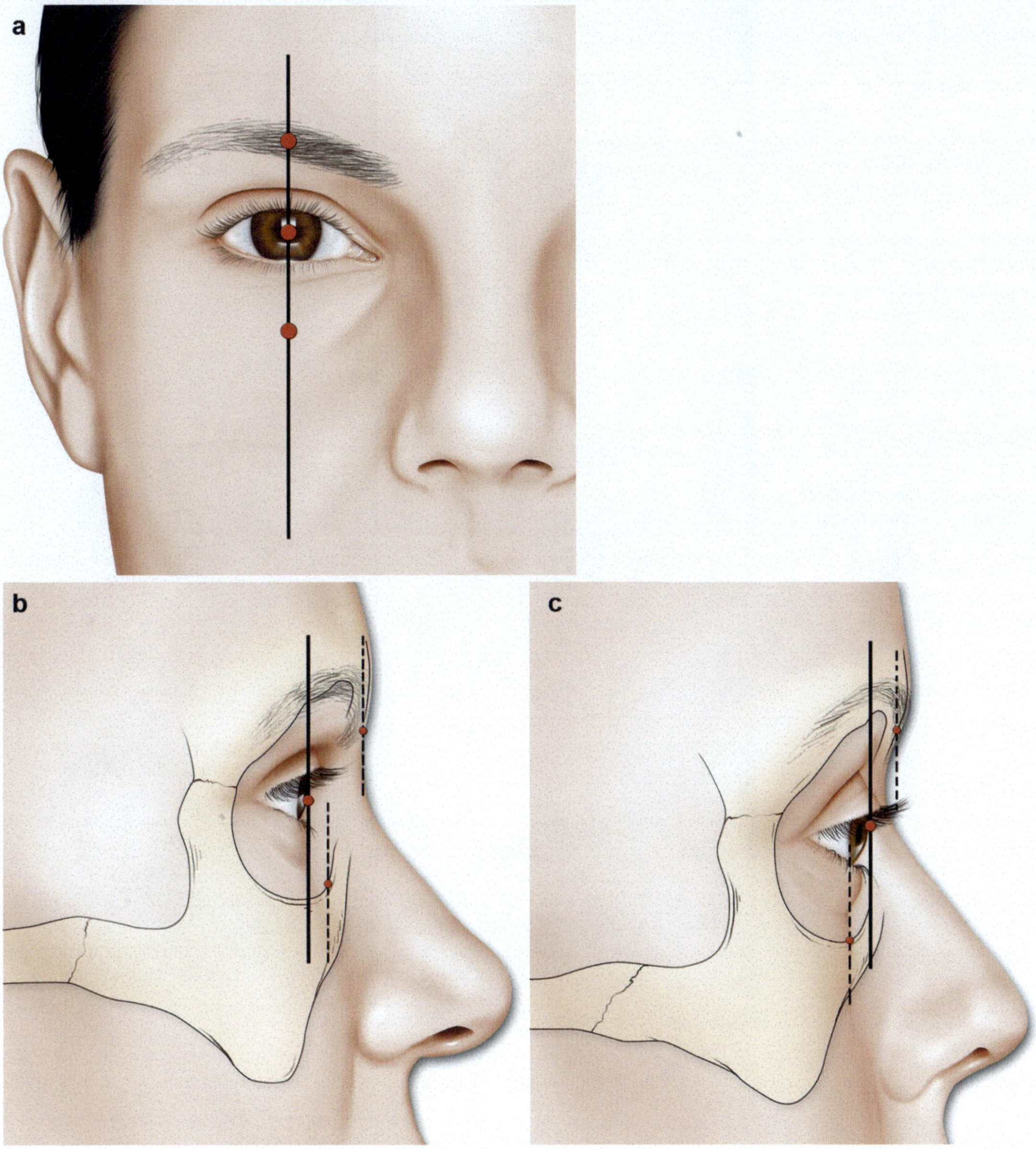

Fig. 6.2 The corneal plane line, the upper orbital rim line, and the lower orbital line coincide in the frontal view (**a**). In the case of a normally positioned eye globe, the upper orbital rim line lies anterior to the corneal plane line, whereas the lower orbital rim line can be anterior (**b**) or posterior (**c**) to it

- The lower orbital rim line. Its position can vary widely from posterior to anterior with respect to the corneal plane line. A protrusive lower orbital rim is associated with good lower lid support and a youthful aspect (Fig. 6.2b), whereas a recessive lower orbital rim line is a sign of infraorbital and midface hypoplasia, which is associated with inadequate support of the lower lid and poor aesthetics (Fig. 6.2c).

The oblique views, examining the upper portion of the ogee curve,[1] are also extremely useful in the evaluation of the skeletal support offered to the lower lid by the inferior and lateral traits of the orbital rim.

[1]See Sect. 5.2.3.

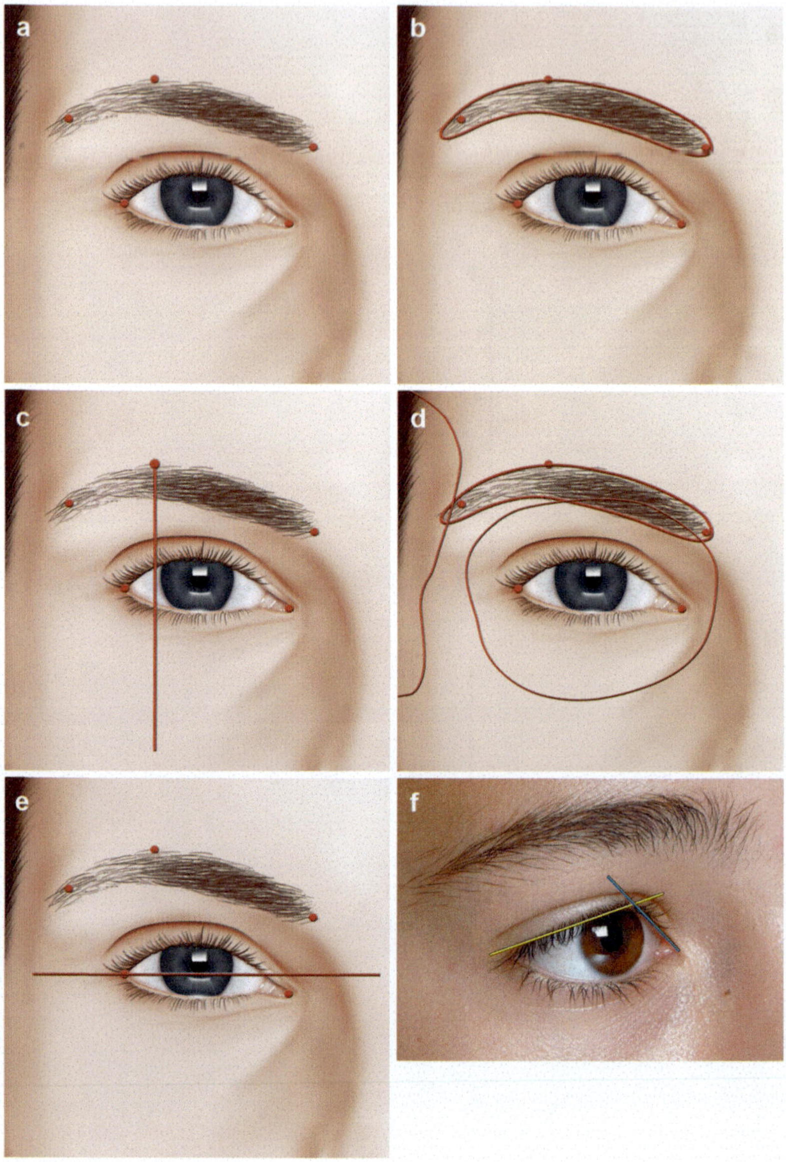

Fig. 6.3 The female attractive eye. The eyebrow shape forms a gentle curve without angularity or interruptions (**a**); the medial and central portions are wider than the lateral (**b**). The eyebrow peak is located on a vertical plane passing lateral to or touching the lateral limbus (**c**). The medial third of the brow lies on the orbital ridge or partially inferior to it, the central third is on the ridge, and the lateral third just above the ridge (**d**). The intercanthal axis should be inclined slightly upward from medial to lateral, producing an upward lateral canthal tilt (**e**). The medial portion of the upper lid margin should be more vertically oriented than the lateral one (**f**)

6.2.1 The Female Attractive Eye

Many authors have studied the attractive female eye and brow, producing the criteria that were assembled and reformulated by Gunter and Antrobus in their article of 1997 [3]. Some of these are:

- Eyebrow shape.[2] This forms a gentle curve without angularity (Fig. 6.3a). The medial and central portions are wider than the lateral portion (Fig. 6.3b).

[2]The size, shape, and spatial position of the eyebrows, in aesthetically pleasing subjects, can vary greatly with age, sex, culture, ethnicity, and fashion trends.

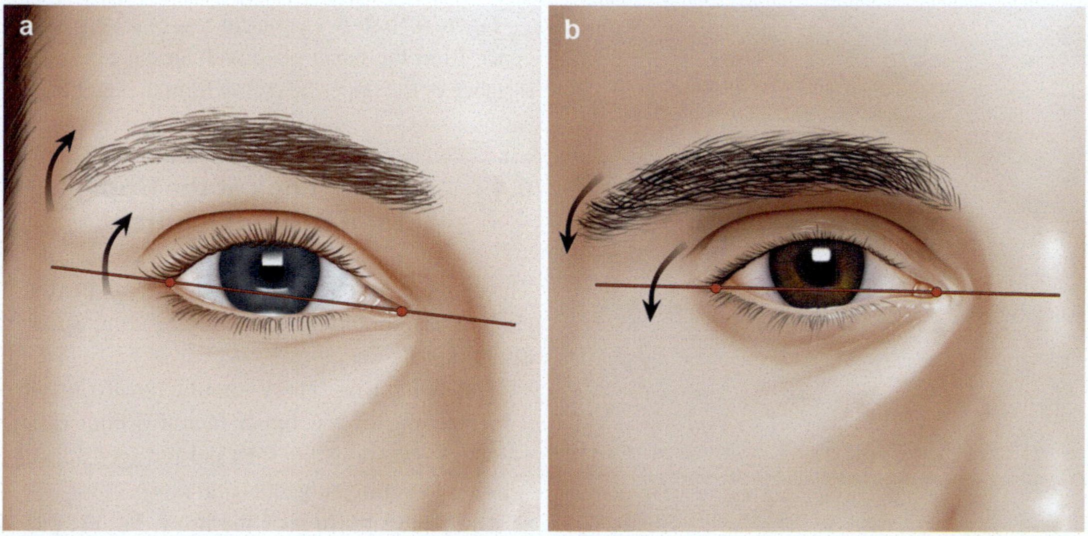

Fig. 6.4 Comparison between the female attractive (**a**) and the male attractive eye (**b**). In male subjects, the intercanthal axis is less inclined upward from medial to lateral, the supraorbital ridge anterior projection is augmented, and the brow is wider, less arched, and more horizontally oriented

- Eyebrow peak. This is located on a vertical plane passing slightly lateral to or touching the lateral limbus (Fig. 6.3c).
- Eyebrow location. The medial end of the eyebrow starts on the same or near the vertical plane of the medial canthus if there is a normal intercanthal distance. The medial third lies on the orbital ridge or partially inferior to it, the central third is on the ridge, and the lateral third just above the ridge (Fig. 6.3d).
- Intercanthal axis. It should be inclined slightly upward from medial to lateral, producing an upward lateral canthal tilt (Fig. 6.3e).
- Upper lid–iris relationship. The upper lid should cover the iris by approximately 1–2 mm.
- Medial and lateral portions of the upper lids margin. The medial portion should be more vertically oriented than the lateral one (Fig. 6.3f).
- Upper lid crease. It should parallel the lash line and divide the upper lid into an upper two thirds and a lower one third.
- Medial and lateral extension of the upper lid crease. The medial extension should not exceed the inner extent of the medial canthus, and the lateral one should not extend beyond the lateral orbital rim.
- Lower lid–iris relationship. There should be minimal, if any, scleral show between the lower lid and iris.[3]
- Lower lid margin. It should bow gently from medially to laterally, with the lowest point between the pupil and the lateral limbus.

The main differences in the attractive male eye are in the intercanthal axis, which is less inclined upward from medial to lateral, in the supraorbital ridge anterior projection, which is augmented, and in the brow, which is wider, less arched, and more horizontally oriented. Figure 6.4 shows a comparison between an attractive female and an attractive male eye.

6.3 Upper Lid Crease Malposition

The vertical position of the upper lid crease must be assessed with precision during clinical examination. It may be related to different conditions

[3]See Figs. 5.14 and 5.15 for more details about the inferior scleral show.

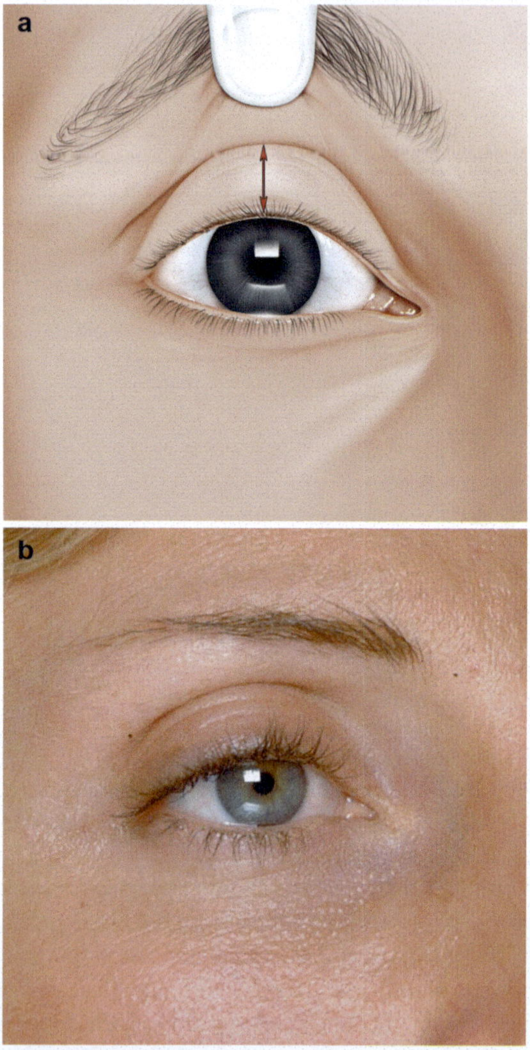

Fig. 6.5 Measurement of the margin crease distance is performed with the eye fold elevated by the examiner and with the patient looking down (**a**). A clinical case of levator dehiscence from the tarsal plate with an increase in the distance of the upper lid crease from the margin (**b**)

such as ethnicity, aging, and levator muscle dehiscence from the tarsal plate [8].

To evaluate the vertical position of the upper lid crease precisely, we can utilize the margin crease distance. It is the distance from the central upper eyelid margin to the tarsal crease measured with the eyelid fold elevated by the examiner and as the patient looks down (Fig. 6.5a). The normal range in occidentals reported by Putterman is 9–11 mm [7], whereas that reported by Wolfort, Baker, and Kanter is 8–10 mm [9].

Figure 6.5b shows a clinical case of levator dehiscence from the tarsal plate with an increase in the distance of the upper lid crease from the margin.

6.4 A Closer Look at the Upper Lateral Orbital Quadrant

The elements of the upper lateral orbital quadrant (Fig. 6.6a) should be inspected, giving special attention to:

- The bony rim. There should be no inferior protruding of the upper lateral orbital ridge, which is responsible for a sad and aged appearance in young subjects (Fig. 6.6b).
- The lateral portion of the brow. Its rest position should not appear to the observer as a sign of sadness, tiredness, or astonishment, as discussed in the following paragraph (Fig. 6.6c).
- The lateral portion of the upper lid crease. It is important to detect a lateral extension over the eyelid and onto the lateral periorbital region of the upper lid crease (Connell's sign), which is a hallmark of forehead ptosis [6] (Fig. 6.6d).
- The presence of a prolapsed lacrimal gland. It can produce an excessive fullness of the lateral third of the upper eyelid (there is no fat in the upper temporal angle of the orbit) (Fig. 6.6e). On the other hand, a moderate fullness of the lateral third of the upper eyelid is aesthetically favorable in women [4].
- The lateral commissure. The laxity of the lateral canthal tendon (lateral canthal bowing) produces an inferior rotation of the commissure (Fig. 6.6f).

6.5 Eyebrow Malposition and Inappropriate Expressions

Eyebrow malposition can produce an unattractive or unwanted look with a negative impact in relationships with others [3, 6]. The surprised–unintelligent look is produced by over-elevation of the eyebrows. Also, the medial placement of the brow peak creates an undesired surprised look. The angry look is due to a low medial brow with a high lateral peak, whereas a large asymmetry in

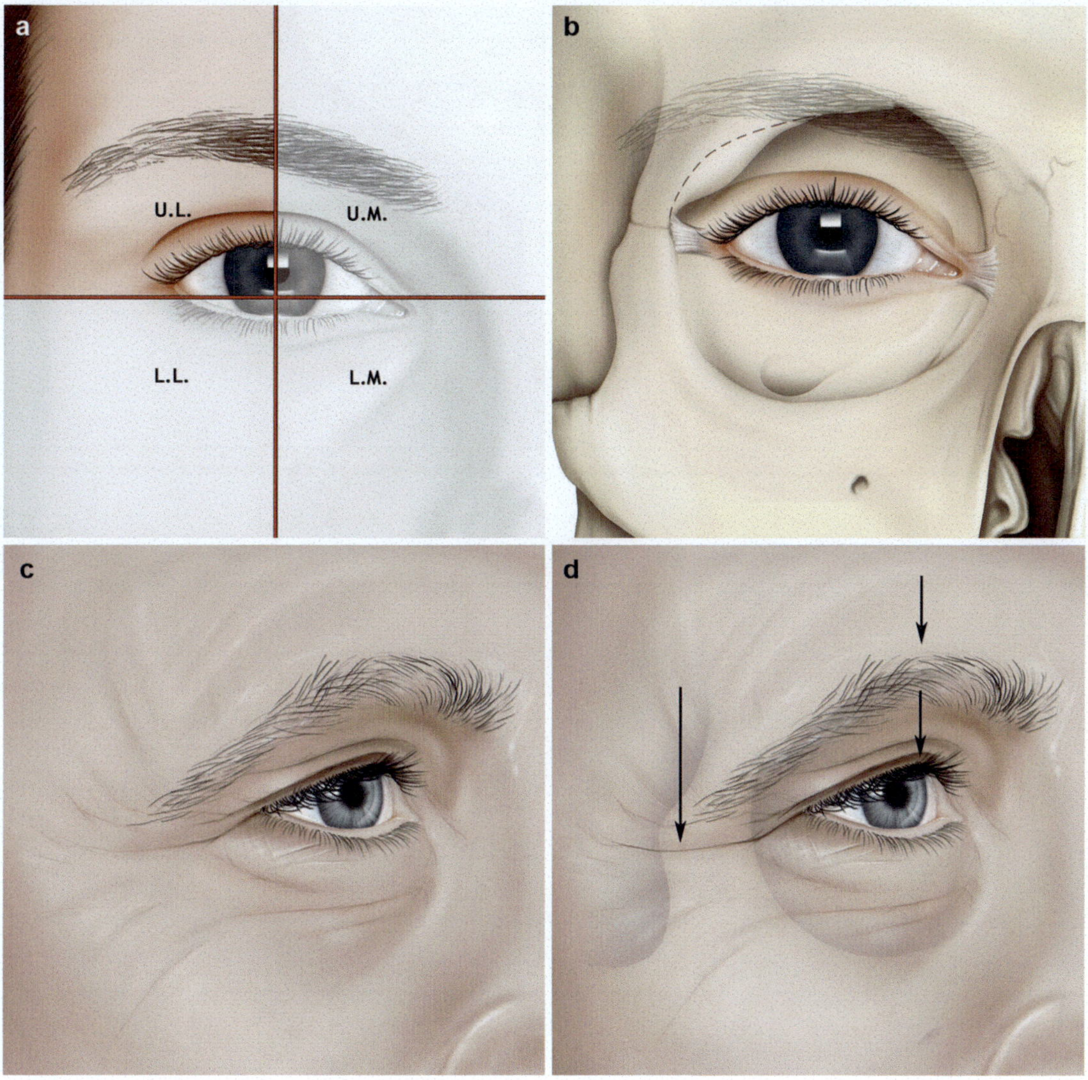

Fig. 6.6 The upper lateral orbital quadrant (**a**). Hanging upper lateral orbital ridge (**b**). Malposition of the lateral brow at rest, resulting in a sad appearance (**c**). Lateral extension of the upper lid crease over the eyelid and onto the lateral periorbital region, or Connell's sign (**d**). Prolapsed lacrimal gland, producing an excessive fullness of the lateral third of the upper eyelid (**e**). Laxity of the lateral canthal tendon, producing an inferiorly rotated commissure (**f**)

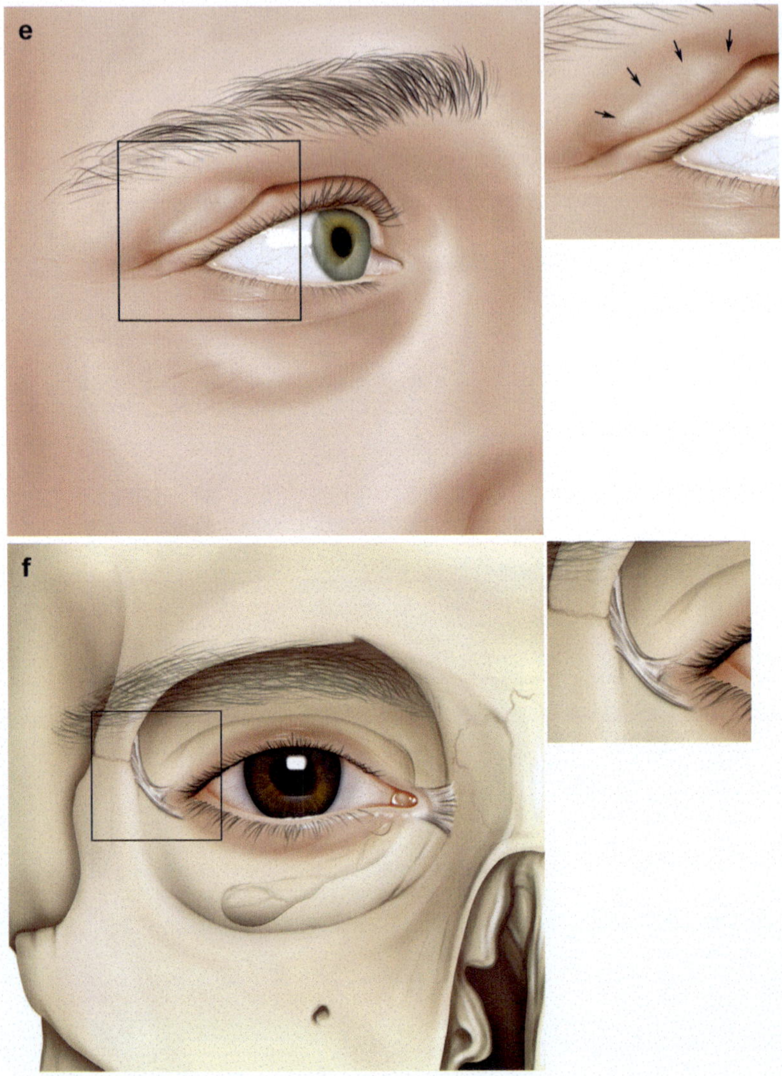

Fig. 6.6 (continued)

the height of the eyebrows gives the inquisitive appearance.

Sometimes the patient is obliged to contract the frontalis muscle to clear the upper visual field obstruction produced by forehead and upper lid ptosis. The result is a bilateral excessive elevation of the medial brows and a corrugated forehead, producing a sad–tired appearance. The surgical removal of upper lid skin excess clears the upper visual field and induces the relaxation of the frontalis with an evident medial brow ptosis and a new, unwanted, angry appearance [6].

During the clinical examination and shooting the photographs, it is fundamental to document these "pseudoexpressions" imposed by the periorbital soft tissue anatomy and dynamics. Some of the eye views, such as the unforced closed view and the looking down view,[4] help to highlight the frontalis muscle contraction, giving a clearer idea of the real vertical position of the eyebrow at rest.

[4]See Figs. 3.18 and 3.19.

6.6 Suspect and Search for the Early Signs of Aging in the Upper Third of the Face

When analyzing a middle-aged subject from the aesthetic point of view, a difficult and at the same time important task is to break up the global problem into its basic elements. These elements are the deformities; which should be considered mainly as a constant factor; any pathology and posttraumatic sequelae, which may or may not be present; and the aging process, which risks being underestimated in that age group.

Sometimes, a deformity of the orbital margins, such as infraorbital hypoplasia, lateral orbital rim overhang, and excessive pneumatization of the frontal sinus, can be mistaken as a sign of premature aging. In other cases, the opposite may happen, and a well-supporting skeleton can positively influence the soft tissue envelope, hiding the aging changes for years.

I always expect and search for the signs of aging in the forehead and orbital region, as it can be detected much earlier than in other facial regions, giving me and my patient the opportunity to deal with these problems with a long-term plan.

Essentially, I look for the following three signs: dermatochalasis, loss of lid tone (eyelid laxity), and herniated orbital fat.

- Dermatochalasis is the excess of eyelid skin. It is usually more relevant in the upper eyelids and is also a frequent condition in middle-aged subjects. The skin excess can be assessed by pinching the excess of eyelid skin with forceps until the eyelashes begin to evert (Fig. 6.7).
- The loss of lid tone is usually more relevant in the lower lid. We refer to lid tone as the ability of the lids to maintain spontaneously and recover (recapture) quickly their normal position against the globe. The presence of horizontal lower lid laxity should be assessed performing the distraction test and the snap test [2]. The lid should not be pulled more than 7 mm away from the inferior limbus (distraction test – Fig. 6.8a) and, after the distraction, should snap back into its normal position immediately (snap test – Fig. 6.8b).

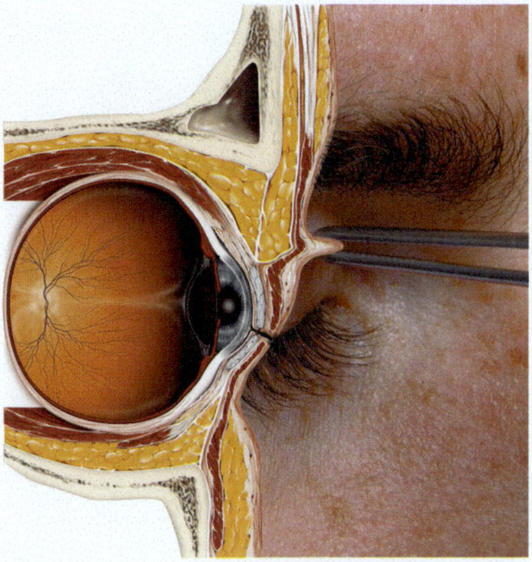

Fig. 6.7 Upper lid early dermatochalasis assessed with the pinch technique. The examiner pinches the excess of eyelid skin with a forceps until the eyelashes begin to evert

- The herniated orbital fat. By gently pressing on the globe, it is possible to produce the protrusion of fat pockets (Fig. 6.9a). The lower lid fat is also assessed with the subject in the upright sitting or standing position and gaze-up eye globes orientation (Fig. 6.9b). In the supine position, the orbital fat, due to its mobility, is spontaneously repositioned into the orbit and is not usually evident in young adults.

Chapter 9 considers further the relationship between skeletal deformities and the aging appearance, whereas Chap. 10 discusses the aging of the upper third of the face in adults and elderly subjects.

6.7 Forehead, Eyebrows, and Eyes Analysis Checklist[5]

- Is the upper third of the face symmetric?
  □ Yes
  □ No, because…

[5]Section 2 on Springer Extra Materials (extras.springer.com).

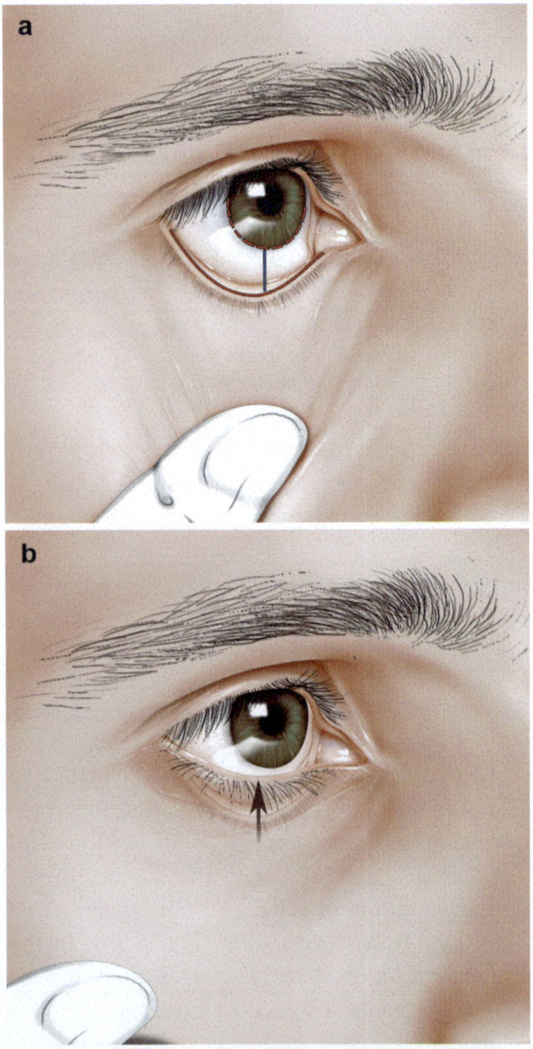

Fig. 6.8 Lower lid horizontal laxity assessment. Distraction test: the lower lid margin should not be pulled more than 7 mm away from the inferior limbus (**a**). Snap test: after distraction, the lower lid should snap back into its normal position immediately (**b**)

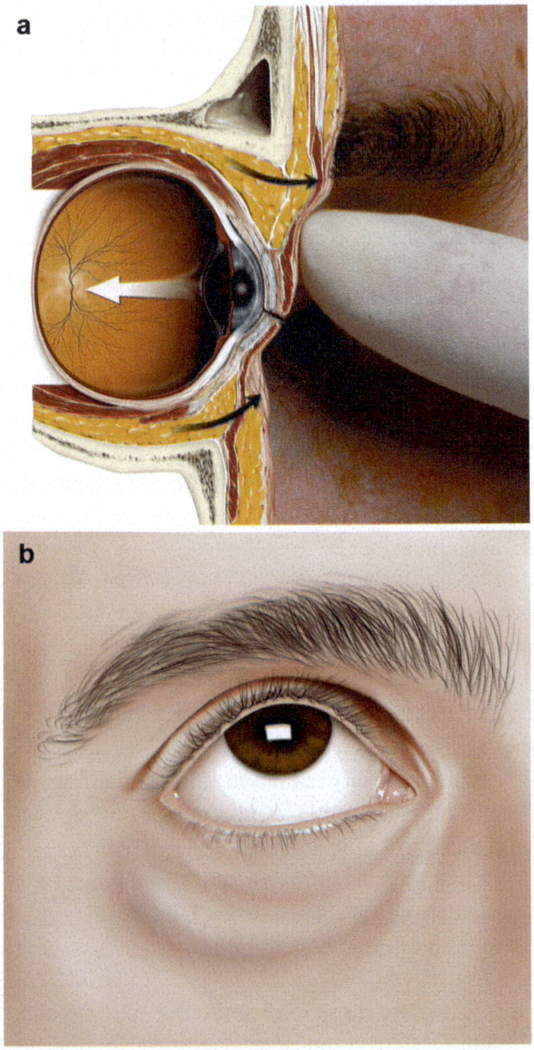

Fig. 6.9 The herniated orbital fat can be highlighted by applying gentle pressure to the eye globe (**a**). Lower lid herniated orbital fat is better assessed with the subject in an upright position and gaze-up eye globe orientation (**b**). In the supine position, the orbital fat, due to its mobility, spontaneously repositions into the orbit and is less evident

- Are the two orbital regions symmetric?
  - □ Yes
  - □ No, because…
- In the frontal view, the forehead is:
  - □ Wide
  - □ Narrow
  - □ Long
  - □ Short
- The trichion is:
  - □ Normally positioned
  - □ Too high
  - □ Too low
- The forehead profile is:
  - □ Flat
  - □ Round
  - □ Presence of inferior concavity (clear definite orbital bar)
- The supraorbital bar is:
  - □ Normally shaped

□ Protruding
□ Recessive

- Skeletal lower lid support:
  □ Poor
  □ Acceptable
  □ Ideal
- Define the malar eminence:
  □ Hypoplastic
  □ Balanced
  □ Pronounced
- Define the symmetry of the eyebrows:
  □ Present
  □ Absent due to…
- Define the symmetry of the eye globes:
  □ Present
  □ Absent due to…
- Define the symmetry of the eyelids:
  □ Present
  □ Absent due to…
- Define the eyebrow position:
  □ Ideal for sex and age
  □ Altered, because…
- Define the upper lid crease position:
  □ Ideal
  □ Too high
  □ Too low
- Define the upper lid margin position:
  □ Ideal
  □ Too high
  □ Too low
- Define the lower lid margin position:
  □ Ideal
  □ Too low
- Define the medial canthus position:
  □ Ideal
  □ Altered, because…
- Define the lateral canthus position:
  □ Ideal
  □ Altered, because…
- Eyelid dermatochalasis:
  □ Absent
  □ Moderate
  □ Marked
  □ Limiting the superotemporal visual field (pathological)
- Upper eyelid ptosis:
  □ Right…
  □ Left…
- Lower eyelid laxity:
  □ Right…
  □ Left…
- Scleral show:
  □ Right (… mm)
  □ Left (… mm)
- Upper lid herniated orbital fat:
  □ Right
  □ Left
- Lower lid herniated orbital fat:
  □ Right
  □ Left
- Prolapsed lacrimal gland:
  □ Right
  □ Left
- Festoons (cheek bags):
  □ Right…
  □ Left…
- Eye globe proptosis (exophthalmos):
  □ Right…
  □ Left…
- Eye globe enophthalmos:
  □ Right…
  □ Left…
- Hypertrophic orbicularis oculi muscle (tarsal portion):
  □ Right…
  □ Left…

6.8 Forehead, Eyebrows, and Eyes: Preferred Terms Checklist[6]

- *Blepharochalasis* – Should be differentiated from dermatochalasis. It is an uncommon condition characterized by episodic edema and erythema of the eyelids. Blepharochalasis is more common in young women and may result in premature relaxation and laxity of the eyelid skin with wrinkling and hooding [2].
- *Blepharoptosis* – Ptosis of the upper lid over the eyeball. The grade of blepharoptosis is evaluated measuring the palpebral aperture in the primary, upward, and downward position of gaze.

[6]Section 3 on Springer Extra Materials (extras.springer.com).

- *Connell's sign* – Lateral extension over the eyelid and onto the lateral periorbital region of the upper lid crease. Connell's sign is considered to be a hallmark of forehead ptosis [6].
- *Crow's feet and eyelid wrinkles* – Fine wrinkles or lines developing on the lower lid and the lateral aspect of the orbital region perpendicular to the fibers of the underlying orbicularis oculi muscle.
- *Dermatochalasis* – Excess of eyelid (redundant) skin, which is usually more prevalent in the upper eyelids. It is a frequent condition in middle-aged subjects and a common one in the elderly.
- *Ectropion* – Eversion of the eyelid margin away from the globe. It is more common in the lower eyelid.
- *Enophthalmos* – The abnormal recession of the eyeball into the orbit.
- *Entropion* – The inward rotation of the eyelid in such a way that the eyelid margin, eyelashes, and skin of the eyelid rub against the globe, resulting in irritative symptoms and possibly abrasion and scarring of the cornea.
- *Epiphora* – The overflow of tears as a result of impeded outflow or excessive secretion.
- *Exophthalmos* – The abnormal prominence or protrusion of the eyeball.
- *Eyebrow ptosis* – The inferior migration of the eyebrow below its natural position over or above the superior orbital rim.
- *Eyelid bags (baggy eyelid)* – The visible bags of the lower eyelid caused by the processes of pseudoherniation of orbital fat and attenuation and lengthening of the orbital septum, orbicularis oculi muscle, skin, and lower canthus (see also festoons).
- *Eyelid laxity* – See lid tone.
- *Eyelid rims (upper and lower)* – The free margins of the eyelids.
- *Festoons (or cheek bags, malar bags)* – Ptosis of the suborbicularis oculi fat. Malar bags can be differentiated from eyelid bags because they occur below the inferior orbital rim.
- *Forehead transverse furrows* – The long horizontal mimetic furrows developing on the forehead perpendicular to the fibers of the underlying frontalis muscle.
- *Glabellar creases (frown lines, vertical glabellar lines)* – The mainly vertically oriented mimetic skin lines developing on the glabella perpendicular to the fibers of the underlying corrugator muscle (see Sect. 10.11.1).
- *Herniated orbital fat (pseudoherniated orbital fat)* – The anterior displacement of the fat located under the orbital septum. It should be examined with the patient in the upright sitting or standing position. The orbital fat pads are classically divided into two upper compartments (medial and central) and three lower compartments (medial, central, and lateral). This is usually due to the attenuation of the orbital septum.
- *Horizontal palpebral aperture* – The distance between the lateral and medial canthus. The average length is 30–40 mm [1].
- *Hypertrophic orbicularis oculi muscle* – A horizontal band or ridge of the pretarsal portion of the lower lid orbicularis oculi muscle that is accentuated by smiling.
- *Inferior scleral show* – See scleral show.
- *Intercanthal axis* – The imaginary line connecting the medial and lateral canthus.
- *Lacrimal gland* – A small gland that normally occupies the lacrimal fossa of the frontal bone inside the upper temporal angle of the orbit (see also prolapsed lacrimal gland).
- *Lagophthalmos* – Incomplete eyelid closure.
- *Lateral canthus* – The lateral angle formed by the junction of the two free margins of the eyelids.
- *Lid tone* – The ability of the lids to maintain spontaneously and recover (recapture) quickly their normal position against the globe when pulled away. The presence of horizontal lid laxity can be assessed performing the snap test and the lid distraction test. The lid should not be pulled more than 7 mm away from the globe (distraction test) and should snap back into its normal position immediately (snap test).
- *Limbus (iris limbus)* – The circular margin of the iris with white sclera.

- *Lower palpebral fissure width* – The distance from the central point of the cornea to the central lower eyelid margin with the patient's eye in straight gaze. It is normally about 5.5 mm and increases with lower lid retraction [7].
- *Malar hypoplasia* – The condition of skeletal flatness of the malar region that is normally prominent.
- *Margin crease distance* – The distance from the central upper eyelid margin to the tarsal crease measured with the eyelid fold elevated by the examiner and as the patient looks down. The normal range reported by Putterman is 9–11 mm [7], whereas that for Wolfort, Baker, and Kanter is 8–10 mm [9]. An elevated upper lid crease may be a sign of disinsertion of the levator aponeurosis.
- *Medial canthus* – The medial angle formed by the junction of the two free margins of the eyelids.
- *Palpebral fissure width (vertical palpebral aperture)* – The distance from the central lower eyelid to the central upper eyelid margins with the patient's eye in straight gaze. Normally, it is about 10 mm [7]. A smaller measurement usually indicates ptosis of the upper lid, whereas a bigger measurement could be a sign of eyelid retraction. It can be divided into the upper and the lower palpebral fissure width.
- *Prolapsed lacrimal gland* – A prolapsed lacrimal gland can produce an excessive fullness of the upper eyelid in the temporal third (there is no orbital fat in the upper temporal angle of the orbit).
- *Scleral show (inferior scleral show)* – The presence of a strip of white sclera between the iris and the lower lid margin with the subject in the natural head position and straight gaze. It may be a sign of exophthalmos, previous trauma, prior surgery, lower lid laxity, or dentofacial deformities with maxillary hypoplasia.
- *Tarsal crease of the upper lid (upper lid crease)* – The horizontal sulcus of the upper lid that normally divides it into an inferior tarsal portion and a superior septal portion. It is frequently hidden in adult and aged subjects by skin redundancy.
- *Trichion* – The hairline midline point.
- *Trichiasis*. The condition in which the eyelashes are in contact with the eye globe.
- *Upper palpebral fissure width* – The distance from the central point of the cornea to the central upper eyelid margin with the patient's eye in straight gaze. The normal range is 4–4.5 mm [7]. A lower value usually indicates ptosis of the upper lid, whereas a larger one could be a sign of upper lid retraction. If a ptotic eyelid covers the central point of the cornea, the number of millimeters that the eyelid must be raised is recorded as a negative number.
- *Vertical palpebral aperture* – See palpebral fissure width.

References

1. Bosniak SL (1990) Cosmetic blepharoplasty. Raven Press, New York
2. Gross SC, Kanter WR (1995) Preoperative assessment for eyelid surgery. In: Wolfort FG, Kanter WR (eds) Aesthetic blepharoplasty. Little, Brown and Company, Boston, pp 53–77
3. Gunter JP, Antrobus SD (1997) Aesthetic analysis of the eyebrows. Plast Reconstr Surg 99:1808–1816
4. Hoefflin SM (2002) The beautiful face: the first mathematical definition, classification and creation of true facial beauty. Steven M. Hoefflin, Santa Monica. ISBN 0–9713445–0–7
5. Marchac D (1991) Aesthetic contouring of the forehead utilizing bone grafts and osteotomies. In: Ousterhout DK (ed) Aesthetic contouring of the craniofacial skeleton. Little, Brown and Company, Boston, p 222
6. Marten TJ, Knize DM (2001) Forehead aesthetics and preoperative assessment of the foreheadplasty patient. In: Knize DM (ed) The forehead and temporal fossa. Anatomy and technique. Lippincott Williams & Wilkins, Philadelphia, pp 91–99
7. Putterman AM (1999) Evaluation of the cosmetic oculoplastic surgery patient. In: Putterman AM (ed) Cosmetic oculoplastic surgery. Eyelid, forehead, and facial techniques. W.B. Saunders Company, Philadelphia
8. Spinelli HM (2004) Atlas of aesthetic eyelid and periocular surgery. W.B. Saunders Company, Philadelphia
9. Wolfort FG, Baker T, Kanter WR (1995) Aesthetic goals in blepharoplasty. In: Wolfort FG, Kanter WR (eds) Aesthetic blepharoplasty. Little, Brown and Company, Boston

Nasal Analysis

7

Contents

The nose, with its central position, plays a major role in facial aesthetics, and the parameters that one must consider in clinical nasal analysis are impressive. For that reason, its evaluation is best done utilizing a practical and comprehensive checklist and writing down, for each clinical case, a list of the features discovered.

As a protruding structure, the nose must be studied trying to envision its composite supporting framework, which is the main determinant of the external shape.

7.1 Points, Lines, and Subunits of the External Nose

As for the whole face, the surface of the nasal pyramid offers some points, lines, and areas for consideration (Fig. 7.1):

1. Alar base width
2. Alar crease junction
3. Alar groove
4. Alar rim
5. Columella
6. Columellar base
7. Columella outline
8. Footplates of the medial crura
9. Glabella
10. Nasal base line
11. Nasal dorsum outline
12. Nasal lobule
13. Nasal lobule outline
14. Nasal radix outline
15. Nasal "unbroken" line

F. Meneghini, P. Biondi, *Clinical Facial Analysis*,
DOI 10.1007/978-3-642-27228-8_7,

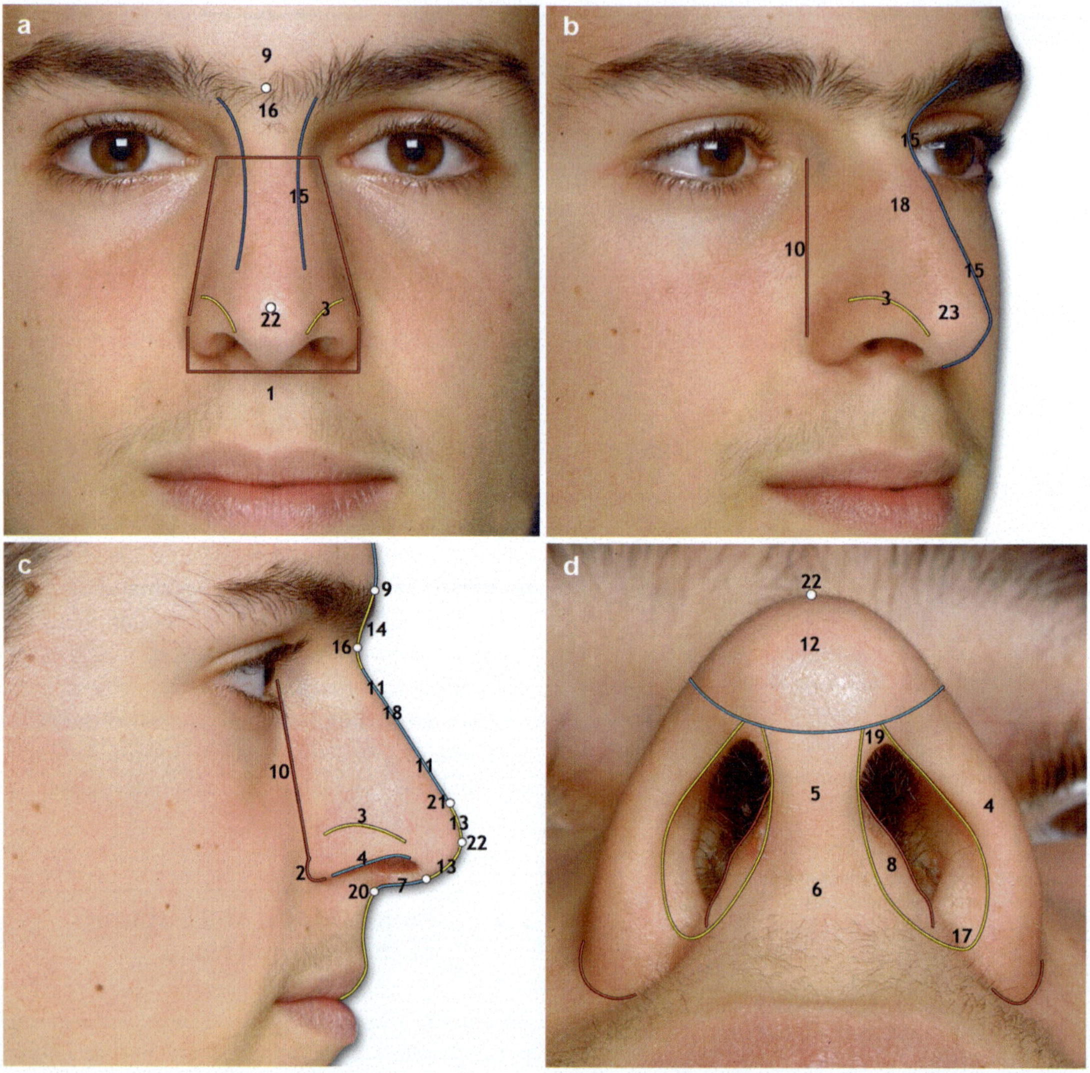

Fig. 7.1 Points, lines, and subunits of the nasal surface in frontal (**a**), oblique (**b**), profile (**c**), and basal view (**d**). The numbers refer to the list in Sect. 7.1

16. Nasion
17. Nostril sill
18. Rhinion (clinically, this is evaluated with direct palpation of the dorsum)
19. Soft triangle or facet
20. Subnasal
21. Supratip area or supratip breakpoint in clinical cases where a clear step over the nasal tip is present
22. Nasal tip
23. Tip-defining points

7.2 Direct and Photographic Clinical Analysis for Nasal Deformities

A note reporting the major findings regarding nasal aesthetics, determined by visual inspection and palpation only, is made during the first consultation. The successive revision and enhancement of the definitive form is written when the photographic documentation, either in a printed form or on a wide monitor, is also available.

Defining a nose as short or long, narrow, or wide should also be related to the sex, height, physique, and primarily to the whole face of the subject. A "balanced" nose exists only for a given face! This assumption points out the necessity of a general facial analysis prior to any specific evaluation of the nasal subunits.

7.2.1 General Considerations

The first step is the assessment of the general symmetry of the face and nose utilizing one reliable horizontal reference line. The most commonly utilized horizontal references are the lines connecting the medial canthus, the upper palpebral folds, or the apex of the eyebrow, which are easy to detect and draw; the next step is the creation of a unique vertical midline that should bisect the glabella, the nasal bridge, the nasal tip, and the Cupid's bow (Fig. 7.2a–d). In a complex case, instead of a unique vertical midline, it is necessary to trace several small midline segments for every facial subunit to evaluate better the role of nasal asymmetry in the context of an asymmetric face (Fig. 7.2e–h).

The skeletal boundaries of the nose must be evaluated in order to recognize the surrounding structures from which the nasal pyramid emerges. Figure 7.3 shows these boundaries in a subject with an adequate supporting base, whereas Fig. 7.4 depicts three cases of depressed paranasal region due to maxillary hypoplasia and a case of a too protruding anterior nasal spine that greatly influences how the observer sees the shape and the projection of the nose. The reader can find the clinical and instrumental assessment of skeletal midface deformities in Chap. 9.

Utilizing the oblique views, the entire nasal outline must be evaluated, searching for the presence of a bilateral symmetric "unbroken" line [11]. In the attractive nose, this line descends gracefully from the supraorbital ridge onto the nasal dorsum and the nasal tip (Fig. 7.5). In the case of a deviated nose, dorsal irregularities, a dorsal hump, or a dorsal saddle, this line is "broken," creating one or two steps or a strong curve as depicted in Fig. 7.6. Utilizing the nasal outline obtained from the oblique view helps in the assessment of the type, grade, and location of the deformity.

The nasal profile slope should be assessed clinically and utilizing the fullface profile view for a better comparison with the whole facial profile. In many cases, identifying and drawing the dorsal line is an easy task, and the difficulties that can remain lie only in the construction of a correct facial plane (Fig. 7.7).

In some nasal and dentofacial deformities, the assessment of nasal slope can be difficult. In a posttraumatic nose with dorsal irregularities, as in a combination of bone hump and cartilage saddle, more than one dorsal line can be considered (Fig. 7.8). Furthermore, none of these lines can be utilized as guidance for the visualization of the treatment goals as they reflect the actual situation measured at different levels (bony nasal dorsum, cartilaginous nasal dorsum, and nasal lobule outline) and not the ideal slope for this subject.[1]

The difficulty in assessing the nasal slope increases in the case of obvious nasal deformity combined with an equally obvious dentofacial deformity. Tracing some reference points and lines helps the observer to distinguish and grade the severity of each deformity (Fig. 7.9). In the sections dedicated to specific nasal regions, such as radix and lobule, more of the factors affecting the real and perceived nasal slope are explored.

The next step consists of the appreciation of nasal widths. It should be done considering eight different basic parameters:

- Whole nasal width
- Radix width at the level of the base
- Radix width at the level of the profile
- Dorsal width at the level of the base
- Dorsal width at the level of the profile
- Alar base width
- Nasal tip width
- Columellar base width

[1]The complete clinical facial photographic documentation of this case is available in Sect. 4 on Springer Extra Materials (extras.springer.com) (clinical case no. 3).

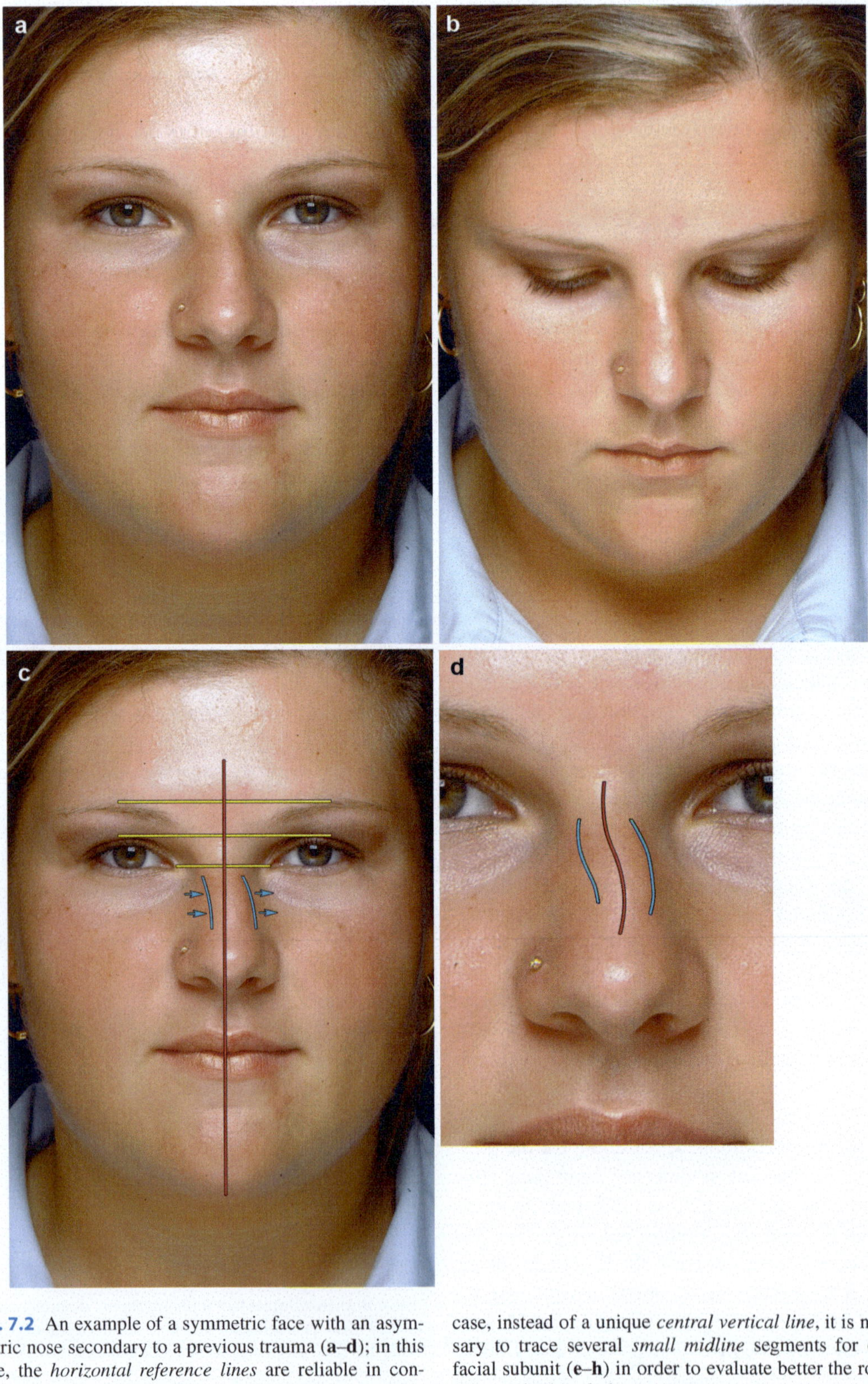

Fig. 7.2 An example of a symmetric face with an asymmetric nose secondary to a previous trauma (**a–d**); in this case, the *horizontal reference lines* are reliable in constructing the *vertical midline*. In a complex asymmetric case, instead of a unique *central vertical line*, it is necessary to trace several *small midline* segments for every facial subunit (**e–h**) in order to evaluate better the role of the nose in the whole asymmetry

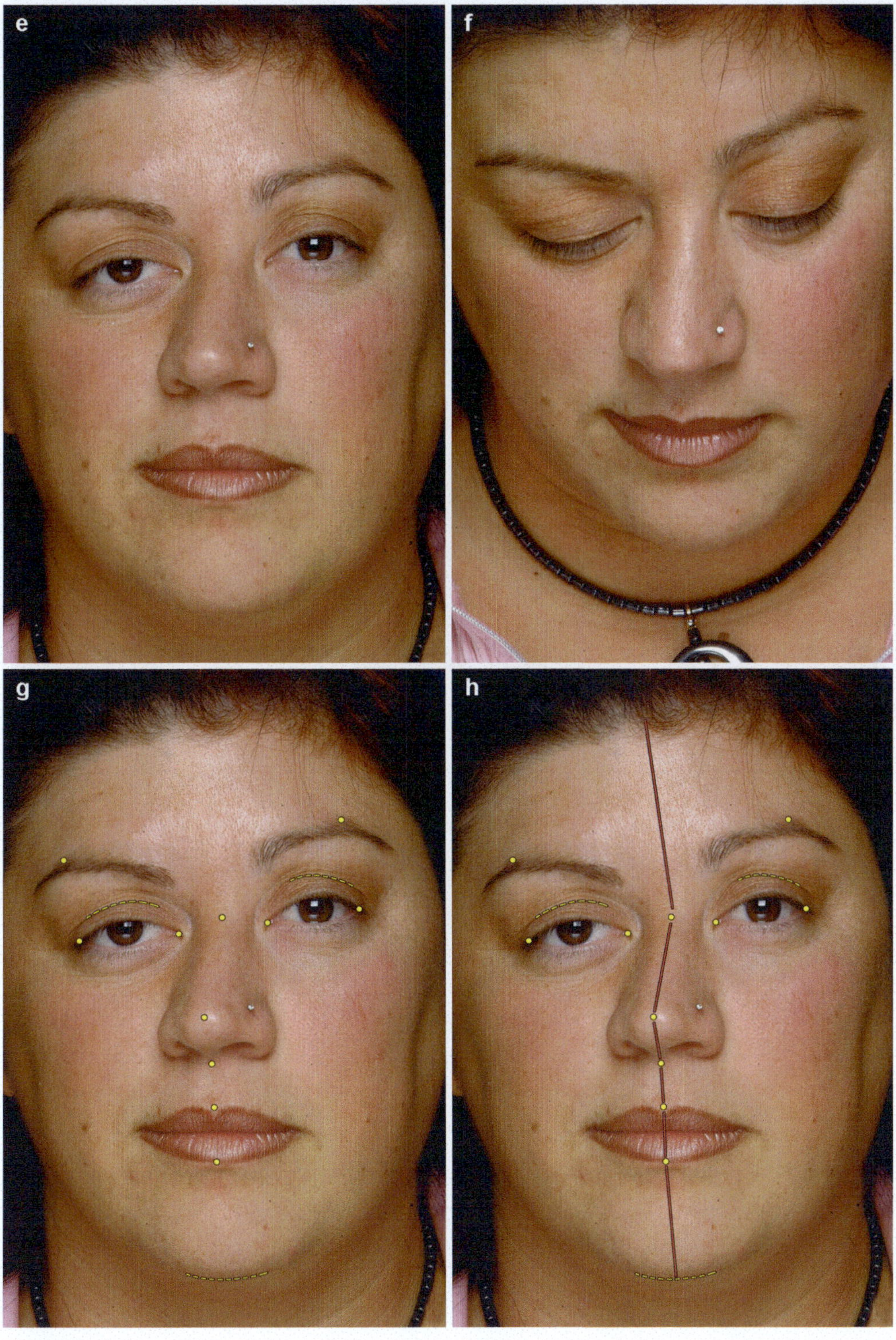

Fig. 7.2 (continued)

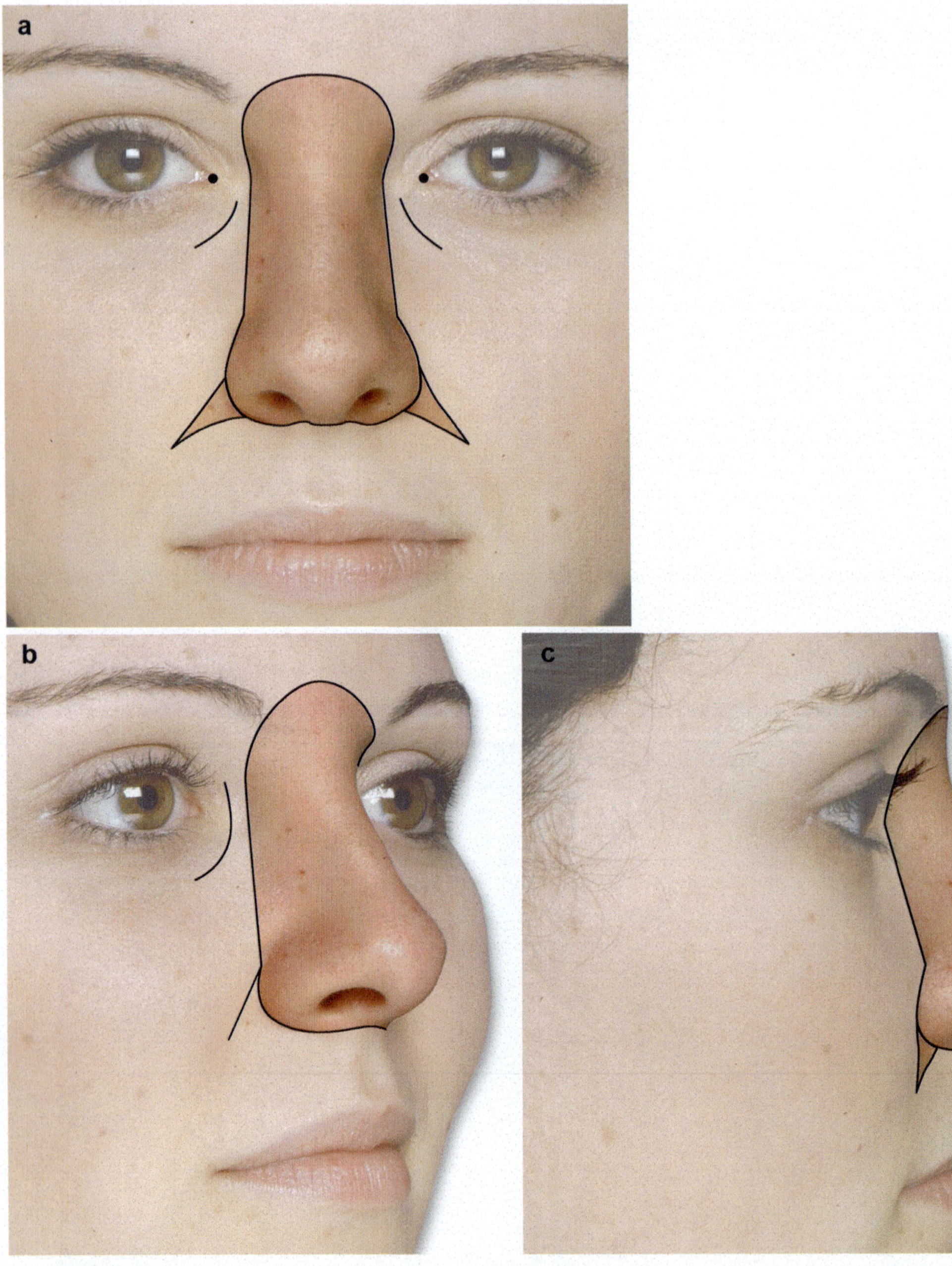

Fig. 7.3 The skeletal boundaries of the nasal pyramid in frontal (a), oblique (b), and profile view (c)

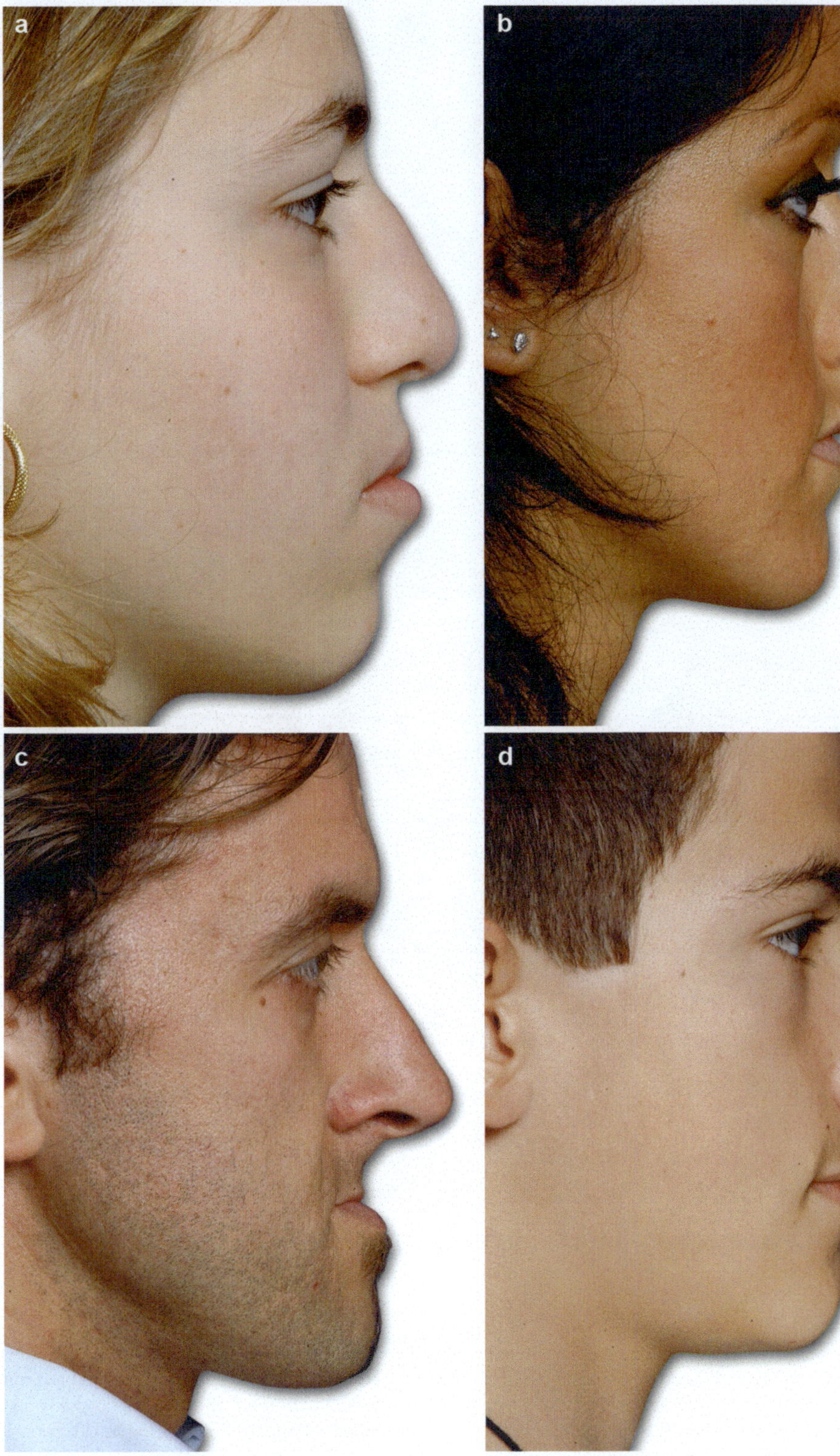

Fig. 7.4 Three cases of depressed paranasal region due to maxillary hypoplasia (**a**–**c**) and a case of a too protruding anterior nasal spine (**d**) that greatly influences how the observer sees the shape and projection of the nose

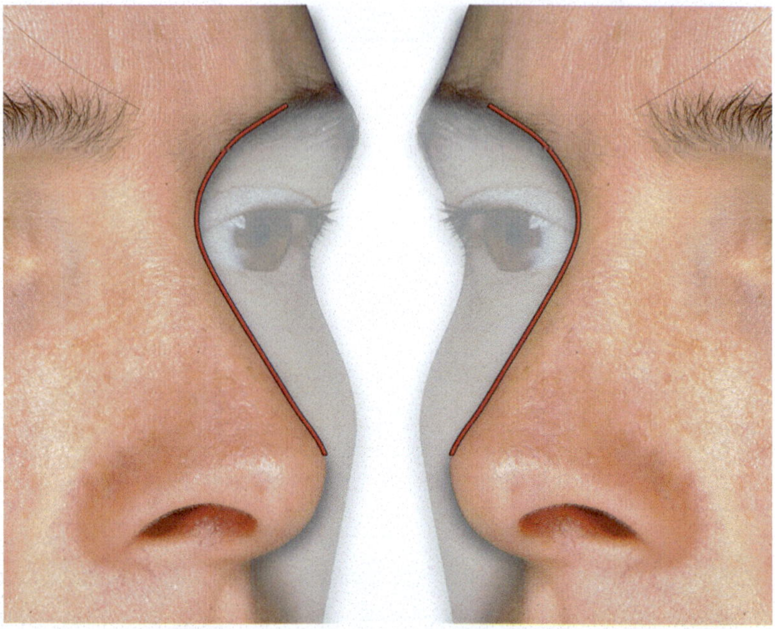

Fig. 7.5 The nasal *unbroken line* is the outline of the nasal pyramid in oblique view. In the attractive nose, this line descends gracefully and symmetrically from the supraorbital ridge onto the nasal dorsum and the nasal tip

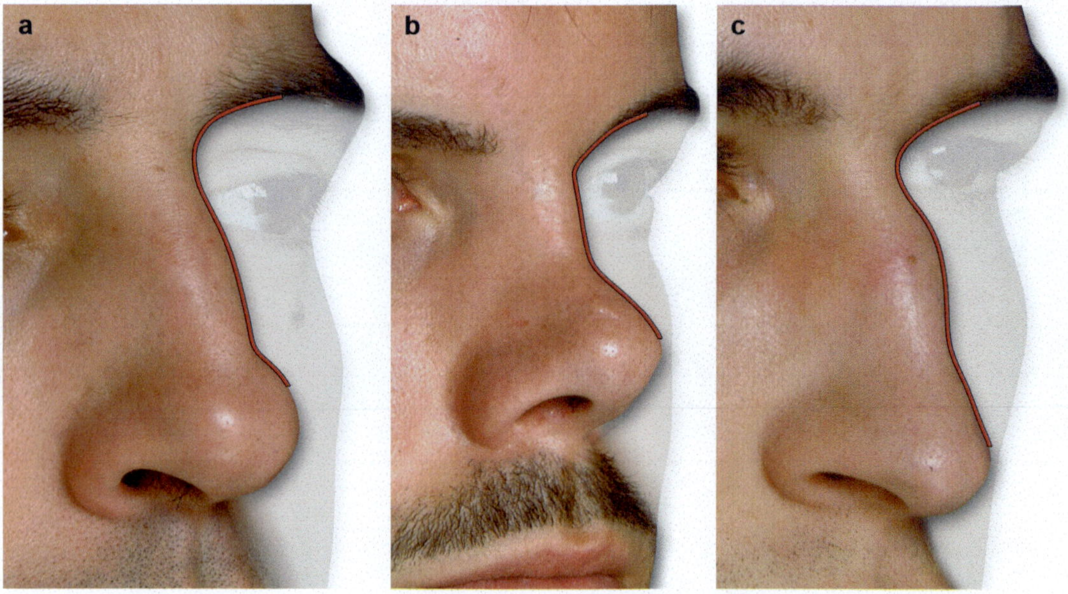

Fig. 7.6 The nasal outline in oblique view of a dorsal hump (**a**), a dorsal saddle (**b**), and a crooked nose (**c**)

Fig. 7.8 A case in which the outcome of nasal trauma results in a bone hump and a cartilaginous saddle (**a**). The construction of the dorsal profile line can be done in different ways (**b**) *line 1* is superimposed on nasal bone outline, *line 2* is superimposed on lobule outline, and *line 3* is superimposed on cartilaginous dorsum outline. None of these lines can be utilized as guidance for the visualization of the treatment goals as they reflect the actual situation measured at different levels (bony nasal dorsum, cartilaginous nasal dorsum, and nasal lobule outline) and not the ideal slope for this subject

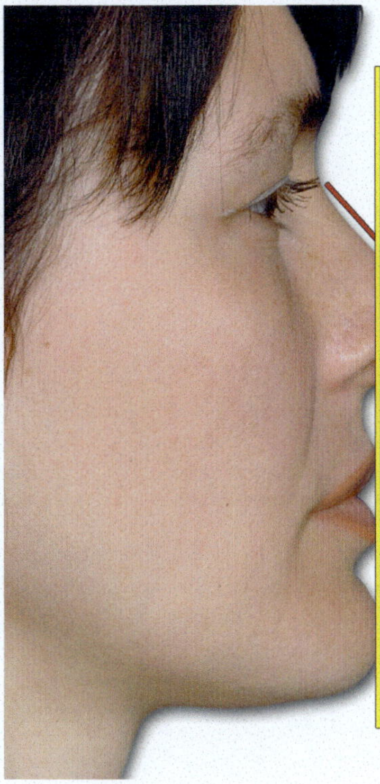

Fig. 7.7 Identifying and tracing the *dorsal line* can be relatively easy to do in the case of a straight dorsal outline. In this patient, the main difficulty is recognizing the projection of the chin that alters the facial plane. A *vertical reference line* passing through the subnasal point helps in the visualization of the excess chin projection

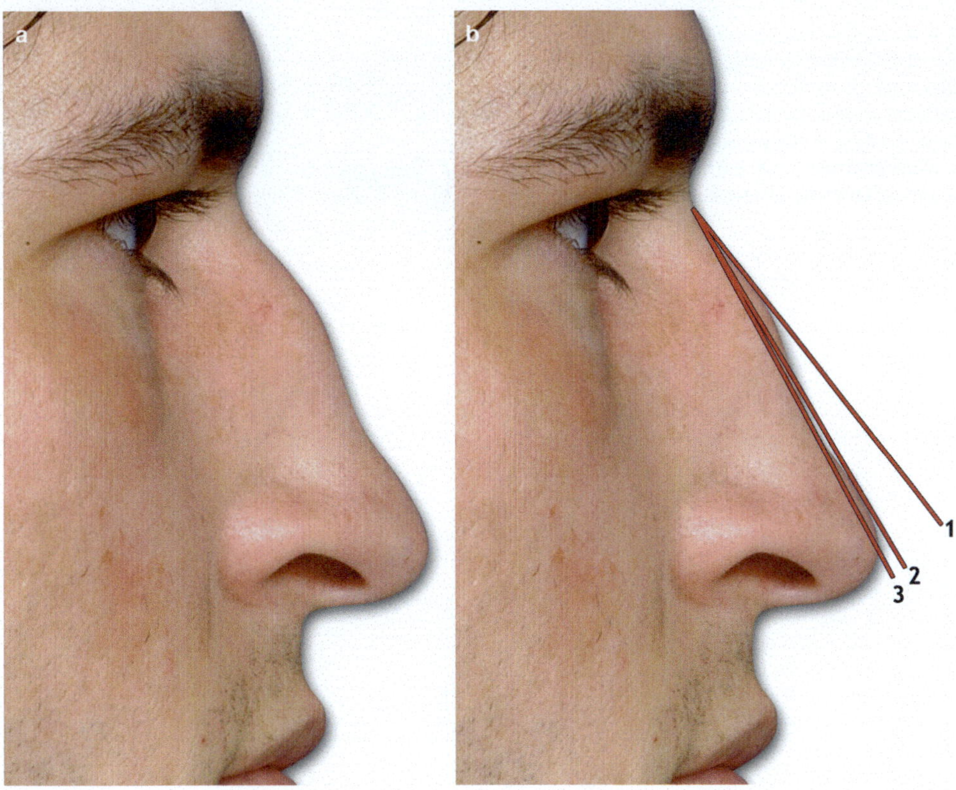

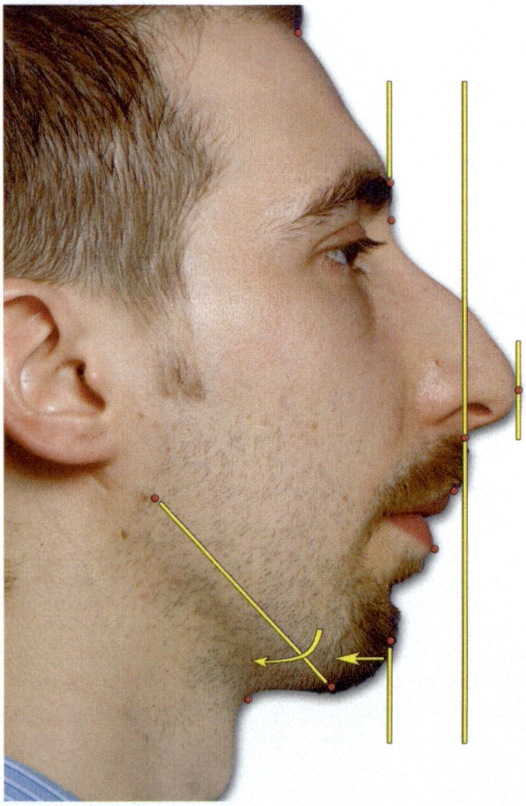

Fig. 7.9 A clinical case combining a clear nasal and dentofacial deformity. Tracing of some *reference points* and *lines* helps to distinguish and grade the severity of each deformity. On understanding the degree of the microgenia and mandibular clockwise rotation, the extent of the counterclockwise rotation of the nasal slope is not as great as may appear on initial examination

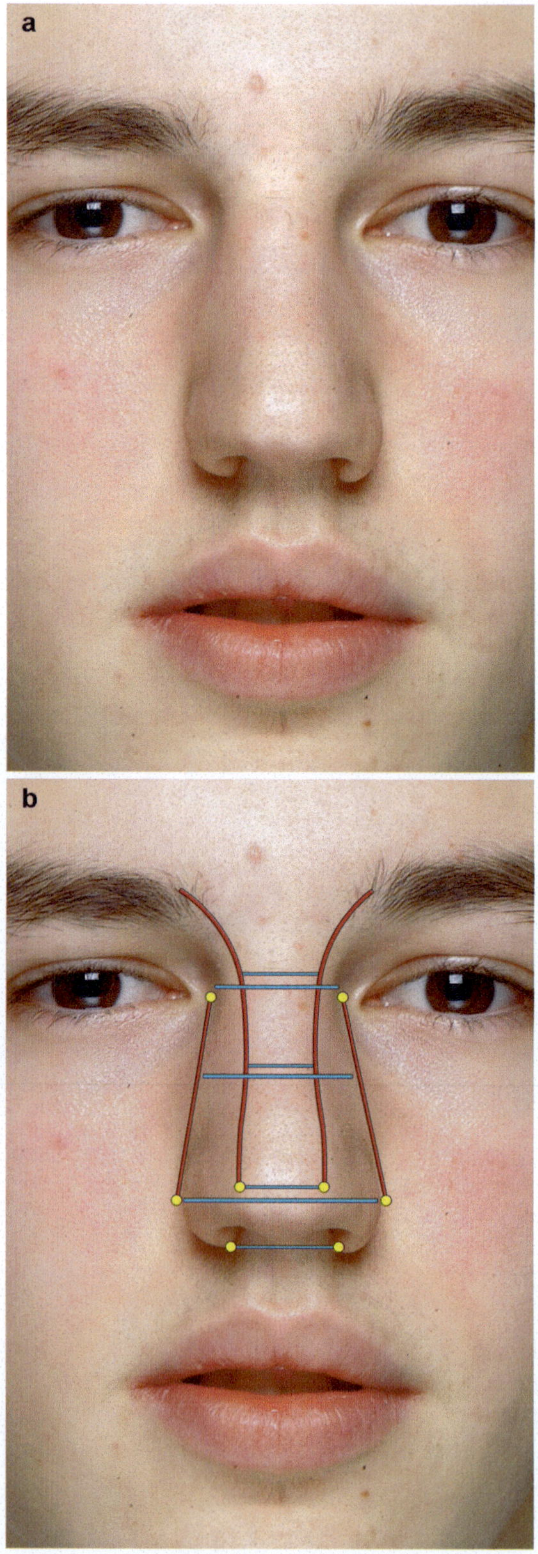

Fig. 7.10 Frontal view of a "large nose" in a teenager (**a**). The analysis of nasal width should consider eight different basic parameters (**b**) whole nasal width, radix width at the level of the base, radix width at the level of the profile, dorsal width at the level of the base, dorsal width at the level of the profile, alar base width, nasal tip width, and columellar base width

Figure 7.10 shows a case of a large nose in which all eight widths are depicted.

The general nose assessment is not finished without examining the overlaying skin and without the information obtainable by palpation. The skin assessment is a very important step; from radix to tip, along the midline, the thickness of the soft tissue envelope is thick over the glabella and radix breakpoint, thinner over the rhinion, and thick again at the supratip area (Fig. 7.11a). Moving from the midline to the nasal base line, at the level of the radix and osteocartilaginous dorsum, the skin thickness increases (Fig. 7.11b). The skin thickness at the level of the lobule and the base of columella is highly variable and must be assessed precisely in each case (Fig. 7.11c–f).

Utilizing the thumb and the index finger of the dominant hand (Fig. 7.12), the nose is palpated in order to establish:

- The length of the nasal bones (Fig. 7.12a).
- The presence of any bony or cartilaginous irregularities (Fig. 7.12b–c).
- The level of the most anterior–inferior aspect of the septal cartilage profile with respect to the most projecting point of the lobule (Fig. 7.12d).
- The resistance offered by the cartilaginous dorsum and nasal tip to posterior displacement by pressure as well the speed with which the tip returns to its normal configuration upon release (Fig. 7.12e, f).
- The grade of passive mobility of the skin over the skeletal framework. Other points to consider regarding the nasal soft tissue envelope are the presence of scars, the grade of elasticity and atrophy, as well the presence of telangiectasias.

7.2.2 Nasal Upper Third Assessment

Identifying the spatial location of the radix breakpoint and the definition of the nasofrontal angle is a fundamental part of nasal analysis.

The radix breakpoint is the most posterior point of the outline between the nasal dorsum and the frontal bone. Any change in the radix breakpoint influences how the observer judges the length as well as the slope of the entire nose. It is best assessed utilizing the corneal plane, the glabella, and the superior palpebral fold[2] as references (Fig. 7.13).

The nasofrontal angle is not necessarily measured and can be assessed simply by drawing (or imaging) two lines on the profile. The upper line is based on the mean inclination of the outline from glabella to the radix breakpoint, whereas the lower one is based on the mean inclination of the outline from the radix breakpoint to the supratip area. Figure 7.14 shows the nasofrontal angle of the three clinical cases presented in Fig. 7.13.

The profile of the bony portion is usually one third of the entire nasal dorsum and should be palpated to identify the real length of the nasal bones. Any convexity–concavity, symmetry–asymmetry, unilateral–bilateral lateral hump must be assessed visually.

7.2.3 Nasal Middle Third Assessment

The clinical analysis of the central portion of the nasal pyramid considers the symmetry, outline, slope, volume, and shape of the cartilaginous dorsum. A particular mental exercise that of correlating the external aspect of the nasal dorsum at every level with the corresponding structural bony or cartilaginous architecture can be very helpful (Fig. 7.15).

The separation between bony and cartilaginous dorsum has its value in that the surgeon needs to treat these two "materials" differently at the time of surgery; however, from the point of view of any other observer, such as the patient, the dorsum is best considered as a unique, highly visible structure connecting the radix to the tip.

The great difficulty in assessing the dorsum often lies in the visual influence of the radix and the tip, which are rarely ideal. So, after the general assessment, it is preferable to reconsider the analysis of the dorsum, when the "construction" of the correct radix and tip is done.

[2]Each of these references is also critically checked for its reliability.

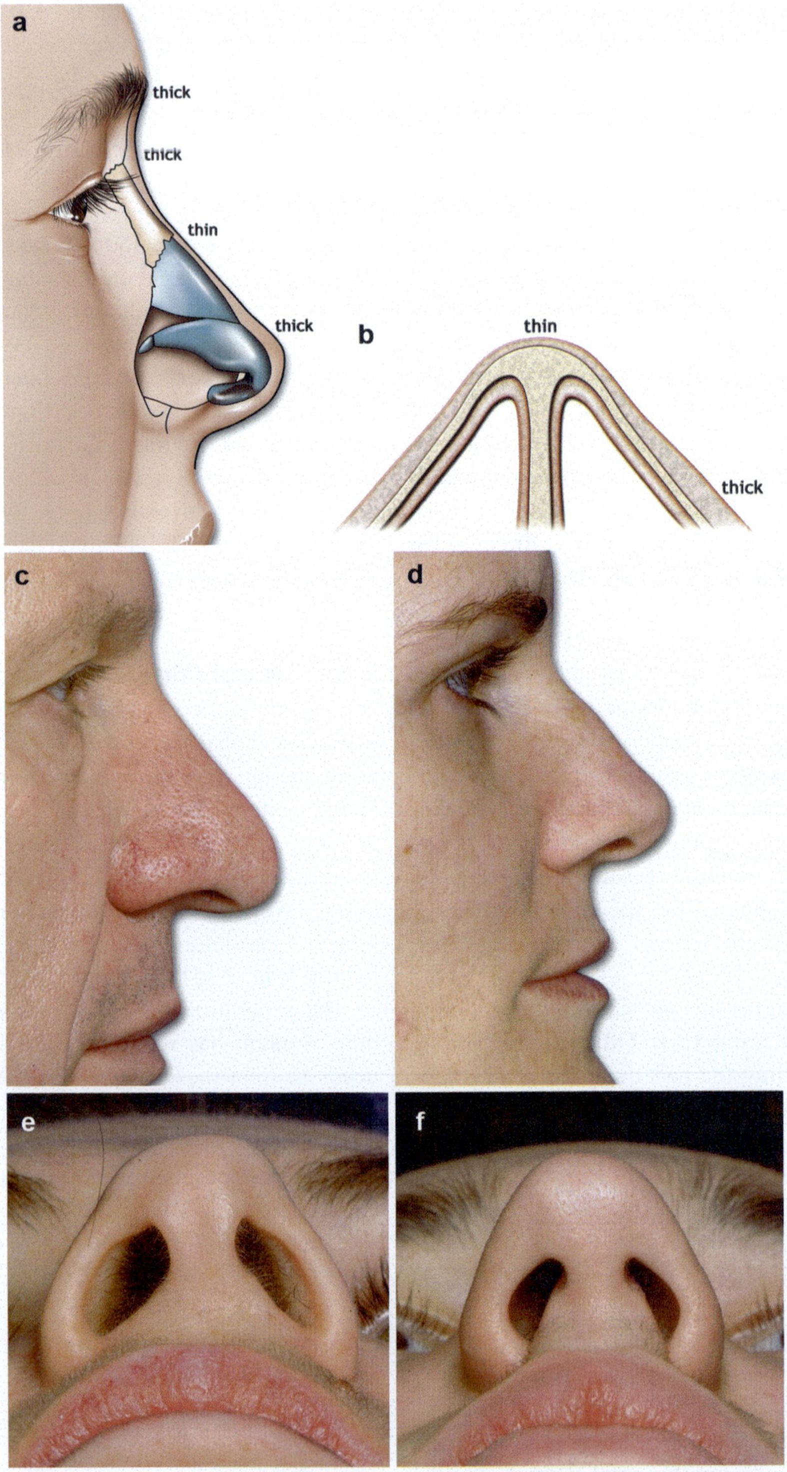

Fig. 7.11 From radix to tip, along the midline, the thickness of the soft tissue envelope is thick over the glabella and radix breakpoint, thinner over the rhinion, and thick again at the supratip area (**a**). Moving from the midline to the nasal base line, at the level of the radix and osteocartilaginous dorsum, the skin thickness progressively increases (**b**). A case of thick sebaceous skin that hides the underlying cartilaginous skeleton of the nasal tip (**c**) and the opposite condition in which the shape and volume of the lower lateral cartilage are easily assessed through the skin (**d**–**e**). A clinical case presenting a large columellar base due to increased soft tissue envelope thickness (**f**)

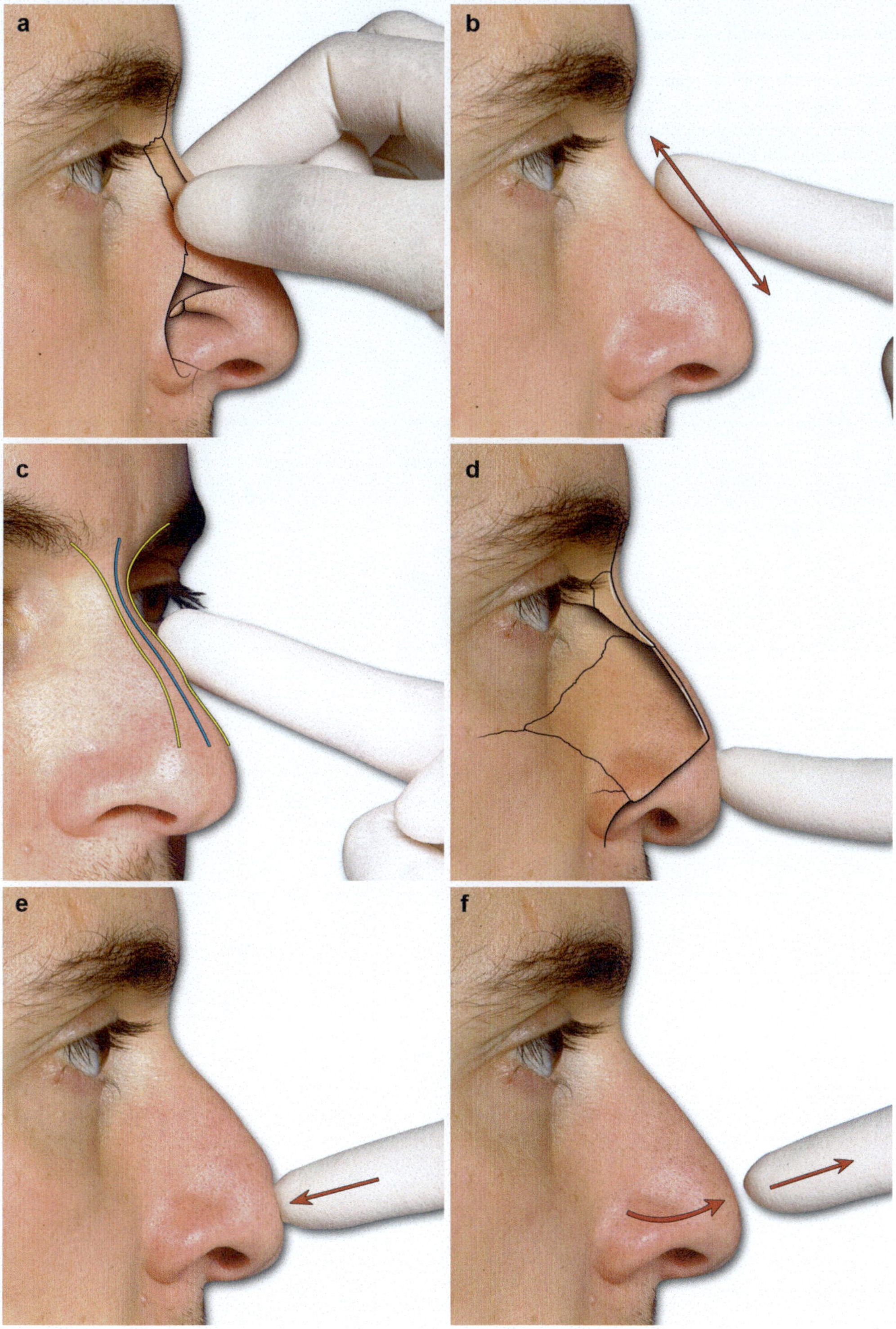

Fig. 7.12 Utilizing the thumb and the index finger of the dominant hand, the examiner can feel the distal end of the paired nasal bones (**a**), detect any bony or cartilaginous irregularities on the midline or the lateral aspects of the dorsum otherwise not evident (**b**, **c**), evaluate the distal portion of the septal cartilage outline normally hidden between the two domes (**d**), feel the amount of resistance offered by the cartilaginous dorsum and nasal tip to posterior displacement, and also observing the speed of the tip to return to its normal configuration upon release (**e**, **f**)

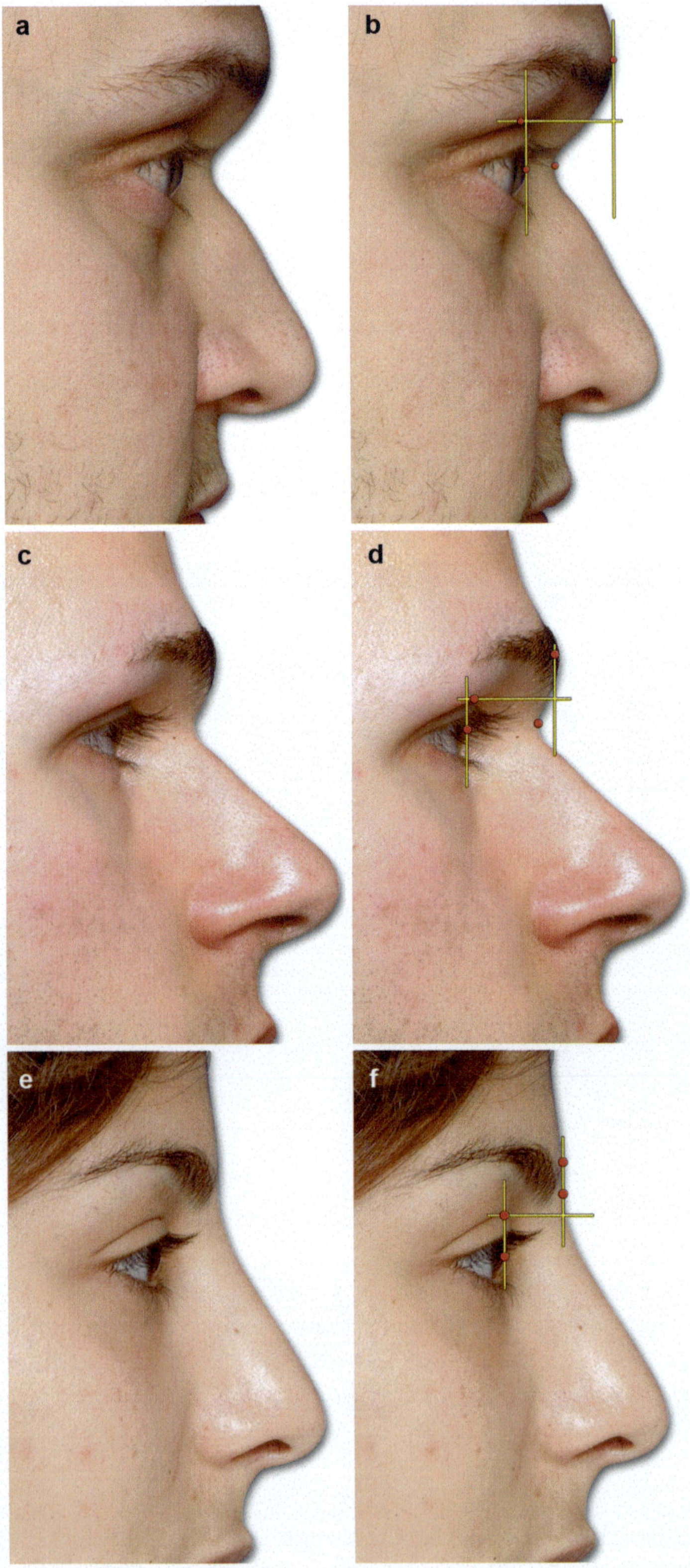

Fig. 7.13 Profile views of three different clinical examples of nasal radix. A too posterior and inferior nasal radix near the corneal plane and well below the superior palpebral fold; the anteriorly positioned glabella is in part secondary to the pneumatization of the frontal sinus (**a**, **b**). An inferior-positioned radix breakpoint, clearly below the superior palpebral fold, which can be mistakenly judged as being too posterior; in this case, the distance between the corneal plane and the nasal outline is not reduced (**c**, **d**). A shallow nasal upper third outline with a too anterior and superior radix breakpoint, which makes the nose appear too long (**e**, **f**)

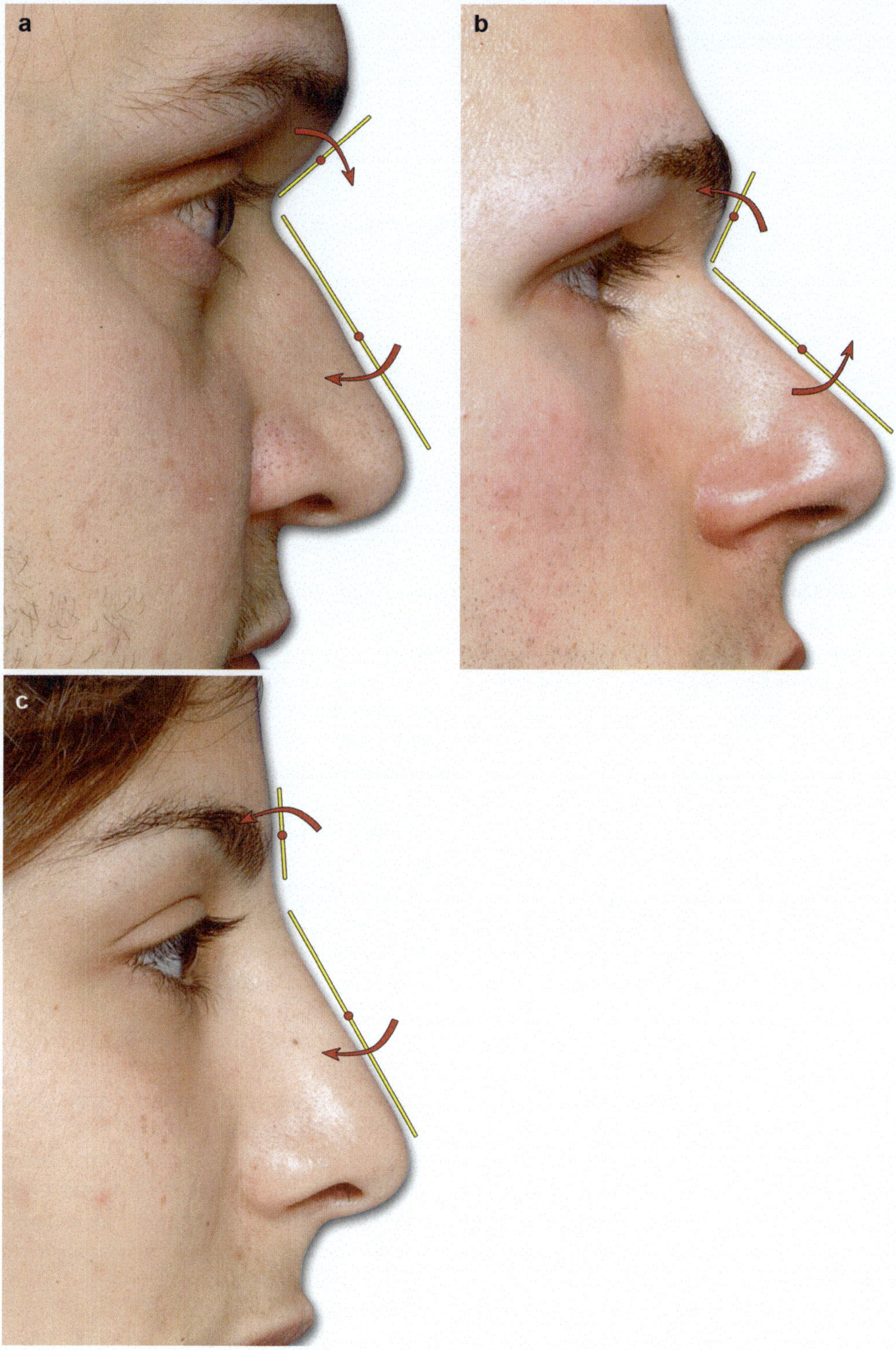

Fig. 7.14 The construction of nasofrontal angle can be simply done by drawing (or imaging) two lines. The *upper line* is based on the mean inclination of the outline from glabella to the radix breakpoint, whereas the *lower one* is based on the mean inclination of the outline from the radix breakpoint to the supratip area. Nasofrontal angles of similar degrees can be rotated clockwise (**a**) or counterclockwise (**b**) resulting in very different nasal patterns. In the case of a wide nasofrontal angle, the transition from the forehead to the nose is not so evident (**c**)

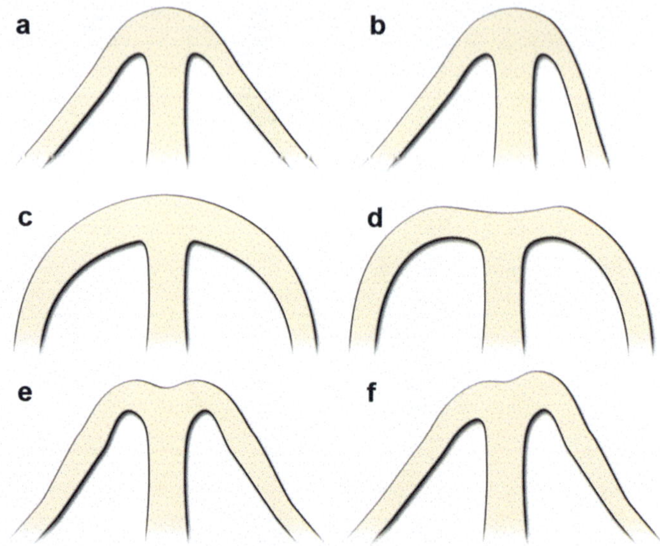

Fig. 7.15 Various types of structural bony and cartilaginous architecture of the nasal dorsum (**a**–**f**)

7.2.4 Nasal Lower Third Assessment

The clinical assessment of the nasal tip must consider these parameters [4]:

- Projection
- Rotation
- Position
- Volume
- Definition
- Width
- Shape

The tip projection is measured from the alar crease junction (ACJ) to the most anterior point of the nasal tip (T) and can be divided into intrinsic and extrinsic projection. The intrinsic projection is related to the lobule portion of the tip, whereas the extrinsic projection is related to the length of the ala and the columella (Fig. 7.16).

The angle of tip rotation is measured between the ACJ–T line and the vertical reference; its normative mean value is 105° for females and 100° for males (Fig. 7.17). The data obtained by this analysis must be added to those emerging from the evaluation of columella incline, the alar profile incline, as well as the incline and the length of the upper lip (see also Sect. 7.3) (Fig. 7.18).

The tip position refers to the location of the tip along the dorsal line (Fig. 7.19). This assessment helps in judging the actual length of the nose, as well as any planned surgical modification of the dorsal profile (shortening or lengthening) varying the tip.

The tip volume, definition, width, and shape are considered intrinsic characteristics of the nasal lobule [4]. The tip volume refers to the size of the lobule and is primarily related to the shape, dimension, and orientation of the lateral crura of the lower lateral cartilage (Fig. 7.20a).

The tip definition is related to the transition between the most anterior-projecting section of the lower lateral crura, the domal segment, and the nearest portion of the lateral crura. In particular, at surgery, the convexity of the dome should turn into a concavity on the lateral crura to create a well-defined tip (Fig. 7.20b).

The tip width refers to the distance between the paired domes (Fig. 7.20c).

The classification of the nasal tip based on its external form has produced many shape-related terms such as boxy tip, bulbous tip, and pinched nose. In the basal view, the shape considered to be ideal resembles a triangle (Fig. 7.20d).

Figure 7.21 shows a case of a "boxy" tip deformity that is apparent only in frontal and basal views, whereas Fig. 7.22 illustrates a secondary deformity concerning the whole nose, with a tip defined in the literature as "pinched."

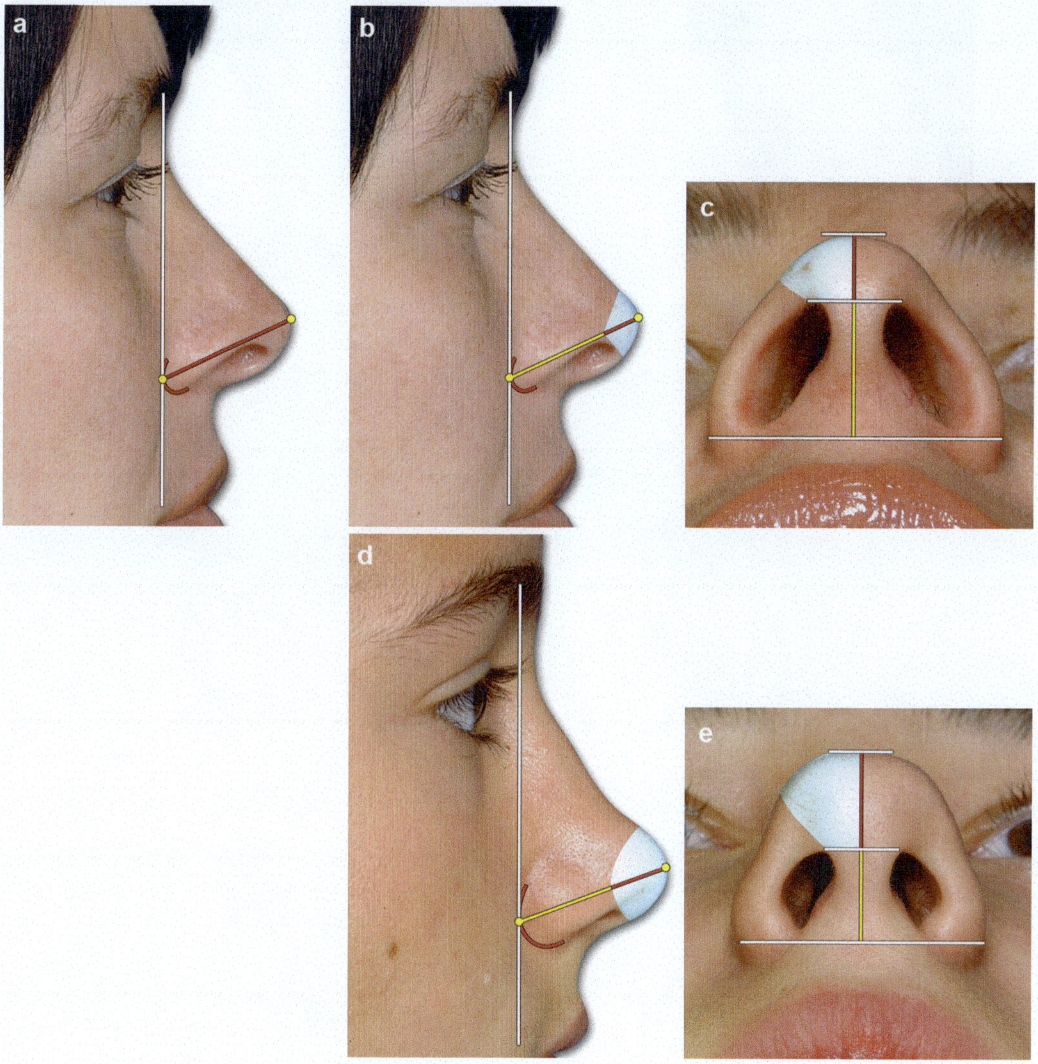

Fig. 7.16 The tip projection is the distance between the alar crease junction (ACJ) and the most anterior point of the nasal tip (T) and can be divided into intrinsic and extrinsic projections. The intrinsic projection is related to the lobule portion of the tip, whereas the extrinsic projection is related to the length of the ala and the columella (**a–c**). A clinical case in which the total tip projection is mainly sustained by the lobule portion (**d**, **e**)

The columellar show is the area of visible columella under the alar rim (Fig. 7.23a). It is best evaluated in profile view, and its normal range is between 2 and 4 mm; as well as the measurement, however, the ala and columellar profile should be analyzed in depth, considering the different combinations of the relationship between ala and columella categorized by Gunter et al. [5]. A reduced columellar show can be produced by a hanging ala (Fig. 7.23b), a retracted columella (Fig. 7.23c) or the combination of these two conditions, whereas an increased columellar show can be produced by a retracted ala (Fig. 7.23d), a hanging columella (Fig. 7.23e) or the combination of these two conditions. The ideal outline of the paired nasal alar rims and the columella, in frontal view, should resemble the figure of a gull in flight (Fig. 7.23f). A different condition, similar to the retracted ala, is the notched alar rim, in which the gentle curvature of the alar outline is lost with the formation of an evident angle (Fig. 7.24).

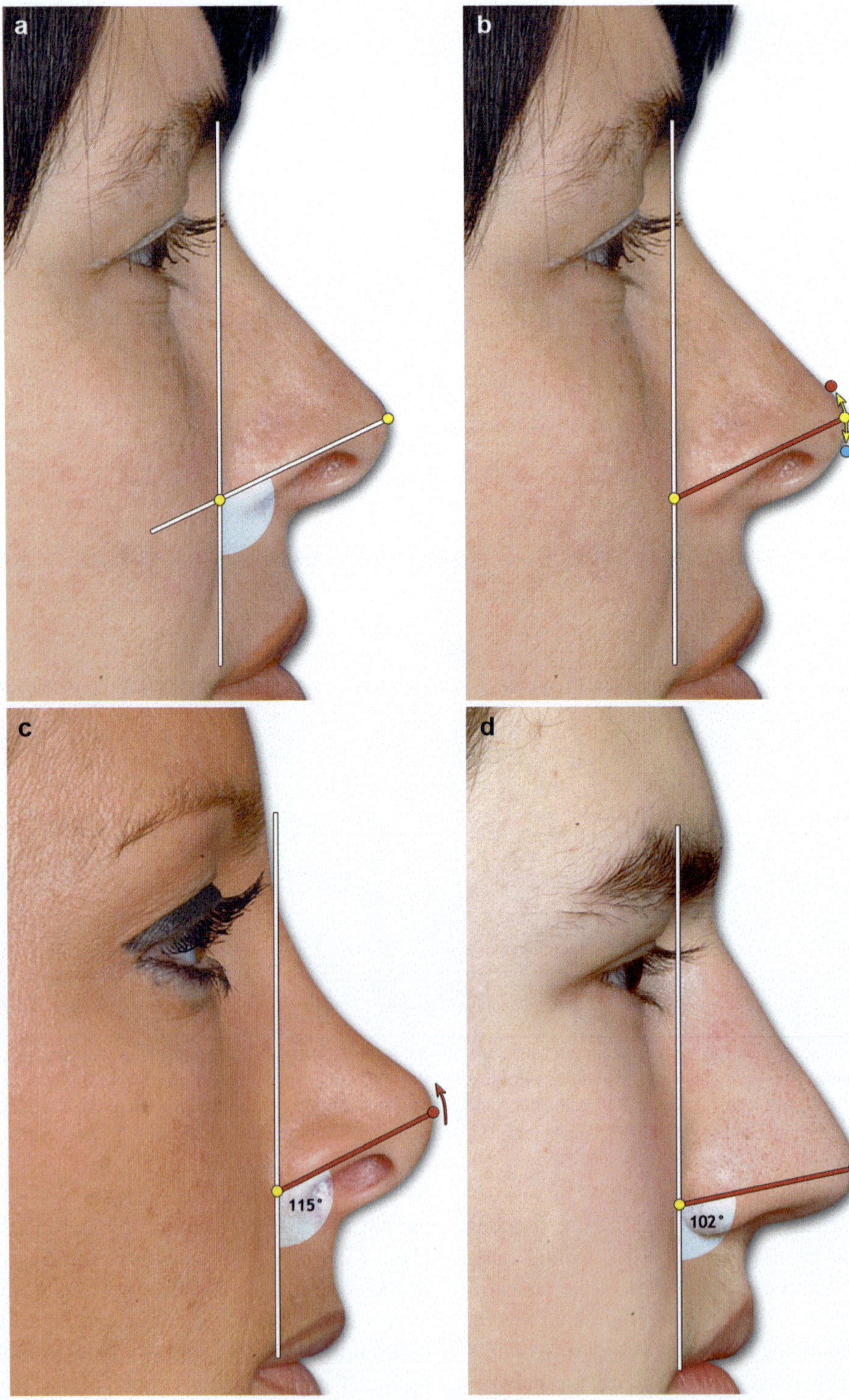

Fig. 7.17 The angle of tip rotation is measured between the *ACJ–T line* and the *vertical reference* (**a**, **b**); its normative mean value is 105° for females and 100° for males. A clinical case of an excessive upward rotation in a secondary nasal deformity (**c**) and a normally rotated tip in a male teenager (**d**)

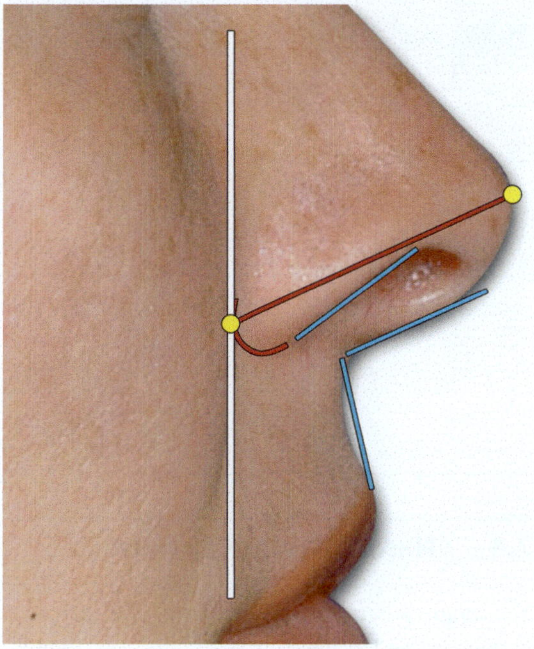

Fig. 7.18 The tip rotation line compared with the profile lines of the columella, nasal ala, and upper lip

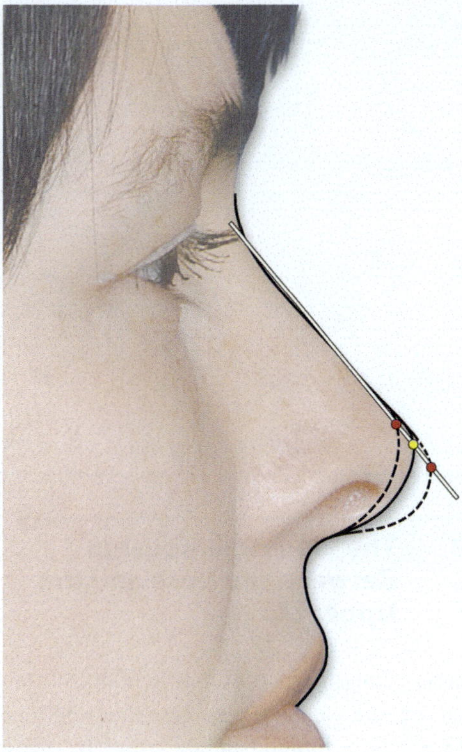

Fig. 7.19 The tip position assessment refers to the location of the nasal tip along the dorsal line

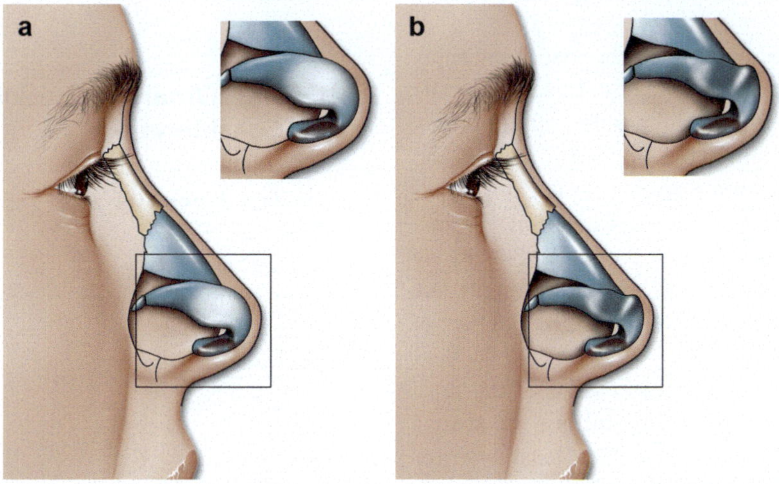

Fig. 7.20 The tip volume refers to the size of the lobule and is primarily related to the shape, dimension, and orientation of the lateral crura of the lower lateral cartilage (**a**). The tip definition is related to the transition between the most anterior projecting section of the lower lateral crura, the domal segment, and the nearest portion of the lateral crura; to create a well-defined tip the convexity of the dome should turn in a concavity on the lateral crura (**b**). The width of the tip refers to the distance between the paired domes (**c**). In the basal view, the nasal shape considered ideal resembles a triangle (**d**)

Fig. 7.20 (continued)

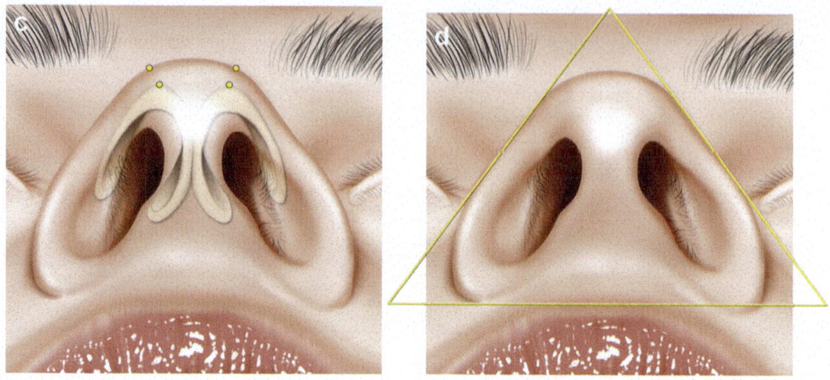

7.3 The Close Relationship Between the Nose and the Upper Lip

Simply changing the observer's point of view in front of the subject changes the relationship between the columella and the upper lip, the nostril show, and also the light reflex over the tip.

Every change in the volume, length, slope, and shape of the lower third of the nose influences how we see the volume, length, slope, and shape of the upper lip. The opposite is also true.

The basic knowledge of the visual interplay between the nasal tip, the columellar–lobule profile and length, the subnasale point or curve, the alar rim profile, the upper lip profile and length, and the labral superior point can be simplified by altering one parameter at a time. Figure 7.25 shows the visual effects of changing the nasal tip rotation, the upper lip length, the upper lip projection, and the profile contour at subnasal.

The mobility of the lower third of the nose and the upper lip when smiling is always assessed and documented with at least two profile photographs. With a range of movement that differs between cases, the tip of the nose is displaced down and posterior, revealing the inferior dorsal profile of the cartilaginous septum, whereas the ala, at the alar crease junction, rises (Fig. 7.26).

7.4 Nasal Analysis Checklist[3]

To obtain a better analysis of the several nasal parameters and to avoid errors of omission, John B. Tebbetts suggests the use of a checklist [12]. The following one is a good tool for a comprehensive nasal analysis and should be based on the direct clinical assessment along with the 11 basic and the five nasal photographic views, described in Chap. 3. It is subdivided into four sections: general considerations, upper third of the nose, middle third of the nose, and lower third of the nose.

7.4.1 Nasal Analysis Checklist: General Considerations

- Is the face symmetric?
  □ Yes
  □ No, because…
- In frontal view, the facial shape is:
  □ Wide
  □ Narrow
  □ Long
  □ Short
- The facial profile is:
  □ Straight
  □ Concave
  □ Convex

[3]Section 2 on Springer Extra Materials (extras.springer.com).

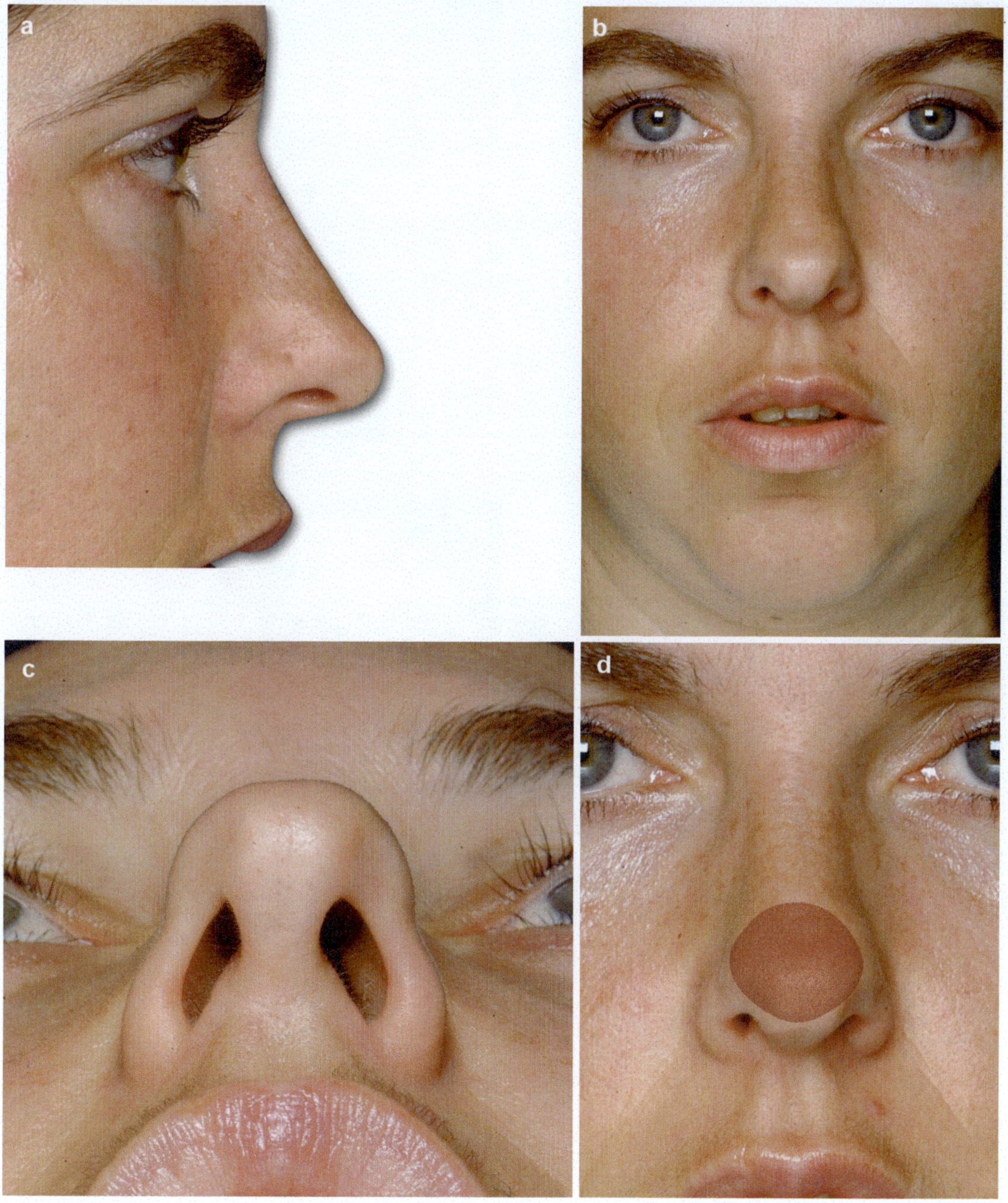

Fig. 7.21 A clinical case of intrinsic tip deformity. In close-up profile view, the nasal outline appears to be quite good (**a**), but the frontal and basal views (**b**, **c**) show a large nasal tip. The increased volume of the lobule (**d**), the lack of definition and angularity (**e**), the increased interdomal distance (**f**), and a shape, recognized as "boxy" (**g**), characterize this nasal lobule. The fullface profile view permits the surgeon to understand the whole facial imbalance due to the severe class II dentofacial deformity (**h**)

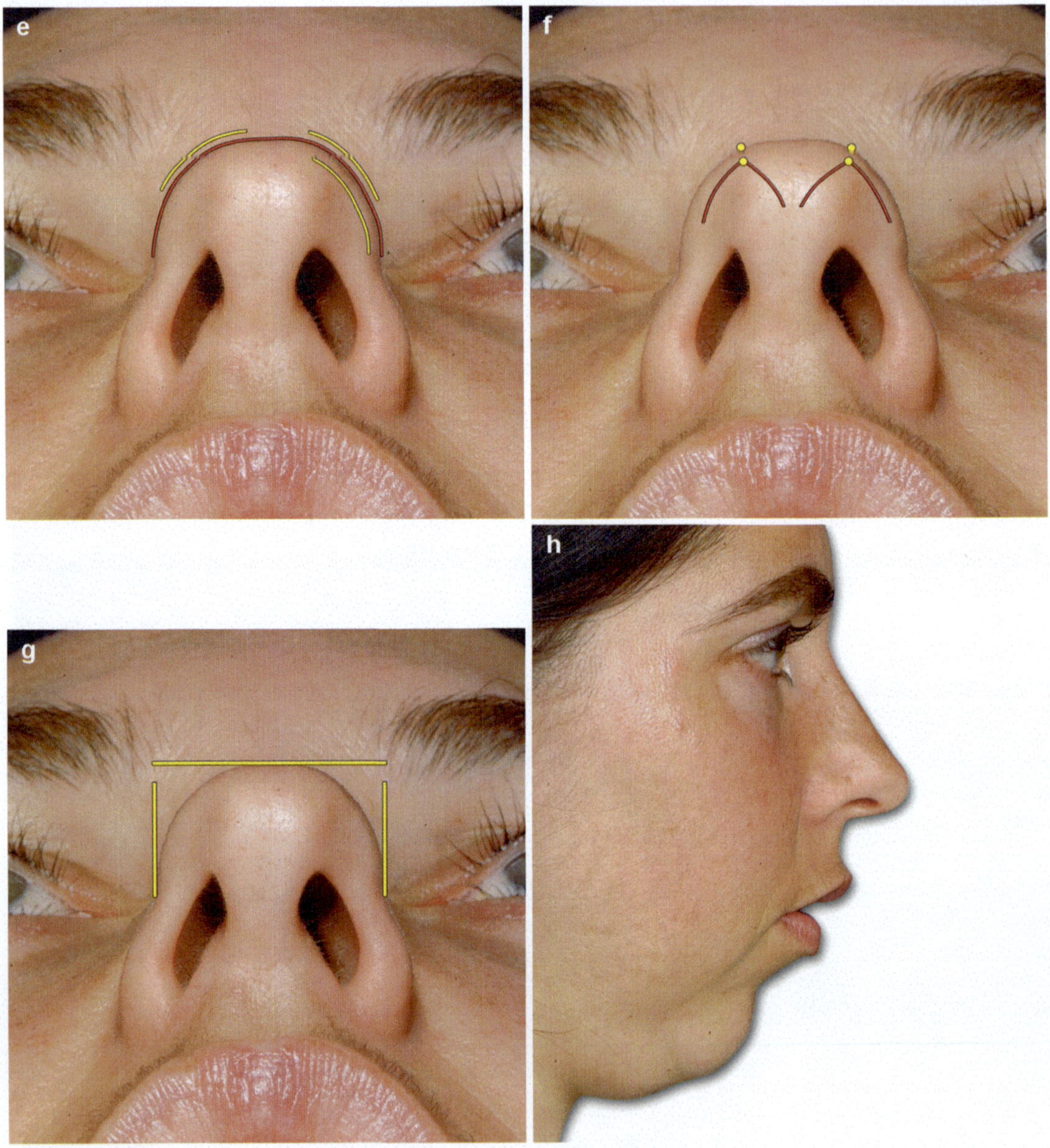

Fig. 7.21 (continued)

- Define the paranasal region (pyriform aperture):
  □ Correct
  □ Hypoplastic (retrusive)
- Is there a dimensional–volumetric balance between the nose and the whole face?
  □ Yes
  □ No, because…
- Is the nose generally proportioned (balanced) by itself?
  □ Yes
  □ No, because…
- Define the whole nose:
  □ Large nose
  □ Narrow nose
  □ Long nose
  □ Short nose
- Is the nose symmetric?
  □ Yes
  □ No, because…
- Are there two symmetric and continuous gentle dorsal curves from the eyebrows to the domal area (nasal "unbroken" lines)?
  □ Yes
  □ No, because…

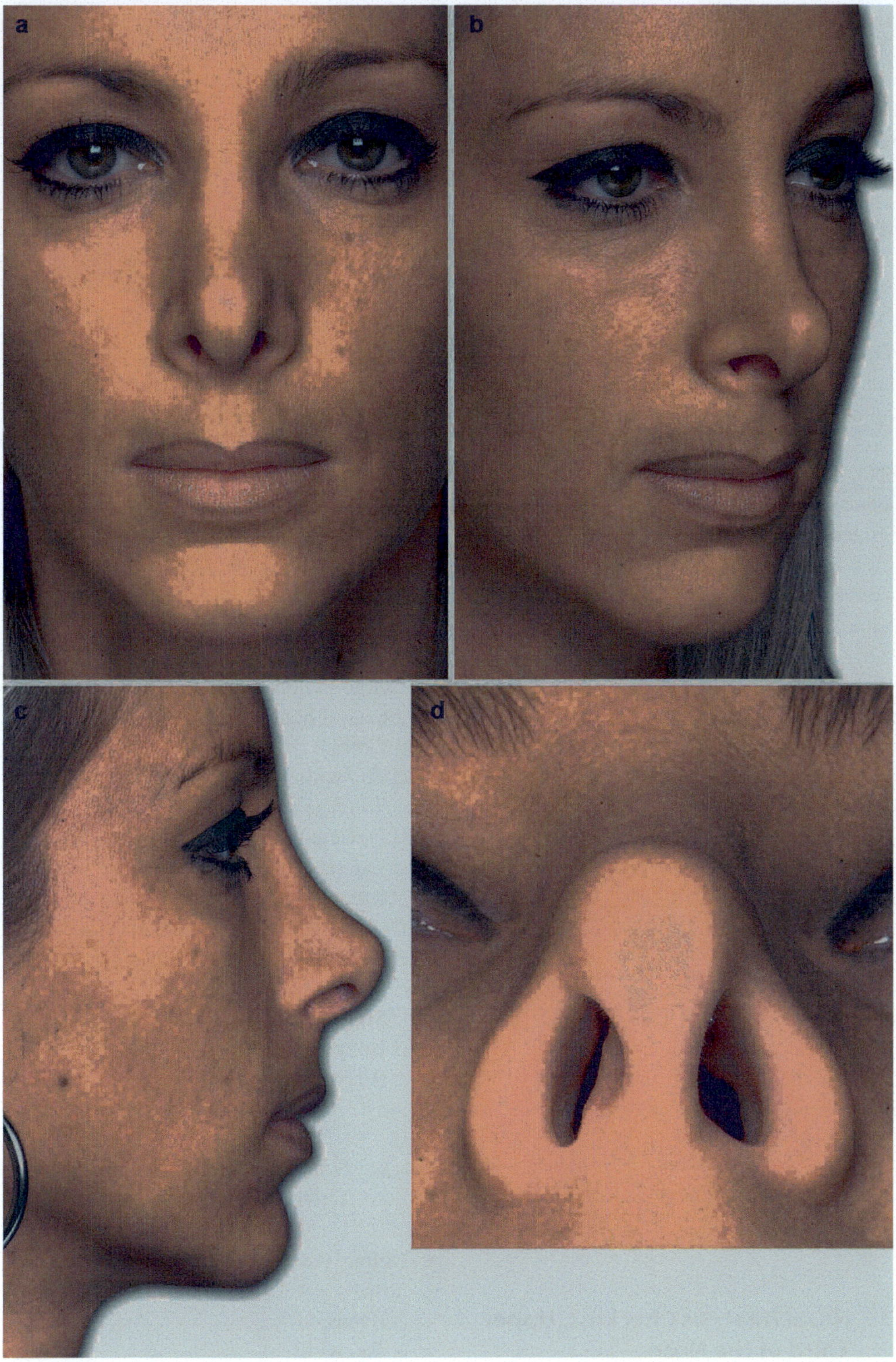

Fig. 7.22 A secondary deformity following aggressive nasal surgery. In the frontal view, the bilateral dorsal lines are interrupted at the level of the cartilaginous dorsum, the nostril show is increased on each side, and the lobule appears bilaterally pinched (**a**). The oblique right view confirms the distortion of the left "unbroken" line due to the dorsal saddle (**b**). In the profile view, the absence of a radix breakpoint, the excessive concave dorsal outline, the overrotated and overprojected intrinsic tip, the retracted right ala, and the long upper lip are evident (**c**). The basal view confirms the pinched aspect of the lobule and reveals the reduction of the right nostril aperture (**d**)

- Define the nasal profile slope:
  □ Ideal (balanced with the face)
  □ Slightly downward rotated
  □ Downward rotated
  □ Slightly upward rotated
  □ Upward rotated
- Is the alar base width similar to the intercanthal distance?
  □ Yes
  □ Wider
  □ Narrower
- In the profile view, are the forehead slope, the chin projection, the submental, and cervical region balanced with the nose?
  □ Yes
  □ No, because…
- Define the upper lip:
  □ Balanced with the nose
  □ Too long
  □ Too short…
- Define the nasal skin:
  □ Oily
  □ Sebaceous
  □ Thin
  □ Thick
- This nose matches one or more of these definitions:
  □ Tension nose
  □ Polly beak
  □ Crooked
  □ Saddle
  □ Greek
  □ Pinched
  □ Inverted-V deformity (see Sect. 7.8, at the end of this chapter)
- Describe the resilience and strength of the supporting tip cartilages (by palpation):
  □ Good
  □ Poor,…
  □ Describe any other findings obtained by palpation:…

7.4.2 Nasal Analysis Checklist: Upper Third of the Nose

- Define the radix width:
  □ Correct
  □ Too wide
  □ Too narrow
- Define the radix breakpoint in the horizontal plane:
  □ Correct
  □ Too anterior (absent)
  □ Shallow
  □ Deep
- Define the glabella in the horizontal plane:
  □ Correct
  □ Too anterior (due to frontal sinus pneumatization)
  □ Shallow
  □ Deep
- Define the corneal plane anteroposterior location:
  □ Correct
  □ Too anterior (exophthalmos)
  □ Too posterior (enophthalmos)
- Define the radix breakpoint in the vertical plane:
  □ Correct
  □ Too high
  □ Too low
- Define the nasal dorsum width at the level of the nasal bones:
  □ Correct
  □ Too wide
  □ Too narrow
  □ Deviated to R–L side
  □ Lateral hump on the R–L side
  □ Bilateral lateral hump (double bridge)
- Define the profile over the nasal bones:
  □ Straight
  □ Slight concave
  □ Slight convex
  □ Bony hump
  □ Bony saddle

7.4.3 Nasal Analysis Checklist: Middle Third of the Nose

- Define the base of the middle third of the nose:
  □ Balanced
  □ Too wide
  □ Too narrow
- Define the dorsum of the middle third of the nose:
  □ Ideal
  □ Too wide

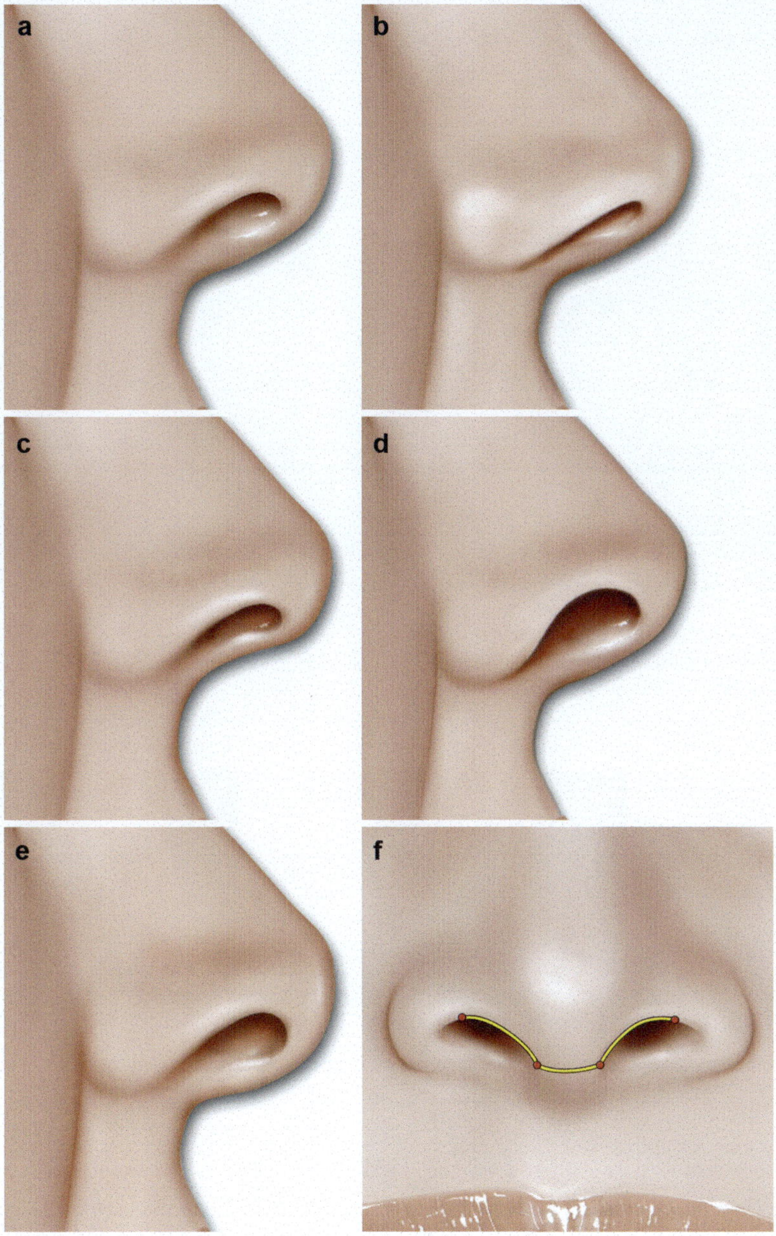

Fig. 7.23 The columellar show is the area of visible columella under the alar rim (**a**). A reduced columellar show can be produced by a hanging ala (**b**), a retracted columella (**c**), or the combination of these two conditions, whereas an increased columellar show can be produced by a retracted ala (**d**), a hanging columella (**e**), or the combination of these two conditions. The ideal outline of the paired nasal alar rims and the columella, in frontal view, should resemble the figure of a gull in flight (**f**)

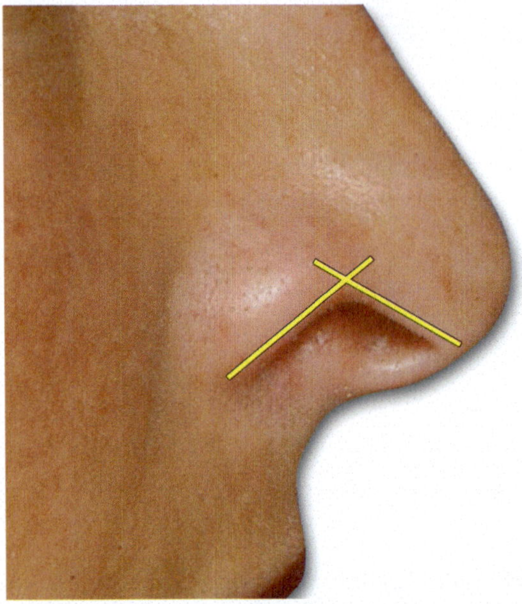

Fig. 7.24 A clinical case of right notched alar rim. The gentle curvature of the alar outline is lost with the formation of an evident angle

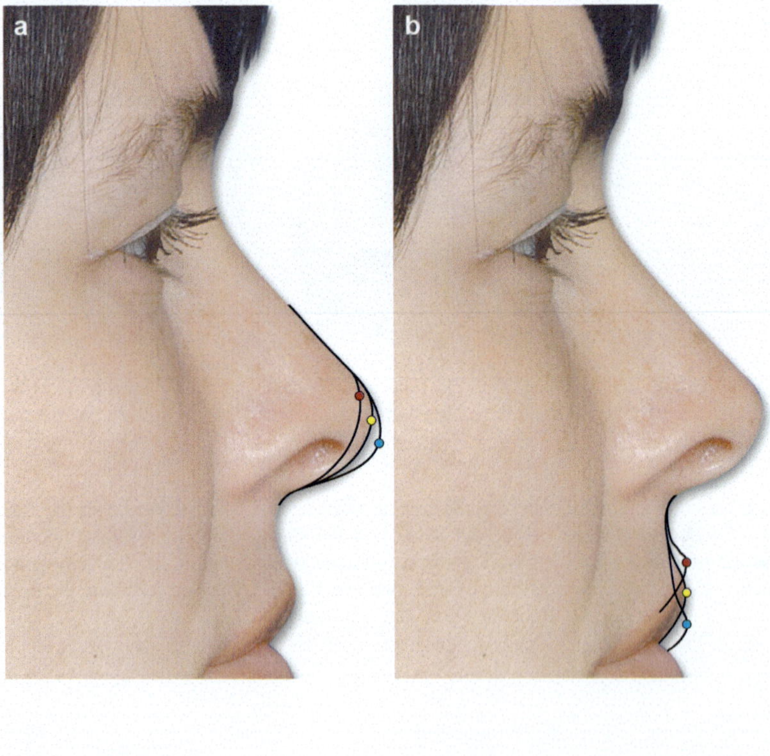

Fig. 7.25 The visual effects of changing the nasal tip rotation (**a**), the upper lip length (**b**), the upper lip projection (**c**), and the profile contour at subnasale (**d**)

Fig. 7.25 (continued)

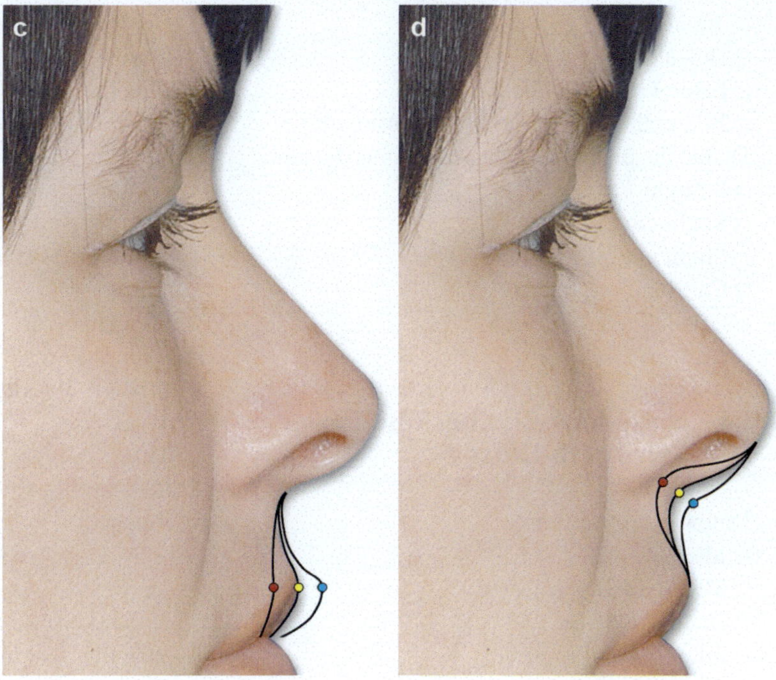

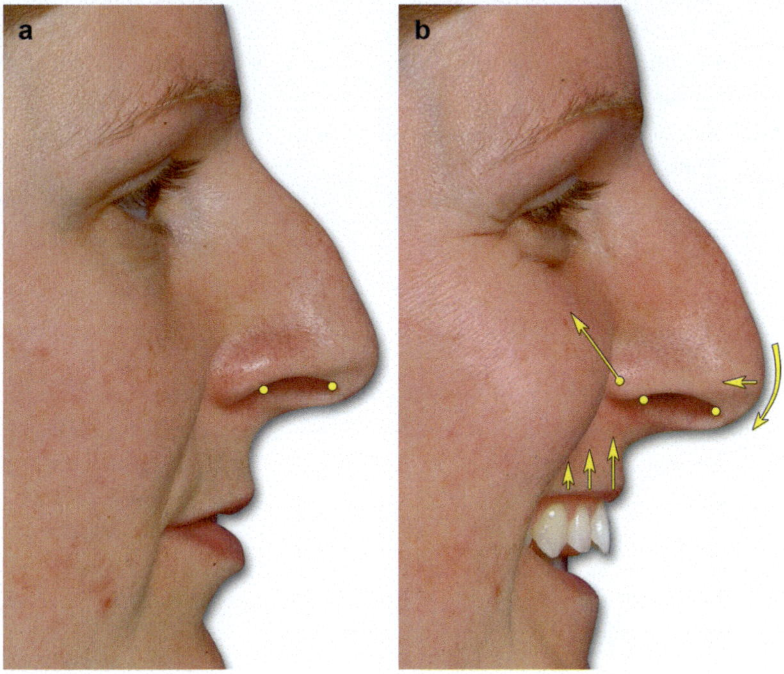

Fig. 7.26 The act of smiling produces a specific pattern of movements on the face and nose. From the relaxed position (**a**) to the smiling one (**b**), the characteristic downward displacement of the lobule is associated with the rising up of the ala at the alar crease junction

□ Too narrow
□ Deviated to R–L side
□ Lateral hump on the R–L side
□ Bilateral lateral hump (double bridge)

- Define the profile of the cartilaginous dorsum:
  □ Straight
  □ Slight concave
  □ Slight convex
  □ Cartilaginous hump
  □ Cartilaginous saddle

7.4.4 Nasal Analysis Checklist: Lower Third of the Nose

- Define tip projection:
  □ Ideal
  □ Slightly underprojected
  □ Underprojected
  □ Slightly overprojected
  □ Overprojected
- Define tip rotation:
  □ Correct
  □ Slightly downward rotated
  □ Downward rotated
  □ Slightly upward rotated
  □ Upward rotated
- Define tip shape (utilizing the basal view):
  □ Triangular
  □ Boxy
  □ Broad
  □ Bifid
  □ Pinched
  □ Deviated to the R–L
  □ Asymmetric…
- Define the alar cartilages – interdomal distance:
  □ Normal
  □ Ideal
  □ Wide
  □ Narrow
  □ Asymmetry…
- Define the alar cartilages – lateral crus width:
  □ Normal
  □ Large
  □ Small
- Define the alar cartilages – lateral crus rotation:
  □ Normal
  □ Cephalad rotated
  □ Caudal rotated
- Define the alar cartilage – lateral crus shape:
  □ Normal
  □ Deformed…
  □ Asymmetric…
  □ R–L differences…
- Define the nostril show on frontal view:
  □ Correct
  □ Excessive
  □ Reduced
- Define the alar rim:
  □ Thick
  □ Thin
  □ Collapsed
  □ Pinched
- Are the alar rims symmetric?
  □ Yes
  □ No, because…
- Define the right alar rim arch:
  □ Correct
  □ Hanging
  □ Retracted
  □ Notched
- Define the left alar rim arch:
  □ Correct
  □ Hanging
  □ Retracted
  □ Notched
- Define the columellar show in lateral view:
  □ Ideal
  □ Hanging
  □ Retracted
- Define the columellar–lobule angle:
  □ Ideal
  □ Increased
  □ Decreased
  □ Too anteriorly positioned
  □ Too posteriorly positioned
- Define the columellar length:
  □ Normal
  □ Long
  □ Short
- Define the columellar–lobule ratio:
  □ Correct
  □ Excessive (long columella and short lobule)
  □ Reduced (short columella and long lobule)
- Define the columellar width:
  □ Normal

  - □ Wide
  - □ Narrow
- Define the medial crus footplates flare (base of the columella):
  - □ Normal
  - □ Too wide
  - □ Too narrow
  - □ Asymmetric…
- Define the nostril aperture shape and orientation in basal view:
  - □ Normal
  - □ Too vertical
  - □ Too horizontal
  - □ Asymmetric…
- Define the alar base width:
  - □ Normal
  - □ Wide
  - □ Narrow
- Define the caudal septum–nasal spine complex:
  - □ Normal
  - □ Overdeveloped
  - □ Underdeveloped (retracted)
  - □ Deviated to the R–L
- Define the depressor septi muscle action on the nasal tip:
  - □ Normal
  - □ Excessive

7.5 The Nasal Analysis Sheets

There are three ways to create the definitive written nasal aesthetic general assessment.

The first is to utilize a preformed and standardized sheet, like the checklist reported above. The advantages of this tool are: first, it guarantees none of the steps are forgotten, and second, one can use the same comparable method to collect data for every patient, for easy future utilization. It also does not require a computer with printer and relative software.

The second requires the printing of the main photographic views onto large sheets to obtain the necessary extra space around every picture for writing the observations (Fig. 7.27). The goal is to correlate the written notes with the photographic images of the patient.

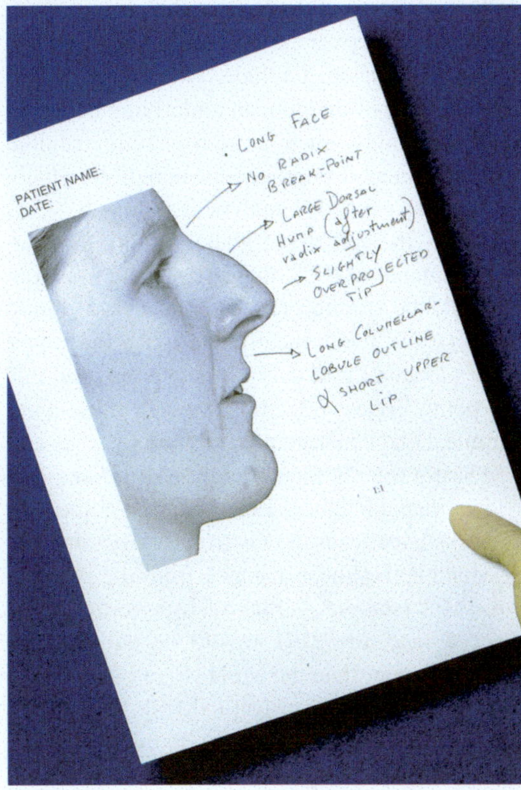

Fig. 7.27 An example of written analysis made directly on the photograph sheet

The third and more complete combines the previous two. It offers the possibility of applying the clinical image to an electronic preformed sheet and thus obtains a printed personalized sheet for every patient.

7.6 Cephalometric Nasal Analysis

7.6.1 The Method of Byrd and Hobar

In 1993, H. Steve Byrd and P. Craig Hobar published a useful nasal analysis method for rhinoplasty [2, 3]. The main purpose was to determine the aesthetically proportioned nasal length, tip projection, and radix projection in relationship to the patient's facial height. The measurements can be made directly on the patient or, better, utilizing life-size photographs in frontal and profile views.

The main steps of the Byrd and Hobar method are as follows:

- Check occlusion. Exclude, with the intraoral and general evaluation, an underlying dentofacial deformity, such as retrognathic maxilla and retrognathic or prognathic mandible, which require an expanded analytical approach.
- Identify the soft tissue glabella (Gs), the alar base plane (ABP), the soft tissue menton (Mes), the stomion (S), the alar crease junction (ACJ), the corneal plane (CP), the superior palpebral fold (SPF), the R point, and the T point. Figure 7.28 illustrates all these anatomical and constructed landmarks.
- Measure the midfacial height (MFH) and the lower facial height (LFH). The first is the linear distance from the Gs to the ABP, and the second is the linear distance from the ABP to the Mes (see Fig. 7.28a, b). In a vertical balanced face, the LFH should be equal to or 3 mm greater than the MFH (Fig. 7.28b).
- Measure the chin vertical (SMes). This is the distance from the stomion (S) to the soft tissue menton (Mes) (Fig. 7.28b).
- Measure the actual nasal length (RT) (Fig. 7.28a, b).
- Calculate and draw the ideal nasal length (RTi) utilizing two different procedures: RTi = 0.67 × MFH or RTi = SMes.
- Choose between these two measurements the one that is closest to the actual nasal length (RT).
- Measure the actual tip projection (ACJ–T) (Fig. 7.28c).
- Calculate the ideal tip projection, deriving it from the ideal nasal length: ideal tip projection = RTi × 0.67.
- Measure the actual radix projection, the distance from the corneal plane to the radix plane (CP–RP) (Fig. 7.28c).
- Calculate the ideal radix projection, deriving it from the ideal nasal length: ideal radix projection = RTi × 0.28. The range is from 9 to 14 mm.
- The ideal radix projection, the ideal tip projection, and the ideal nasal length are used to draw the ideal R point and the ideal T point on the profile view. In this way, it is possible to envision the "boundaries" of the ideal nose.
- Plan, in agreement with the patient, the desired dorsal profile. As reported by the authors, variation may include a slight dorsal convexity, a straight dorsum between the radix and the tip, and a straight dorsum reduced to a level of 1–2 mm below the tip, creating retrousse with a supratip break. In the same papers the authors presented a further step dedicated to the assessment of chin projection [2, 3].

7.7 Nasal Airway Assessment

The external aesthetic analysis must be associated with a complete medical "nasal" history and an anterior rhinoscopy to detect problems related to the nasal airway (see Sect. 13.6). It is interesting that many of the external details found during

Fig. 7.28 The landmarks utilized in the Byrd and Hobar method on frontal (**a**) and profile views (**b**, **c**). *Gs*, soft tissue glabella, the clinically palpable and usually visible anatomic midline point in the lower forehead; this is the most prominent point on the curve of the frontal bone before the nasal–frontal junction. *ABP* alar base plane, is a plane running through the alar base and utilized as a division between the midface and the lower face. *S* stomion, is the midline point at the junction of the upper and lower lip vermillion. *Mes* soft tissue menton, is the most inferior midline point on the inferior border of the chin. *ACJ* alar crease junction, is the most posterior point of the curved line formed by the alar crease as seen in profile view; it is utilized as a landmark for measuring tip projection. *CP* corneal plane, is a coronal plane tangential to the surface of the cornea in profile view; it is utilized as a landmark for measuring the radix projection. *SPF* superior palpebral fold, is the vertical reference landmark utilized to identify the *R* point in the midline of the nasal dorsum (the *R* point is constructed and may differ with the existing radix breakpoint). The *T* point is the midline point on the nasal tip taken at the level of the dome projecting points of the lower lateral cartilages

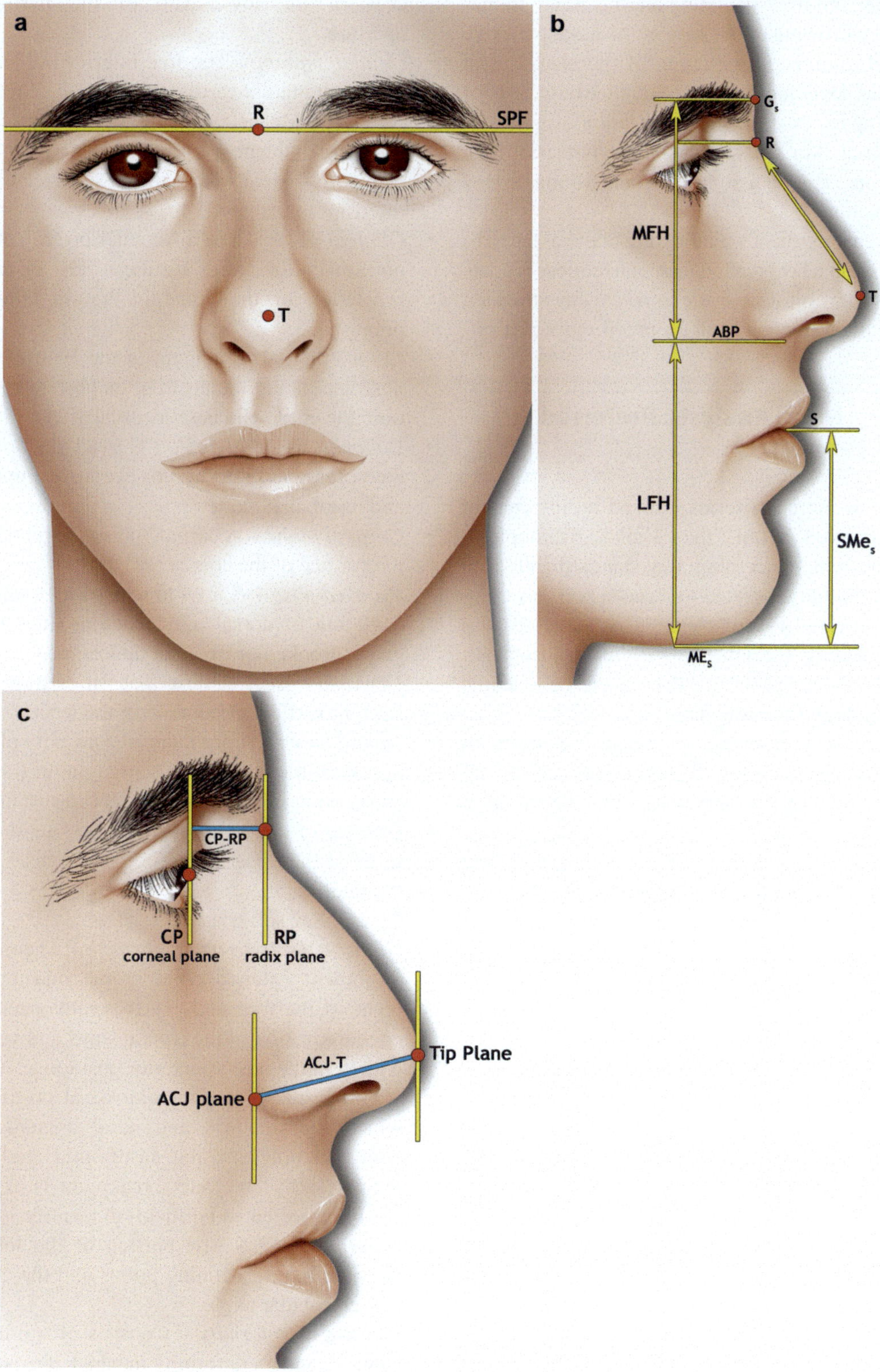
a
R
SPF
T
b
Gs
R
T
MFH
ABP
S
LFH
SMes
MEs
c
CP-RP
CP
corneal plane
RP
radix plane
ACJ-T
Tip Plane
ACJ plane

the aesthetic analysis, such as crooked or saddle dorsum, midline deviation of the nasal framework, narrowing of the base of the nasal pyramid, nostril asymmetry, pinching of the alae, caudal septum deviation, broad columellar base, loss of tip support, excessive down rotation of the nasal tip, nasal skin scars, maxillary hypoplasia, long face, etc., can be a sign of an underlying airway obstruction.

Even if a patient wanting rhinoplasty assures the clinician that her breathing through the nose is good, every effort must be made to reveal any structural cause of obstruction in all the preoperative phases.

7.8 Nasal Analysis: Preferred Terms[4]

Many of the nasal terms utilized in this chapter are derived from the Dallas Rhinoplasty Symposium concerning the standardization of the terminology related to nasal surgery. A complete vocabulary for rhinoplasty surgeons was published by Rohrich et al. [10] and is also available on the web [7]. This list reports the essential terminology for nasal analysis.

- *Accessory cartilages* – Small cartilages of nasal alae found in the space between the lateral ends of the lateral crura and the pyriform aperture edge.
- *Alae* – The lateral wall of the nostril that extends from the tip to join the upper lip.
- *Alar crease junction* – The most posterior point of the curved line formed by the alar crease as seen in profile view.
- *Alar base width* – The width of the nose measured at the alar–cheek junction.
- *Alar groove* – The external, oblique skin depression that follows the caudal margin of the lateral crus as it leaves the alar rim to run in a more cephalic direction. It separates the tip from the thickened portion of the ala that joins the face at the superior cheek–lip junction.
- *Anatomic dome* – The junction of the medial and lateral crus.

[4]Section 3 on Springer Extra Materials (extras.springer.com).

- *Anterior nasal spine* – The median bony process of the lower rim of the pyriform aperture.
- *Caudal septum* – The free inferior border of the quadrangular cartilage.
- *Caudal* – Means the same as inferior when referring to the nose.
- *Cephalic* – Means the same as superior when referring to the nose.
- *Clinical dome* – The most anterior-projecting portion of the lower cartilage. The external projection of the dome is the tip-defining point.
- *Columella* – The column at the base of the nose separating the nostrils. Its posterior portion, the columella base, is usually wider.
- *Columellar–labial angle* – Curved junction of the columella with the lip. See also subnasal and nasolabial angle.
- *Corneal plane* – A coronal plane tangential to the surface of the cornea.
- *Crooked nose* – A nose in which any break or deviation of dorsal nasal contour lines may give a crooked or irregular appearance.
- *Deviated nose* – A nose that varies from the straight vertical orientation of the face.
- *Dorsal hump* – A pronounced convexity of the dorsal profile of the nose. Cartilaginous framework, bony framework, or both can sustain it.
- *Dorsum of the nose* – Where the lateral surfaces of the upper two thirds of the nose join the midline.
- *Facet* – See soft triangle.
- *Glabella* (*soft tissue glabella*) – The most prominent anterior point in the midsagittal plane of the forehead [9]. It is influenced by pneumatization of the frontal sinus and varies widely in the posteroanterior position.
- "*Greek nose*" – A particular nasal profile in which the forehead and nasal dorsum are almost in line and the nasofrontal angle is almost 180°. The radix breakpoint is excessively projected and difficult to identify.
- *Infratip lobule* – The portion of the lobule between the tip defining points and the columellar–lobular angle.
- *Inverted-V deformity* – Consists of a middle vault secondary deformity in which the caudal

edge of the nasal bone is visible in broad relief. It is due to inadequate support of the upper lateral cartilages and/or inadequate nasal bones osteotomy [1].

- *Keystone area* – The junction of the perpendicular plate of the ethmoid with the septal cartilage at the dorsum of the nose.
- *Lower lateral cartilage* – The paired inferior nasal cartilages consisting of the medial, middle, and lateral crura.
- *Nasal base line* – A slightly oblique line on the skin that constitutes the lateral boundaries of the nasal pyramid. The nasal base line starts superiorly near to the medial canthus and ends at the alar crease junction.
- *Nasal lobule* – The lower part of the nose bounded by the anterior nostril edge postero inferiorly, the supratip area superiorly, and the alar grooves laterally.
- *Nasal pyramid* – The bony portion of the nose made up bilaterally of the nasal bone and frontal process of the maxilla.
- *Nasal septum* – The vertical wall that divides the nasal passage into two distinct tunnels. It is composed of a bony (perpendicular plate of ethmoid, vomer, and premaxillary crest), cartilaginous (quadrilateral), and membranous portion.
- *Nasal "unbroken" line* – The outline of the nasal pyramid in oblique view. In the attractive nose, this line descends gracefully from the supraorbital ridge onto the nasal dorsum and the nasal tip.
- *Nasofrontal angle* – Angle of demarcation between forehead and nasal dorsum, best seen in profile.
- *Nasolabial angle* – The angle seen on lateral view formed by a line drawn through the most anterior to the most posterior point of the nostril, intersecting the vertical facial plane. The desired angle is 90–95° in males and 95–100° in females [10]. Other authors identify the nasolabial angle as the angle defined by the columellar point to subnasal line intersecting with the subnasal to labral superior line; the desired angle is 90–120°, more acute in males and more obtuse in females.
- *Nostril sill* – The skin area forming the base of the nostril.
- *Pinched nose (pinched nasal tip)* – A nasal tip deformity secondary to collapse of the alar rims subsequent to loss of lateral crural support from either congenital or acquired causes [6].
- *Piriform aperture* – The pear-shaped external bony opening of the nasal cavity.
- *Polly beak nasal deformity* – Secondary deformity refers to postoperative fullness of the supratip region, with an abnormal tip–supratip relationship [1].
- *Radix* – The area of the junction between the nasal dorsum and the frontal bone, inferiorly to the glabella. The radix break point is the most posterior point of this junction in profile view.
- *Rhinion* – The most caudal point of the intranasal suture [8].
- *Saddle nose* – A pronounced concavity of the dorsal profile of the nose. Cartilaginous framework, bony framework, or both can sustain it.
- *Soft triangle (or facet)* – The thin skin fold between the alar rim and the curved caudal border of the junction of the medial and lateral crura. When this is well defined, it is referred to as a facet.
- *Subnasale* – The point at which the columella merges with the upper lip in the midsagittal plane [9]. It varies widely in relation to caudal septum prominence and nasal spine morphology.
- *Supratip area* – The area just superior to the nasal tip at the inferior aspect of the nasal dorsum.
- *Tension nose (prominent-narrow pyramid syndrome)* – A particular deformity in which the external nasal pyramid is abnormally prominent. The length and the height of the nose are usually greater than normal. The radix breakpoint is shallow, and the nasolabial angle is increased [8].
- *Tip* – The apex of the lobule, but it is frequently used when referring to the lobule.
- *Tip-defining points* – The most projecting area on each side of the tip, which produces an external light reflex.
- *Tip projection* – The horizontal component of the distance from the most anterior point of

the nasal tip and the most posterior point of the nasal–cheek junction.

- *Tip rotation* – Determined by the tip angle as measured from a vertical line at the alar crease to the tip, with the norms being 105° for females and 100° for males [4].
- *Upper lateral cartilage* (*or triangular cartilage*) – The paired superior nasal cartilages and triangular in shape extending laterally from the dorsal septum making up the lateral walls of the middle third of the nose.
- *Weak triangle* (*or converse triangle*) – Area superior to paired domes where the cephalic margins of the lower lateral cartilage separate to travel in a superior–lateral direction.

References

1. Becker DG (2002) Complications of rhinoplasty. In: Papel ID (ed) Facial plastic and reconstructive surgery, 2nd edn. Thieme, New York, pp 452–460
2. Byrd HS, Hobar PC (1993) Rhinoplasty: a practical guide for surgical planning. Plast Reconstr Surg 91:642–654
3. Byrd HS, Burt JD (2002) Dimensional approach to rhinoplasty: perfecting the esthetic balance between the nose and chin. In: Gunter JP, Rohrich RJ, Adams WP (eds) Dallas rhinoplasty. Nasal surgery by the master. Quality Medical Publishing, St. Louis
4. Daniel RK (2002) Rhinoplasty. An atlas of surgical techniques. Springer, New York
5. Gunter JP, Rohrich RJ, Friedman RM (1996) Classification and correction of alar-columellar discrepancies in rhinoplasty. Plast Reconstr Surg 97: 643–648
6. Gunter JP, Rohrich RJ, Hackney FL (2002) Correction of the pinched nasal tip with alar spreader grafts. In: Gunter JP, Rohrich RJ, Adams WP (eds) Dallas rhinoplasty. Nasal surgery by the master. Quality Medical Publishing, St. Louis
7. http://rhinoplastyinfocentral.com/rhinoplasty_glossary_dictionary.htm. Accessed 3 March, 2012
8. Huizing EH, de Groot JAM (2003) Functional reconstructive nasal surgery. Thieme, Stuttgart
9. Jacobson A, Vlachos C (1995) Soft-tissue evaluation. In: Jacobson A (ed) Radiographic cephalometry. From basics to videoimaging. Quintessence Publishing, Chicago, pp 239–253
10. Rohrich RJ, Muzaffar AR, Oneal RM (2002) Preferred anatomic terms for rhinoplasty. In: Gunter JP, Rohrich RJ, Adams WP (eds) Dallas rhinoplasty. Nasal surgery by the master. Quality Medical Publishing, St. Louis
11. Sheen JH (1978) Aesthetic rhinoplasty. Mosby, St. Louis, p 51
12. Tebbetts JB (1998) Primary rhinoplasty. A new approach to the logic and technique. Mosby, St. Louis, pp 50–51

8 Lips, Teeth, Chin, and Smile Analysis

Contents

The analysis of the lower third of the face must be conducted considering the following three points:

- Patients' main concerns regarding their facial aesthetics are usually related to the perioral area.
- Lips, teeth, and chin are of interest to different specialists, increasing the need for a team approach to diagnosis and treatment planning.
- Documentation and analysis of the lower third of the face must include the action of smiling.

8.1 Dental Occlusion: Basic Assessment

The basic elements of dental occlusion need to be known because of the important role played by the dental structures in supporting and shaping the lower third of the face. The sagittal, vertical, and transversal relationship of the two arches during occlusion, as well as any crowding, loss, or abnormal shape of the teeth should be noted as a matter of routine during the direct facial lower third examination. Figure 8.1 shows the dental cast of a subject with optimal dental occlusion [3, 4].

Figure 8.2 shows the three basic sagittal relationships between the incisors (overjet). In the case of ideal overjet (Fig. 8.2a), the upper incisors are in front of the lower ones with little or no space between them. The increased overjet (Fig. 8.2b) consists of an excessive horizontal distance between the teeth, whereas the reverse

F. Meneghini, P. Biondi, *Clinical Facial Analysis*,
DOI 10.1007/978-3-642-27228-8_8, © Springer-Verlag Berlin Heidelberg 2012

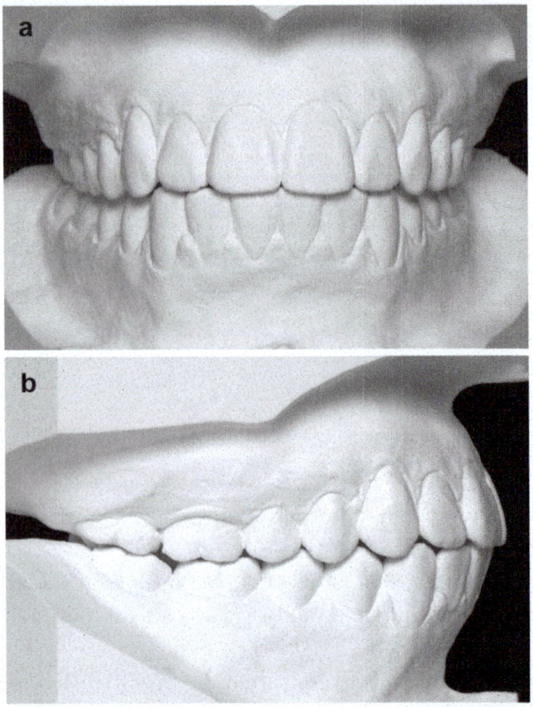

Fig. 8.1 Frontal (**a**) and profile right (**b**) views of the dental cast of a subject with optimal dental occlusion. Note that the upper arch is wider than the lower one, there is no space between adjacent teeth (diastema), there is no space between the two arches (normal overbite and absence of open bite), the upper incisors are in front of the lower incisors (normal overjet), the upper and lower dental midlines coincide, and there is no teeth rotation or abnormal teeth inclination

overjet (Fig. 8.2c) requires that the lower teeth are in front of the upper ones.

The sagittal relationships between the dental arches can be divided into three main classes. Class I presents the ideal posteroanterior relationship between the two dental arches (Fig. 8.3a). Class II is a too anterior upper dental arch and/or a too posterior lower dental arch (Fig. 8.3b). Class III is a too posterior upper dental arch and/or a too anterior lower dental arch (Fig. 8.3c).

Figure 8.4 shows the three basic vertical relationships between the upper and lower incisors (overbite). In the case of ideal overbite, the upper incisors are in front of the lower ones with a limited overlap between them of 1–2 mm (Fig. 8.4a). The deep bite consists of an excessive overlap between the teeth (Fig. 8.4b), whereas the open bite (Fig. 8.4c) requires the presence of a vertical separation between the teeth.

Assessment of the occlusal transversal relationships considers the presence of a midline deviation between the dental arches, a crossbite between opposite teeth, and/or a cant of the occlusal plane (Fig. 8.5).

One important task of the examiner is to correlate the intraoral findings with the external facial appearance of the subject in order to establish the role of dental occlusion on the facial

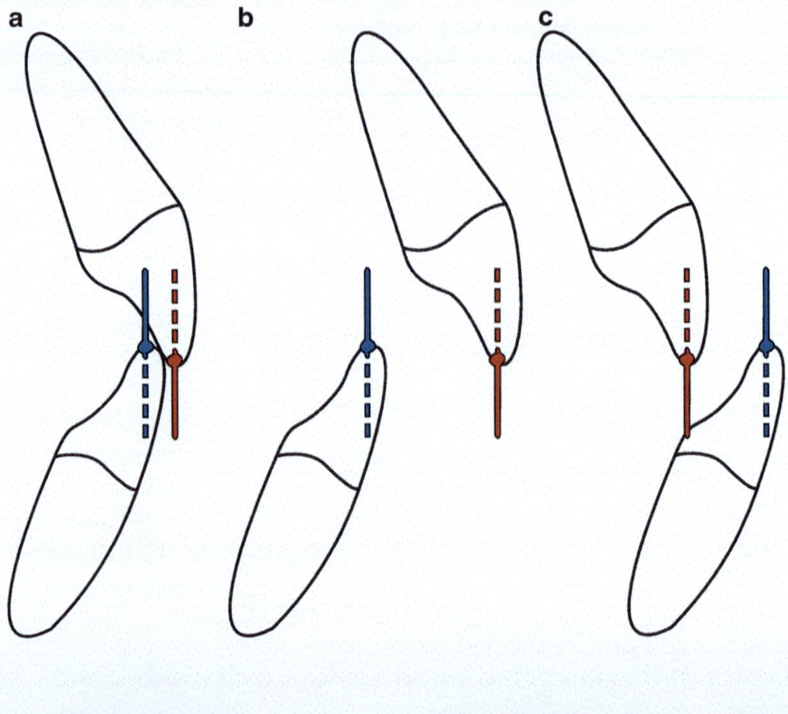

Fig. 8.2 Sagittal relationship between the incisors. Ideal overjet with the upper teeth in front of the lower ones (**a**), increased overjet with excessive horizontal distance between the teeth (**b**), reverse overjet with the lower teeth in front of the upper ones (**c**)

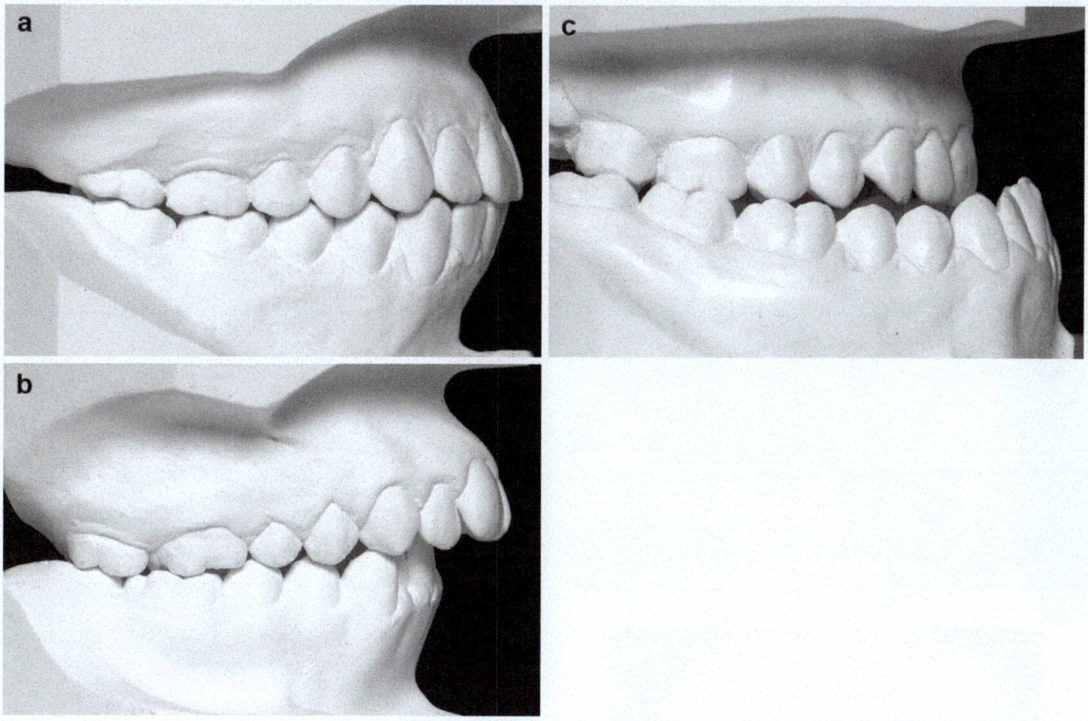

Fig. 8.3 Sagittal classification of dental occlusion. Class I: ideal posteroanterior relationship between the two dental arches (**a**). Class II: too anterior upper dental arch and/or too posterior lower dental arch (**b**). Class III: too posterior upper dental arch and/or too anterior lower dental arch (**c**)

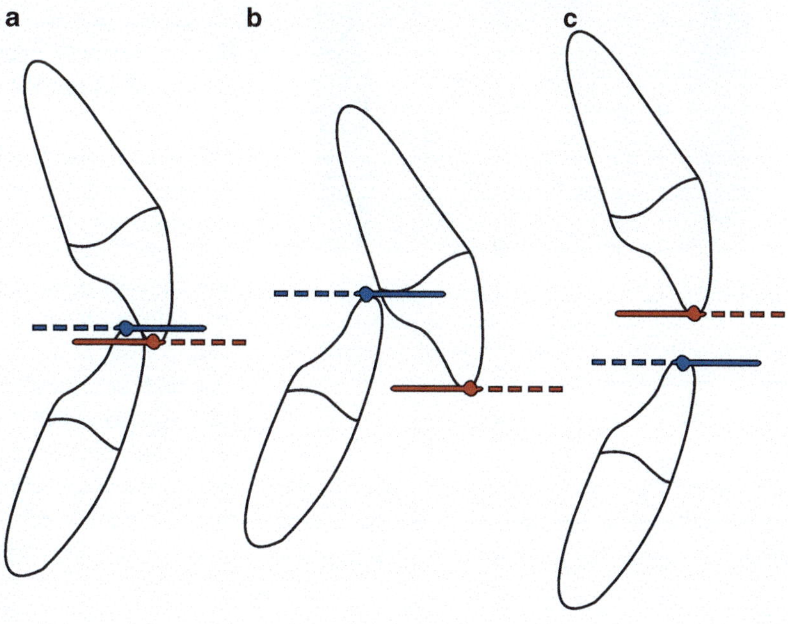

Fig. 8.4 Vertical relationships between the upper and lower incisors. Ideal overbite with a limited overlap of 1–2 mm between the incisors (**a**). Deep bite or excessive overlapping between the incisors (**b**). Open bite or excessive vertical distance between the margins of the incisors (**c**)

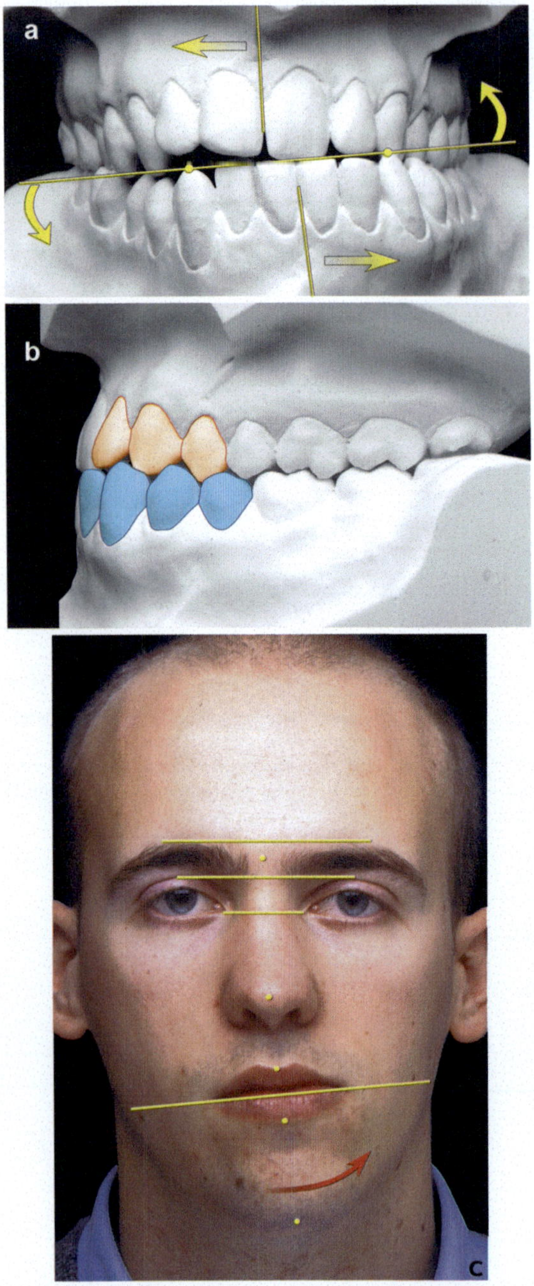

Fig. 8.5 Dental malocclusion with mandibular deviation on the left cant of the occlusal plane (**a**), dental crossbite of some teeth (**b**) associated with facial asymmetry and cant of the lip commissures (**c**)

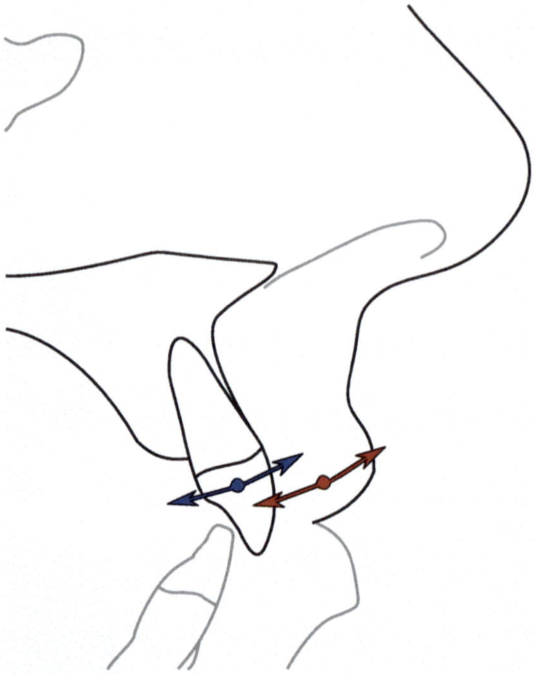

Fig. 8.6 The tracings show the intimate relationship between the inclination of the upper incisors and the upper lip position

aesthetics. The long-term support effect of particular teeth on the lips and cheeks is also considered. With aging, the soft tissue envelope aesthetic is progressively more dependent on the skeletal support offered by well-aligned and correctly inclined frontal teeth and the surrounding alveolar bone (Fig. 8.6).

8.2 Upper Frontal Teeth Assessment

The upper frontal teeth need special attention in all patients, even if they are not mentioned in the patient priority list. Their role in overall facial aesthetics is so important that a qualitative and sometimes quantitative analysis can add many details that help in planning treatment. The upper frontal teeth consist of the four incisors, the two canines, and the four premolars; these teeth should occupy the larger part of the smile. The teeth shape, color, alignment, and symmetry must be evaluated, as well as the architecture and color of their gingival margin. Figure 8.7 shows the detail of well-proportioned and aligned upper frontal teeth.

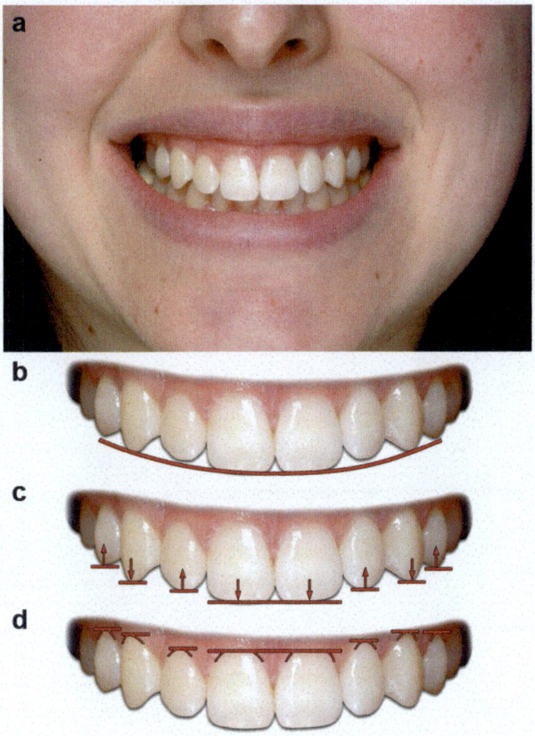

Fig. 8.7 Smiling view of a well-proportioned and aligned upper frontal teeth group (**a**). It can be noted that the outline created by the occlusal margin forms a gentle curve (**b**), adjacent teeth have different marginal vertical positions (**c**), and the gingival margins also have a different shape and position (**d**)

One of the most difficult and at the same time most important aspects to assess is the anteroposterior projection of the upper teeth relative to the facial profile. The orthodontic literature has called this topic "anterior limit of dentition." Clinically and using photographs, the full facial profile view at rest must be compared with the same during a posed smile. Figure 8.8 shows the assessment of the anterior projection of the upper incisors in three different clinical cases.

Two particular aesthetic problems of the upper incisors are the midline diastema and the black triangle. The midline diastema is represented by a space between the two upper incisors (Fig. 8.9b), whereas the so-called black triangle is a base-up triangular space bounded by an excessive mesial inclination of the two upper first incisors (Fig. 8.9c). In both cases, the observer and the patient usually perceive the dark shadow between the teeth as an aesthetic problem.

The spatial position and inclination of the incisors are discussed further in Sect. 9.6.

8.3 Lips Assessment

The first problem in the assessment of the lips is to obtain a truly relaxed position from the patient. When reviewing a complete set of photographs of a clinical case, it is not unusual to discover that the lip position is not constant but changes from a complete seal, most frequently at the start of the photographic session, to a more relaxed (habitual!) one with the presence of a more or less wide space between the two lips (Fig. 8.10). A partial nasal obstruction should be suspected when the subject has the habit of maintaining a space between the lips and breathing through the mouth.

Figure 8.11 shows a case of lip incompetence with absence of lip seal at rest due to an increased overjet with mandibular hypoplasia. In these cases, maintaining perfect lip closure requires a voluntary contraction that results in the flattening of the lip profile curves.

8.3.1 The Attractive Female Lips

Knowing a prototype of younger, "healthy," and attractive female lips helps us to understand the roles and effects of intrinsic lip problems and any possible correlation with a dentofacial deformity, the aging process, or an acute lip trauma; it also helps to define the younger, "healthy," and attractive male lips.

Figures 8.12 and 8.13 show this prototype in frontal and profile views, as well as the preferred anatomical terms of the perioral region. The characteristics of attractive female lips can be summarized as follows:

- Mouth width or distance between the two lip commissures can be measured utilizing the close-up view of the lip at rest with a ruler. It is of paramount importance for facial aesthetics and can rarely be modified with surgical

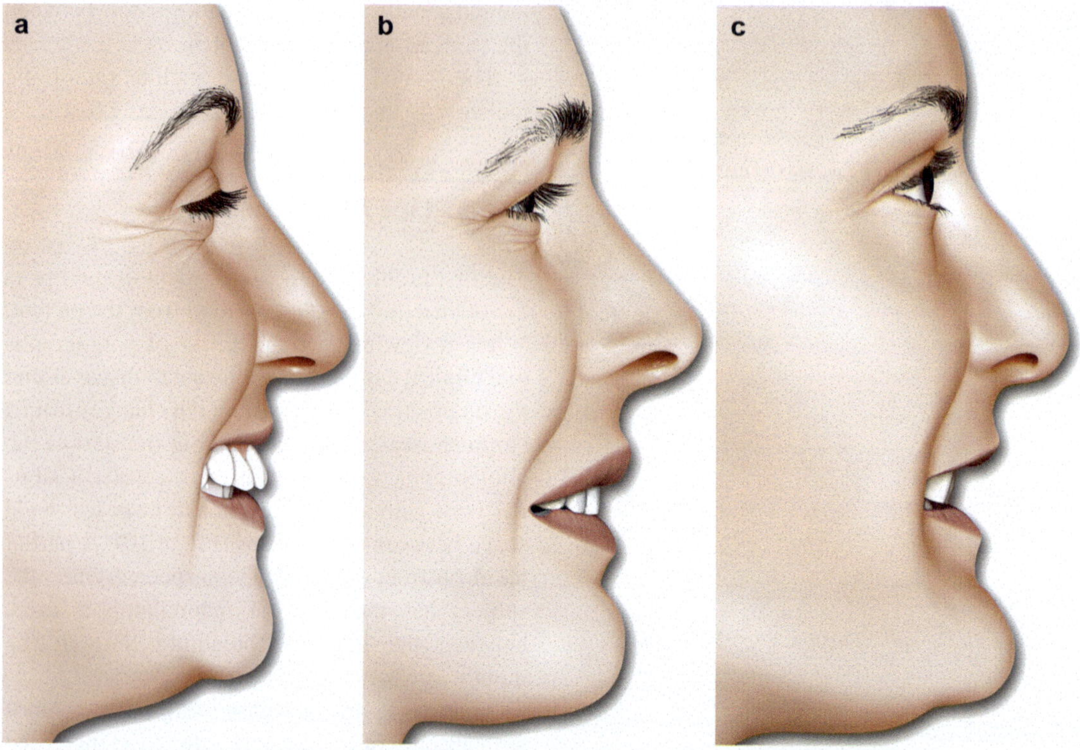

Fig. 8.8 Full facial profile view during smiling. Clinical examples of excessive (**a**), ideal (**b**), and reduced (**c**) sagittal projection of the upper anterior teeth relative to the facial profile

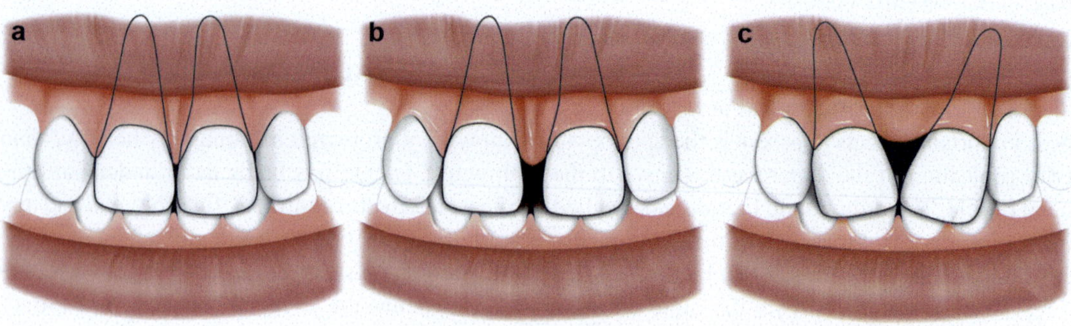

Fig. 8.9 The most favorable aesthetic relationship between the upper incisors, as well as other teeth, requires considerable contact between the two parallel structures (**a**). The presence of a *midline dark shadow* between upper central incisors may be a diastema (**b**) or a "black triangle" (**c**)

treatment. In particular, a reduced mouth width greatly affects the aesthetics of the lower third of the face (Fig. 8.14). The mean value, as reported by Farkas [5], measured in a group of attractive, young, adult North American Caucasian females is 50.9 mm.

- The nasolabial sulcus is almost undetectable when the patient is in the rest position.
- The skin linear reliefs of the philtrum columns, the Cupid's bow, and the upper and lower lip rolls are all present and well defined.

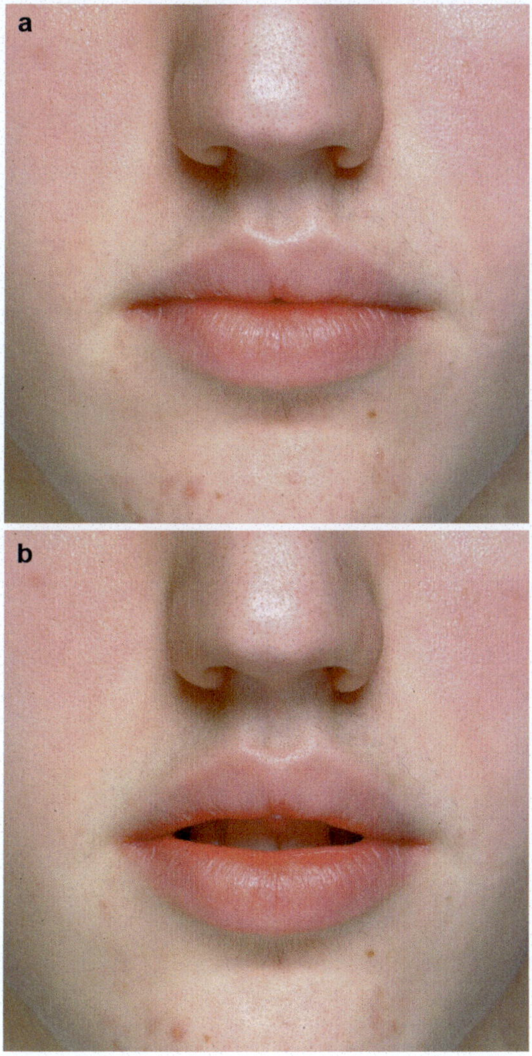

Fig. 8.10 These photographs were taken in sequence during the same sitting without requesting the patient to take a particular lip position. After a few seconds in which the patient maintained a lip seal sustained with some muscular contraction (**a**), he returned to his habitual relaxed position with loss of contact between the lips (**b**)

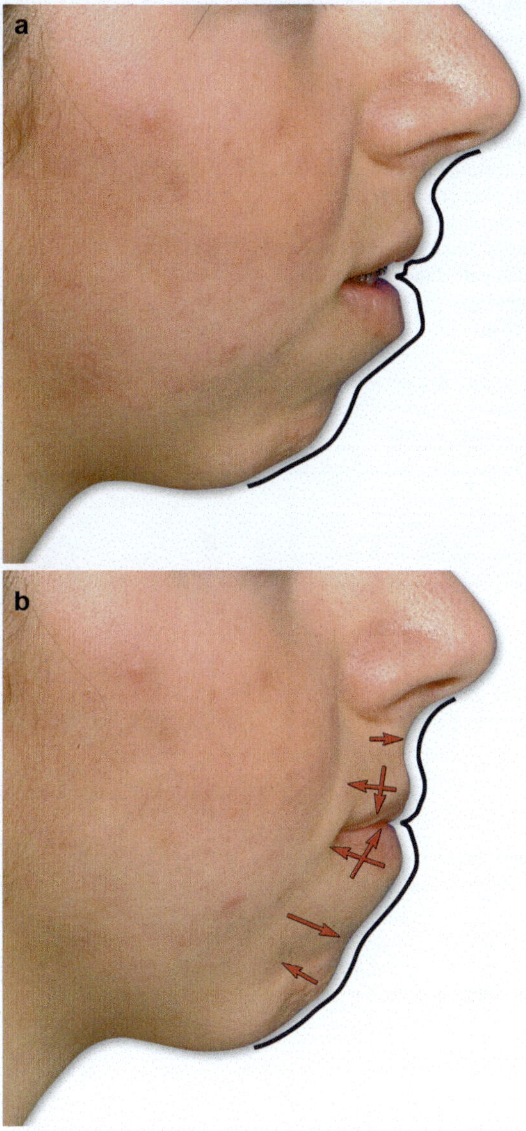

Fig. 8.11 A case of lip incompetence with absence of lip seal at rest due to an increased overjet with mandibular hypoplasia (**a**). In these cases, maintaining perfect lip closure requires a voluntary contraction that results in the flattening of the lip profile *curves* (**b**)

- The vermillion area and volume of the lower lip exceed those of the upper lip.
- The most anterior lower lip points in the profile view (labrale inferior) lie slightly anterior to the upper ones (labrale superior).
- The upper lip profile from subnasale to labrale superior is never vertically or posteriorly oriented but forms a gentle concave curve anteriorly projected.
- From the nasal tip to the soft tissue menton, there is a series of gentle curves, without straight traits, and a unique well-defined angle at the stomion (Fig. 8.13).
- The Ricketts' E-line, the reference line connecting the tip of the nose with the soft tissue pogonion (Fig. 8.13), passes about 4 mm in

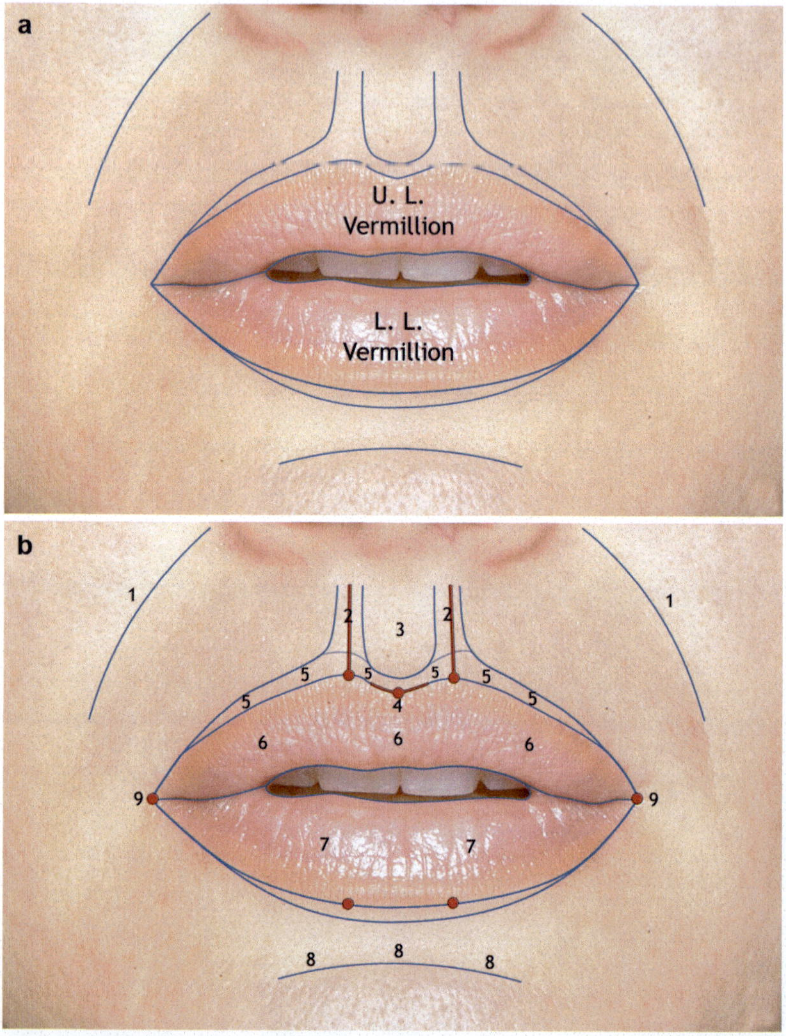

Fig. 8.12 Frontal views of younger, "healthy," attractive female lips (**a**, **b**). Perioral soft tissue determinants (**b**): *1* nasolabial sulcus, *2* philtrum columns, *3* philtrum, *4* Cupid's bow, *5* lip white roll, *6* upper lip vermillion (its central and more projecting portion is also called the upper lip tubercle), *7* lower lip vermillion, *8* labiomental sulcus, *9* lip commissures (the distance between the two commissures is defined as mouth width)

front of the upper lip and 2 mm in front of the lower lip [6].

For comparison, the main differences in the attractive male lips are:

- The upper lip is higher and less anteriorly inclined. The height of the vermillion portion is reduced compared with that of the skin portion.
- The profile from the nasal tip to the soft tissue menton may show the presence of angles instead of gentle curves, in particular a more defined passage from lower lip to chin (labiomental fold).
- The distances between the lips and the Ricketts' E-line are greater with a flatter profile.

8.4 Smile Analysis

The smile may be either posed or spontaneous. The differences between the two are important because the posed smile is voluntary, not elicited by an emotion, static, unstrained, and fairly reproducible. The unposed (spontaneous) smile is

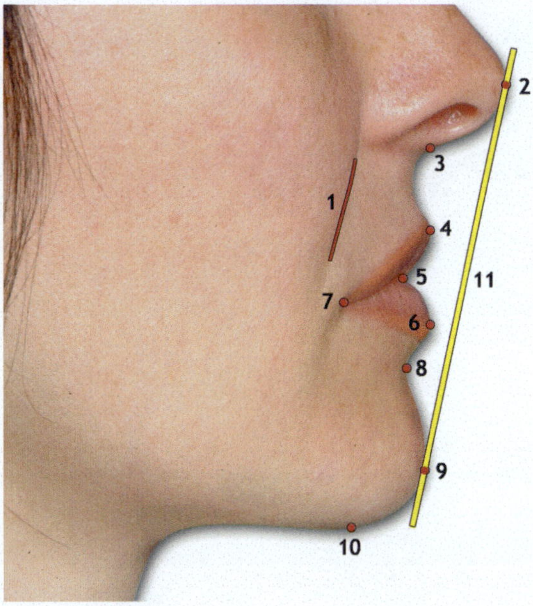

Fig. 8.13 Profile view of younger, "healthy," attractive female lips. Reference points and Ricketts' lips projection reference E-line: *1* nasolabial sulcus, *2* nasal tip, *3* subnasale, *4* labrale superior, *5* stomion, *6* labrale inferior, *7* lip commissure, *8* labiomental sulcus, *9* soft tissue pogonion, *10* soft tissue menton, *11* Ricketts' E-line. The series of gentle curves from nasal tip to soft tissue menton characterize the lips profile

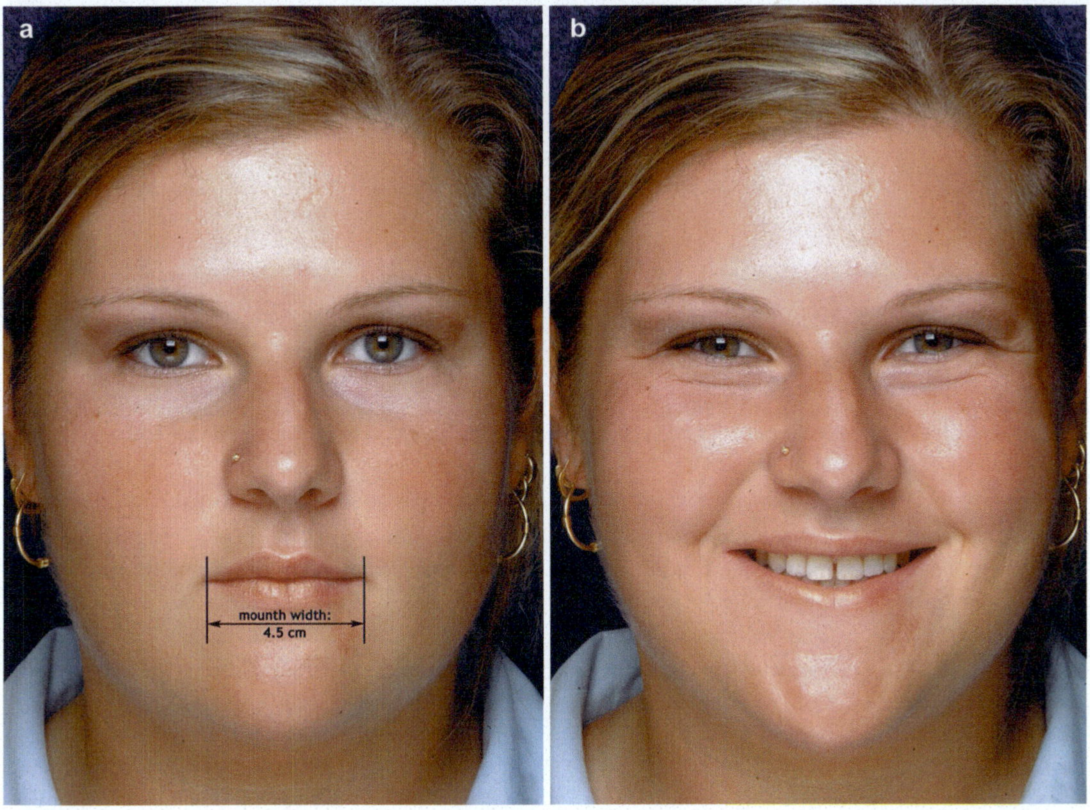

Fig. 8.14 A clinical case of absolute (4.5 cm) and relative (large face) reduction of the mouth width (**a**). Fortunately, the action of smiling reverses this situation to a more pleasing proportion (**b**)

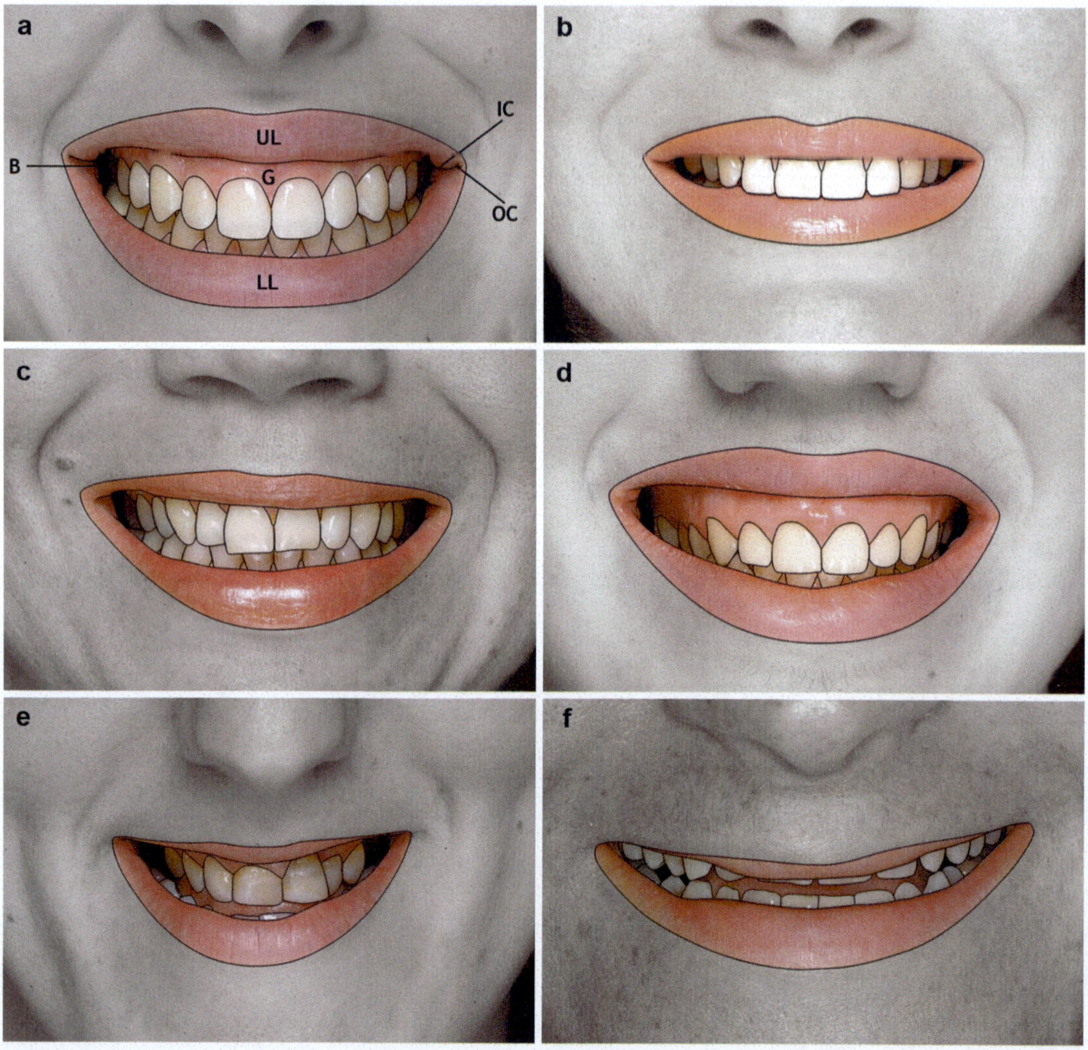

Fig. 8.15 The smile components and the display zone. *B* buccal corridors, *OC* outer commissure, *IC* inner commissure, *G* gingival, *UL* upper lip vermillion, *LL* lower lip vermillion (**a**). Display zones of five different subjects (**b–f**)

involuntary, induced by joy or mirth, and is not sustained (it is dynamic). It is often characterized by more lip elevation than the posed smile. When a subject is forced to mimic an unposed smile, this cannot be sustained and will appear strained and unnatural [1]. So, we mainly conduct the analysis utilizing the posed smile because of the need for reproducible features.

The upper and lower lips frame the display zone that contains the teeth and the gingival scaffold [1]. The soft tissue determinants of the display zone are lip thickness and marginal profile, intercommissure width (mouth width during smiling), smile index (width/height), and gingival architecture (Fig. 8.15a) [2]. Figure 8.15b–f shows the variability in the shape and total area of the display zone, utilizing five clinical examples.

An important characteristic of the smile is the presence of the buccal corridors, the so-called negative space described in the orthodontic literature (Fig. 8.15a), which are the bilateral dark shadows situated between the buccal (vestibular) surface of the posterior teeth and the inner commissure of the lips. The perceived dimensions and depth of the shadows in this space depend on several factors, such as the width of the dental arches, the sagittal position of the dental arches, the range of horizontal movements produced at the lip commissure, and the type of lighting utilized during the assessment and photographic session. Both the absence and the enlargement of the buccal corridors negatively affect the aesthetics of the face. The smile with a lack of buccal corridors is called a "denture smile."

The assessment of a smile is not complete without evaluation of the smile arc. This is the relationship between the curvature of the incisal edges of maxillary incisors and canine to the curvature of the lower lip in the posed smile. It is defined as "consonant" when the maxillary incisal curve is parallel to the curvature of the lower lip on smiling, as in Fig. 8.15a, and "nonconsonant," or flat, when the incisal curvature is flatter than the curvature of the lower lip on smiling, as in Fig. 8.15b [2, 7].

8.4.1 The Attractive Female Smile

The characteristics of the attractive female smile can be summarized as follows:

- Generous display of upper anterior teeth.
- Noticeable lip movement from the relaxed position of the lips to the smiling one.
- Prevalence of the transverse dimension of the display zone of the smile over the vertical one.
- Absent or limited display of inferior teeth.
- Presence of a variable amount of upper gingival display (this is also correlated with the age of the subject).
- Presence of a moderate amount of buccal corridors.
- The presence of a consonant smile arc, Fig. 8.16 shows two clinical cases of attractive female smiles with less and more gingival display.

8.4.2 The "No-Smile Patient"

An uncommon but serious facial deformity is the inability to produce a smile. An example of this is

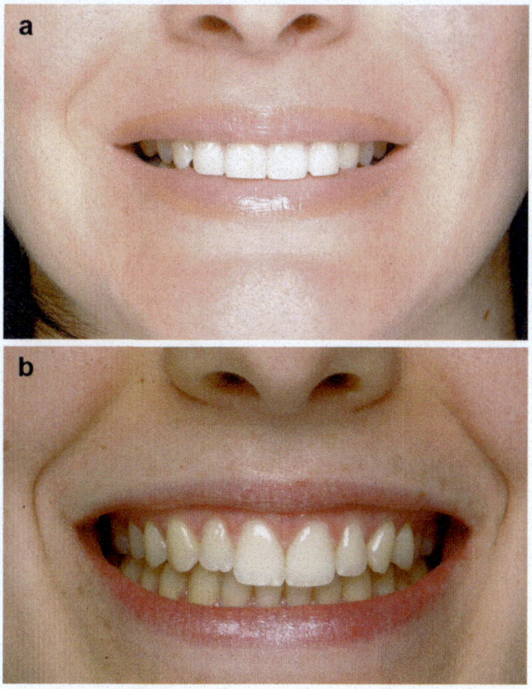

Fig. 8.16 Frontal view of attractive female smile (**a**). An increased display of gingival tissue (**b**) gives a more youthful appearance

shown in Fig. 8.15f, where the outline of the upper anterior teeth is barely visible even though the subject is trying to elevate the upper lip as high as possible. The factors involved in this dynamic deformity, which is evident to observers only during smiling, are multiple and can be classified as follows:

- Vertically long upper lip at rest, due to an increment of the skin area only (the vermillion area is frequently reduced)
- Poor upper lip elevation during smiling
- Small size of upper anterior teeth or loss of anterior teeth
- Posterior positioned upper incisors
- Posterior inclined upper incisors
- Posterior positioned maxilla (maxillary deficiency)
- Vertically short maxilla (short middle third of the face)

It is clear that the "no-smile patient" facial deformity is a mix of soft tissue, dental, and skeletal problems, which needs a team approach to diagnose and treat completely (Fig. 8.17a–f).

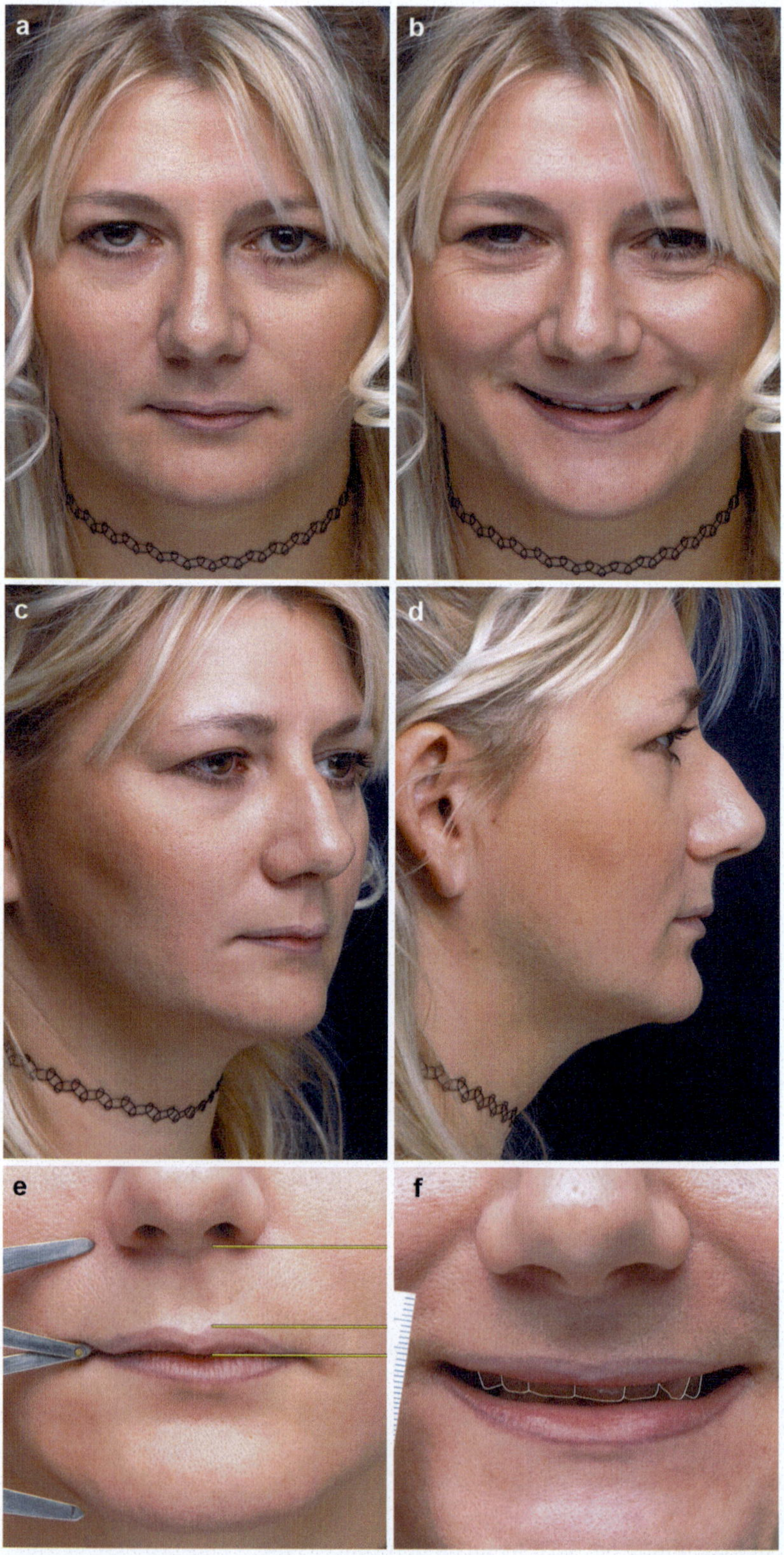

Fig. 8.17 A clinical case of a "no-smile patient." The frontal (**a**), frontal during smiling (**b**), oblique right (**c**), and profile right views (**d**) show the vertically long upper lip at rest, the poor upper lip elevation during smiling, the clockwise rotation and the flattening of the upper lip profile. The frontal lips' close-up view at rest (**e**) highlights that the skin area of the upper lip greatly exceeds the small vermillion area, whereas the close-up frontal smile (**f**) demonstrates that the upper incisors are hidden under the upper lip

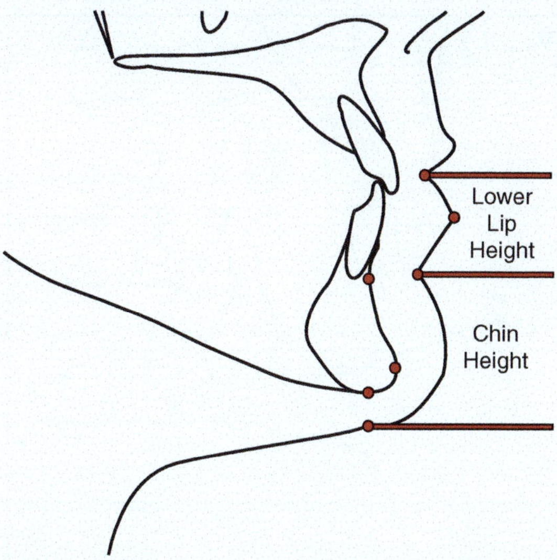

Fig. 8.18 The bony and soft tissue parameters to consider in chin cephalometric tracing are the vertical position of the labiomental fold, which determines the height of the lower lip and chin pad segments, the thickness of the tissue around the bony chin, and the shape of the chin profile

8.5 Chin Assessment

An in-depth direct and photographic study of the chin should be done with the lips in a relaxed position (in many clinical cases, this means without contact between the lips), lips in an unforced contact position (lip seal), and during smiling.

The first step considers the balance of the chin with the other facial subunits, mainly the nose, the lips, the submental, and the neck; it is essential to distinguish between an isolated chin deformity and one that is combined with dentofacial or nasal deformities. The chin shape must also be related to the sex, the general proportion of the face, and the height of the subject.

Discerning between the underlying skeletal bony contour and the thickness of the soft tissue envelope must be done by palpation. The soft tissue thickness must also be palpated off the midline because the chin soft tissue is thinnest at the center; the normal thickness of the chin pad soft tissue is 8–10 mm [8]. The labiomental fold divides the lower facial height into two distinct segments, the chin pad and the lower lip. As Zide et al. reported [8], a high- or low-positioned labiomental fold changes the lengths and the relationships between the two segments (Fig. 8.18).

The cephalometric analysis of the lateral view can be helpful in distinguishing between skeletal and chin pad deformity. Figure 8.18 shows the basic measurements obtainable from a cephalometric tracing in the lower teeth– mandibular symphysis region, whereas Fig. 8.19 shows different patterns of chin morphology with the relative soft tissue outline.

An asymmetric deformity can also be related to the shape of the bony structure, the thickness of the soft tissue, or an asymmetric muscular contraction (dynamic chin asymmetry).

8.6 Lips, Teeth, Chin, and Smile Analysis Checklists[1]

8.6.1 Dental Occlusion Analysis Checklist

- Is the dental occlusion symmetric with the face?
  □ Yes
  □ No, because…
- Do the upper and lower dental midlines coincide with each other?
  □ Yes
  □ No, because…
- Are the upper incisors in front of the lower incisors (overjet)?
  □ Yes.
  □ Yes, but they are horizontally separated (increased overjet).
  □ No (reverse overjet).
- Is the upper arch wider than the lower one?
  □ Yes
  □ No, because of bilateral dental crossbite
  □ No, because of unilateral dental crossbite (□ right crossbite □ left crossbite)
- Define the vertical relationship between upper and lower incisors (overbite):
  □ Ideal overbite
  □ Deep bite
  □ Open bite

[1]Section 2 on Springer Extra Materials (extras.springer.com).

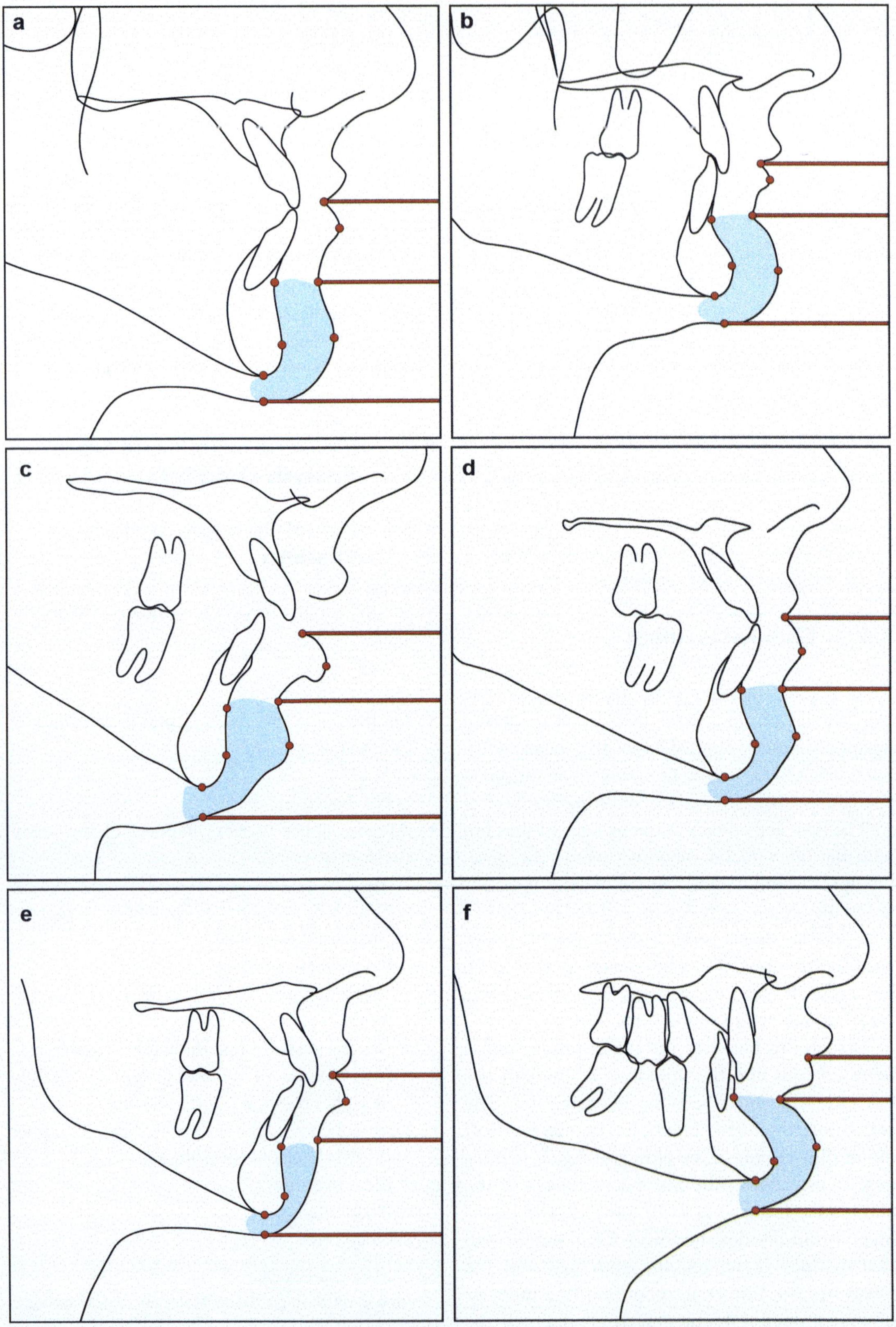

Fig. 8.19 The morphology of the bony chin as well as overlying soft tissue varies greatly (**a**–**f**)

- Is there upper arch dental crowding?
  □ No
  □ Yes, …
- Is there lower arch dental crowding?
  □ No
  □ Yes, …
- Is there any dental diastema?
  □ No.
  □ Yes. Where is it? …
- Are there any missing or lost teeth?
  □ No
  □ Yes, …
- Are there any supernumerary teeth?
  □ No
  □ Yes, …
- The role of the dental arches in supporting the lips and the cheeks is:
  □ Adequate
  □ Excessive
  □ Poor

8.6.2 Upper Frontal Teeth Analysis Checklist

- Is the upper dental midline symmetric with the face?
  □ Yes
  □ No, because …
- The anteroposterior projection of the upper frontal teeth is:
  □ Ideal
  □ Too anterior
  □ Too posterior
- The total width (transverse dimension) of the upper frontal teeth is:
  □ Ideal
  □ Too wide
  □ Too narrow
- The outline created by the upper anterior teeth margins is:
  □ Ideally curved
  □ Too flat
  □ Tilted …
  □ Irregular due to agenesis
  □ Irregular due to …
- The upper frontal teeth are:
  □ Well aligned
  □ Crowded, because …
- The upper central incisors height/ width ratio is:
  □ Ideal
  □ Reduced (vertically short incisors – square incisors shape)
  □ Increased (vertically long incisors – rectangular incisors shape)
- The gingival margins are:
  □ Well positioned
  □ Too high (long teeth appearance)
  □ Too low (short teeth appearance)
- The upper lateral incisors are:
  □ Ideal
  □ Too small compared to the central ones
  □ Too big compared to the central ones
  □ Unilaterally absent (R or L agenesis)
  □ Bilaterally absent (R and L agenesis)
- Recognize the presence of a:
  □ Midline diastema
  □ Midline "black triangle"
  □ Other aesthetic problems …

8.6.3 Lips Analysis Checklist

- Are the lips symmetric?
  □ Yes
  □ No, because …
- Is the lip seal reached with muscular strain?
  □ Yes
  □ No
- Is the lip seal maintained when the perioral musculature is relaxed?
  □ Yes
  □ No
- In frontal view, are the upper and lower vermillion areas balanced?
  □ Yes
  □ No, because …
- In frontal view, the mouth width is:
  □ Ideal
  □ Too large
  □ Too small
- In profile view, is there a series of gentle curves from the nasal tip to the soft tissue

menton, without straight traits, and a unique well-defined angle at the stomion?
□ Yes
□ No, because …

- The upper lip volume is:
  □ Ideal
  □ Excessive
  □ Deficient
- The upper lip vermillion area is:
  □ Ideal
  □ Excessive
  □ Deficient
- The upper lip profile is:
  □ Normally projected
  □ Too anterior
  □ Too posterior
- The lower lip volume is:
  □ Ideal
  □ Excessive
  □ Deficient
- The lower lip vermillion area is:
  □ Ideal
  □ Excessive
  □ Deficient
- The lower lip profile is:
  □ Normally projected
  □ Too anterior
  □ Too posterior

8.6.4 Posed Smile Analysis Checklist

- Is the posed smile symmetric?
  □ Yes
  □ No, because …
- Is the display zone symmetric?
  □ Yes
  □ No, because …
- Width of the display zone is:
  □ Ideal
  □ Limited
  □ Excessive
- Height of the display zone is:
  □ Ideal
  □ Limited
  □ Excessive
- Range of upper lip elevation is:
  □ Ideal
  □ Limited
  □ Excessive
- Maxillary incisor and gingival display:
  □ Absence of incisor display
  □ Poor incisor display
  □ Ideal (slightly above the gingival margin)
  □ Increased (aesthetically acceptable gingival display)
  □ Excessive gingival display
- Mandibular teeth display:
  □ Absence of inferior teeth display
  □ Limited inferior teeth display
  □ Evident inferior teeth display
- Define the buccal corridors:
  □ Absent – "denture smile"
  □ Limited
  □ Ideal
  □ Excessive
  □ Symmetric
  □ Asymmetric, …
- Define the smile arc:
  □ Consonant
  □ Flat

8.6.5 Chin Analysis Checklist

- Is the bony chin symmetric?
  □ Yes
  □ No, because …
- Is the external chin shape symmetric?
  □ Yes
  □ No, because …
- Does the chin maintain its symmetry during smiling?
  □ Yes
  □ Dynamic asymmetry due to …
- In the frontal view, the chin shape is:
  □ Wide
  □ Narrow
  □ Vertically long
  □ Vertically short
- The chin profile is:
  □ Balanced
  □ Too protrusive
  □ Too recessive

- The soft tissue pogonion is:
  - □ Too posterior to labrale inferior
  - □ Slightly posterior (balanced) to labrale inferior
  - □ Vertical to labrale inferior
  - □ Anterior to labrale inferior
- Define the chin shape:
  - □ Pointed
  - □ Large
  - □ Square
  - □ Witch's chin (ptotic chin)
  - □ Cleft chin
  - □ …
- The labiomental fold is:
  - □ Balanced
  - □ Deep
  - □ Shallow
- The vertical lower lip/chin ratio is:
  - □ Balanced
  - □ Long lip and short chin
  - □ Short lip and long chin

8.7 Lips, Teeth, Chin, and Smile Analysis: Preferred Terms[2]

- *Black triangle.* The presence of a dark and unaesthetic triangular space, base-up, between the two upper central incisors caused by midline gingival retraction and/or dental inclination.
- *Buccal corridors (negative space).* The space that is created when a patient smiles, between the buccal (vestibular) surface of the posterior teeth and the commissure of the lips. The perceived dimension of this space depends partially on the type of lighting utilized during the assessment and photographic session.
- *Chin pad.* The thick soft tissue overlying the bony chin.
- *Cleft chin.* The median-depressed vertical skin line of the chin pad characterizing some subjects.
- *Crossbite.* When one or more maxillary teeth are lingually (internally) positioned relative to the respective mandibular teeth. The anterior crossbite is also called reverse overjet.
- *Cupid's bow.* The central linear portion of the upper lip white roll skin relief of the upper lip between the philtrum and the vermillion. It connects the inferior ends of the philtrum columns.
- *Dental agenesia.* The lack of development of one or more teeth.
- *Dental classes.* Classification of the sagittal relationship between the dental arches. Class I: normal posteroanterior relationship between the two dental arches. Class II: too anterior upper dental arch and/or too posterior lower dental arch. Class III: too posterior upper dental arch and/or too anterior lower dental arch.
- *Dental crowding.* The lack of alignment between adjacent teeth. It is usually graded from mild to severe crowding.
- *Diastema.* A space between adjacent teeth. Normally there is no space between adjacent teeth.
- *Display zone.* The area framed by the lips during the act of smiling.
- *E-Line (esthetic line).* A reference line connecting the tip of the nose to the most anterior point of the chin contour (soft tissue pogonion).
- *Gingival scaffold.* The area of gingiva shown during the act of smiling.
- *Lip commissures.* The points at which the upper and lower lips join together. During the act of smiling, the eye of the observer can perceive the inner and the outer commissures, as delineated by the innermost and outermost confluences, respectively, of the vermillion of the lips at the corner of the mouth.
- *Labial commissure.* The point of lateral confluence of the lips. During the act of smiling, it consists of the inner and the outer commissure.
- *Labiomental fold (mandibular sulcus contour).* The horizontal skin depression that separates the chin from the lower lip. It varies from a flat curve to a deep sulcus.
- *Labrale inferior.* The median point in the lower margin of the lower membranous lip in profile view [6].

[2]Section 3 on Springer Extra Materials (extras.springer.com).

- *Lip white rolls.* The linear white skin relief placed around the vermillion border of both lips. It flattens and sometimes totally disappears with aging.
- *Labrale superior.* A point indicating the mucocutaneous border of the upper lip in the profile view. It is usually the most anterior point of the upper lip [6].
- *Mouth width.* The distance between the two lip commissures; it is measured utilizing the close-up view of the lip at rest with ruler. It is not modifiable with surgery. The mean value, reported by Farkas [5], measured in a group of attractive, young, North American Caucasian adults, is 53.9 mm in male subjects and 50.9 mm in female subjects.
- *Overbite.* The vertical overlap of the incisors obtained when the two dental arches occlude together. Deep bite – excessive vertical overlap between upper and lower incisors. Open bite – in this condition, there is no overlap but a vertical separation.
- *Overjet.* The horizontal overlap of the upper incisors in front of the lower incisors. Normally it is 2–3 mm due to the thickness of the edge of the upper incisors; the increased overjet is the excessive horizontal distance between the upper and lower incisors. Reverse overjet (anterior crossbite) – if the lower incisors are in front of the upper incisors.
- *Philtrum.* The central and vertically oriented portion of the upper lip situated between the two skin reliefs of the philtrum columns. There is a gentle concavity on its lower portion, the philtrum dimple.
- *Pogonion.* The most prominent or anterior point on the chin bony profile [6].
- *Soft tissue pogonion.* The most prominent or anterior point on the chin pad profile [6].
- *Pointed chin deformity.* The combination of a reduced width with an increased anteroinferior projection of the chin.
- *Posed smile.* A voluntary smile; it need not be elicited or accompanied by emotion. A posed smile can be sustained, and it is reliably repeatable [1].
- *Smile arc.* The relationship of the curvature of the incisal edges of maxillary incisors and canine to the curvature of the lower lip in the posed smile [2, 7].
- *Stomion.* The point of contact between the two lips in profile view. In the case where contact between the lips is absent, the stomion superior can be considered to be the lowermost point of the vermillion of the upper lip and the stomion inferior to be the uppermost point of the vermillion of the lower lip.
- *Supernumerary tooth.* The presence of an extra tooth over the normal number of teeth.
- *Unposed (spontaneous) smile.* An involuntary smile, induced by joy or mirth. An unposed smile cannot be sustained (it is dynamic) [1].
- *Vermillion.* The red portion of the external surface of the lips.
- *Witch's chin deformity (ptotic chin).* The flattening and the ptosis of the chin pad associated with the deepening of the submental crease. It can be age related or secondary to previous surgery.

References

1. Ackerman JI, Ackerman MB, Brensinger CM, Landis JR (1998) A morphometric analysis of the posed smile. Clin Orthod Res 1:2–11
2. Ackerman MB, Ackerman JI (2002) Smile analysis and design in the digital era. J Clin Orthod 36:221–236
3. Andrews LF (1972) The six keys to normal occlusion. Am J Orthod 62:671–690
4. Andrews LF (1989) Straight wire. The concept and the appliance. L.A. Wells Co., San Diego
5. Farkas LG (1994) Anthropometry of the attractive North American Caucasian face. In: Farkas LG (ed) Anthropometry of the head and face, 2nd edn. Raven Press, New York, p 159
6. Jacobson A (1995) Radiographic cephalometry. From basics to videoimaging. Quintessence Publishing, Chicago
7. Sarver DM (2001) The importance of incisor positioning in the esthetic smile: the smile arc. Am J Orthod Dentofacial Orthop 120:98–111
8. Zide BM, Pfeifer TM, Longaker MT (1999) Chin surgery: I. Augmentation – the allures and the alert. Plast Reconstr Surg 104:1843–1853

Dentofacial Deformities

9

Contents

Dentofacial deformities are of interest to many specializations, even though they are mainly treated by two professional figures who work together: the orthodontist and the maxillofacial surgeon. In the 1960s and 1970s, the prevailing orthodontic view was that "Jaw deformity will inevitably affect the integumental profile of the individual and will lead to a relative imbalance of the nose, lips and chin. Dental occlusion can be used as a reference for defining these distortions" [1]. Such thinking is now xout of date. Today, the dental occlusion is considered as only one component of the deformity, and its normalization with orthodontics and jaw surgery is not synonymous with facial balance and improved

F. Meneghini, P. Biondi, *Clinical Facial Analysis*,
DOI 10.1007/978-3-642-27228-8_9, © Springer-Verlag Berlin Heidelberg 2012

aesthetics. For this and other reasons, in many clinical cases, the preoperative analysis and the treatment planning should also be conducted in collaboration with experts in other fields.

The study of dentofacial deformities is based on three different sequenced analyses:

- Direct and photographic clinical facial analyses, which dictate the need for surgery to change the facial appearance
- Intraoral and dental cast analysis, which is necessary to assess the malocclusion in its two components: intra-arch and interarch relationships
- Cephalometric analysis, which can add new data, measure some parameters, and permit, through the creation of the visualization of treatment objectives, an in-depth study of the effects of jaw surgery on skeletal, dental, and soft tissue spatial position

9.1 The Basic Components of Dentofacial Deformities

Understanding a dentofacial deformity clinical case can be made easier by the identification of its basic components:

- Anterior vertical excess or deficiency
- Class III or II sagittal discrepancy
- Transverse discrepancies and asymmetry

9.1.1 Anterior Vertical Excess

The anterior vertical excess has been given many other terms, such as vertical maxillary excess, hyper divergent skeletal pattern, high-angle case, long face, and skeletal open bite.

Figure 9.1 shows a clinical case[1] in which many of the external morphological and skeletal characteristics of the anterior vertical excess are present. Analyzing the frontal view (Fig. 9.1a), we note a clear elongation of the vertical axis of the face, with a reduction in the facial widths. The mandibular outline is asymmetric at the angles, and a general impression of flatness of the malar, infraorbital, paranasal, cheek, and chin regions is perceived.

The oblique view (Fig. 9.1b) confirms the flattening of the malar, infraorbital, cheek, paranasal, and chin regions. In particular, the ogee curve outline, in all its components, is constituted of long and nearly straight tracts joined together with open angles.

The profile view (Fig. 9.1c) adds the following important diagnostic elements:

- The total anterior facial height is augmented.
- All the anterior facial thirds appear to be augmented.
- The flatness of the malar, infraorbital, paranasal, cheek, and chin regions is confirmed.
- The nose appears to be long.
- The upper lip outline is clockwise rotated with a lack of anterior projection.
- The labiomental fold is flat.
- The mandibular border outline is partially hidden and clockwise rotated.
- The total chin–throat–neck outline length is reduced with an open cervicomental angle.

The intraoral view (Fig. 9.1d), despite the external facial morphology, shows a molar class I, an anterior dental malocclusion with no anterior open bite.

The cephalometric tracing (Fig. 9.1e), obtained from the cephalograms in the lateral view, permits the correlation of the facial profile with the shape and spatial position of some of the dental and skeletal supporting structure.

9.1.2 Anterior Vertical Deficiency

The anterior vertical deficiency is characterized by the opposite features of the vertical excess and is also called vertical maxillary deficiency, hypodivergent skeletal pattern, low-angle case, short face, and skeletal deep bite.

Figure 9.2 shows a clinical case[2] in which many of the external morphological, skeletal, and dental

[1]The complete clinical facial photographic documentation of this case is available in Sect. 4 on Springer Extra Materials (extras.springer.com) (Clinical Case No. 4).

[2]The complete clinical photographic documentation of this case is available in Sect. 4 on Springer Extra Materials (extras.springer.com) (Clinical Case No. 5).

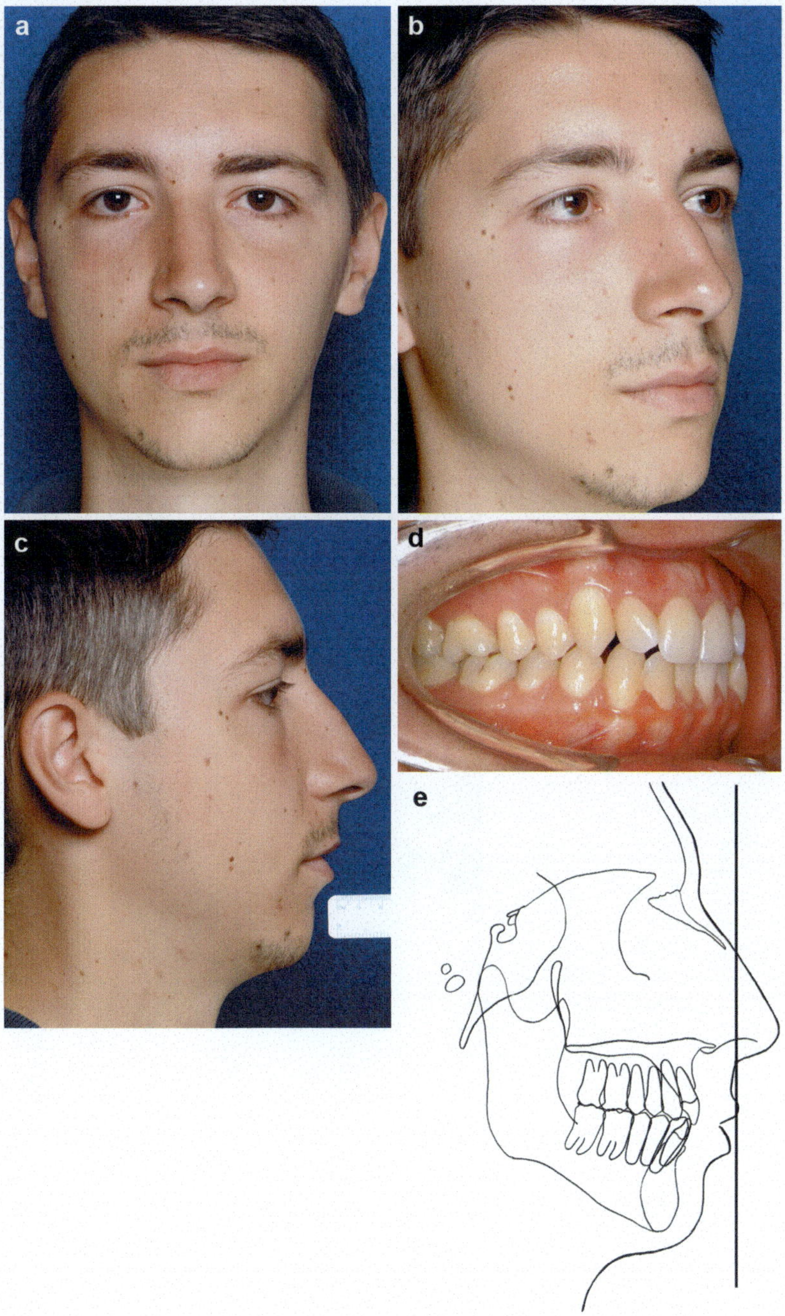

Fig. 9.1 A clinical case of anterior vertical excess. Frontal (**a**), oblique right (**b**), profile (**c**), intraoral right views (**d**), and cephalometric tracing (**e**)

characteristics of the anterior vertical deficiency are present. Analyzing the frontal view (Fig. 9.2a), we note a short vertical axis of the face with a large reduction of the lower facial third height and the relative increase of all facial widths.

The oblique view (Fig. 9.2b) confirms the large reduction of the lower face height, also drawing attention to the long and overprojected nose.

The profile view (Fig. 9.2c) confirms and adds some important diagnostic elements such as:

- Reduction of the lower anterior face height; conversely, the central and upper anterior facial third may appear augmented.

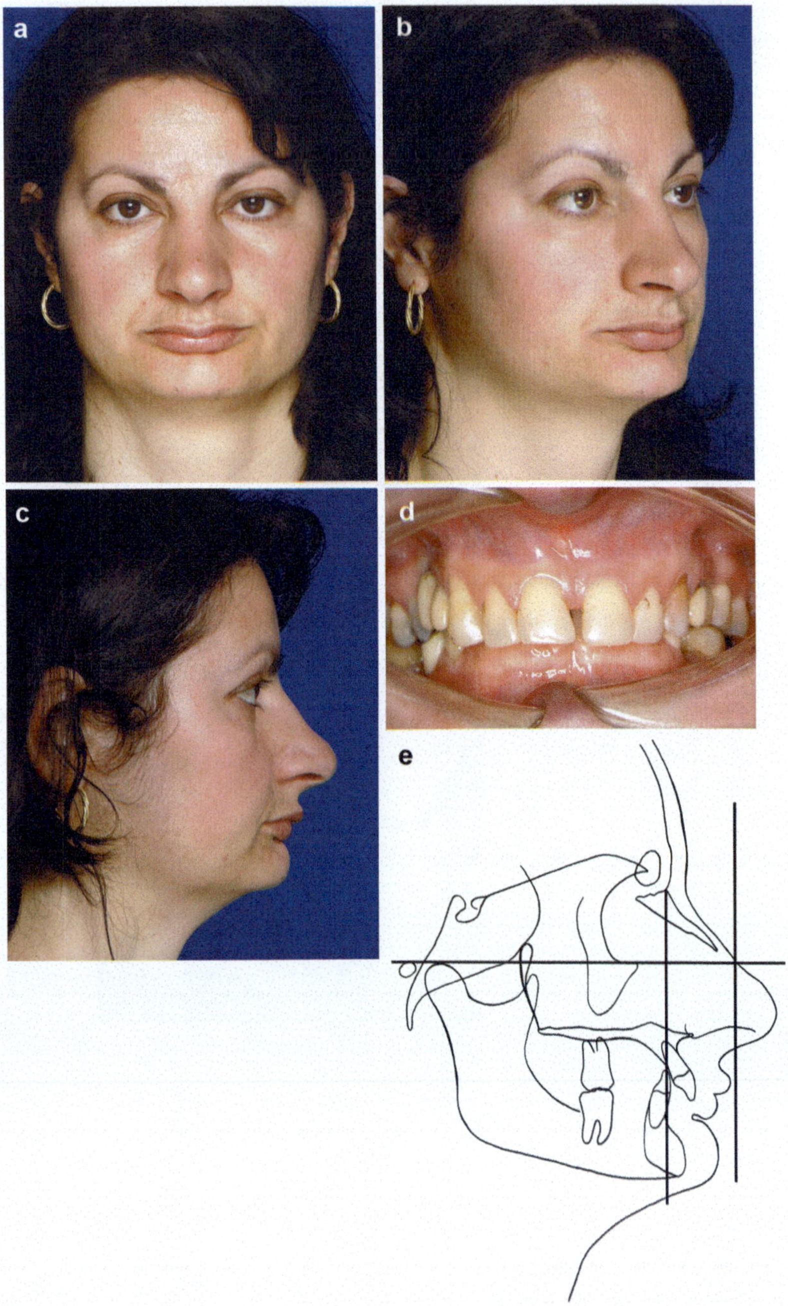

Fig. 9.2 A clinical case of anterior vertical deficiency. Frontal (**a**), oblique right (**b**), profile (**c**), intraoral anterior views (**d**), and cephalometric tracing (**e**)

- The nose appears to be long.
- The upper lip outline is counterclockwise rotated and excessively concave.
- The labiomental fold is extremely deep and unnatural.
- The mandibular border outline is counterclockwise rotated in a nearly horizontal position. This affects the chin projection, which seems to be increased; nevertheless, this is not sufficient to obtain a pleasant cervicomental angle.
- The throat length is extremely short.

The frontal intraoral view (Fig. 9.2d), according to the external facial morphology, shows the anterior dental deep bite (the lower teeth are totally hidden by the upper incisors and cuspids). The cephalometric tracing (Fig. 9.2e), obtained from the cephalograms in the lateral view, permits the correlation of the facial profile with the shape and spatial position of some of the dental and skeletal supporting structure.

9.1.3 Class III Sagittal Discrepancy

The class III sagittal discrepancy brings together many deformities common to an anteriorly positioned lower third of the face and/or a posterior-positioned middle third.

Figure 9.3 shows a clinical case[3] in which many of the external morphological, skeletal, and dental characteristics of the class III sagittal discrepancy are present. Analyzing the frontal view (Fig. 9.3a), we note the depressed infraorbital and paranasal regions with a tendency toward an inferior scleral show. The total facial height and the facial widths seem proportioned, whereas a general impression of flatness of infraorbital, paranasal, and cheek regions is perceived.

The oblique view (Fig. 9.3b) confirms the flattening of the infraorbital, cheek, and paranasal regions; in particular, the ogee curve outline shows the tendency toward a concave face due to midface retrusion.

The profile view (Fig. 9.3c) confirms and adds some important diagnostic elements such as:

- The total anterior facial height appears to be increased.[4]
- The flatness of malar, infraorbital, cheek, and paranasal regions is confirmed.
- The lower third of the nose appears to be normal in spite of the lack of skeletal support.
- The upper lip outline is clockwise rotated.
- The chin is slightly overprojected.
- The labiomental fold is normally shaped.
- The mandibular border outline is well defined and clockwise rotated.
- The total chin–throat–neck outline length, as well as the cervicomental angle definition and degree, are pleasing.

The oblique right intraoral view (Fig. 9.3d) shows a dental malocclusion with molar and canine class III, partial anterior reverse overjet, and anterior dental crowding of the lower anterior teeth.

The cephalometric tracing (Fig. 9.3e), obtained from the cephalograms in the lateral view, permits the correlation of the facial profile with the shape and spatial position of some of the dental and skeletal supporting structure.

9.1.4 Class II Sagittal Discrepancy

The class II sagittal discrepancy brings together many deformities common to a posteriorly positioned lower third of the face (more frequent) and/or an anteriorly positioned middle third (less frequent).

Figure 9.4 shows a clinical case[5] in which many of the external morphological, skeletal, and dental characteristics of the class II sagittal discrepancy are present. Analyzing the frontal view (Fig. 9.4a), we note an evident facial asymmetry, a large and deviated nose, and a reduced chin width.

The right oblique view (Fig. 9.4b) reveals the flat malar, infraorbital, cheek, paranasal, and chin regions. The ogee curve outline, in this particular case, helps the observer to recognize the extreme grade of the chin underprojection.

The profile view (Fig. 9.4c) adds the following important diagnostic elements:

- The facial profile is convex, which is primarily due to the clockwise overrotated mandible.
- The flatness of the malar, infraorbital, cheek, paranasal, and chin regions is confirmed.
- The upper lip outline is slightly clockwise rotated.
- The labiomental fold is flat.
- The chin is severely underprojected.
- The mandibular border outline is clockwise rotated.

[3]The complete clinical photographic documentation of this case is available in Sect. 4 on Springer Extra Materials (extras.springer.com) (Clinical Case No. 6).

[4]This affirmation contradicts the previous one based on frontal view analysis; whenever this happens, it is preferable to follow the indication obtained from the frontal and oblique views because patients principally judge themselves utilizing these projections when looking in the mirror.

[5]The complete clinical photographic documentation of this case is available in Sect. 4 on Springer Extra Materials (extras.springer.com) (Clinical Case No. 7).

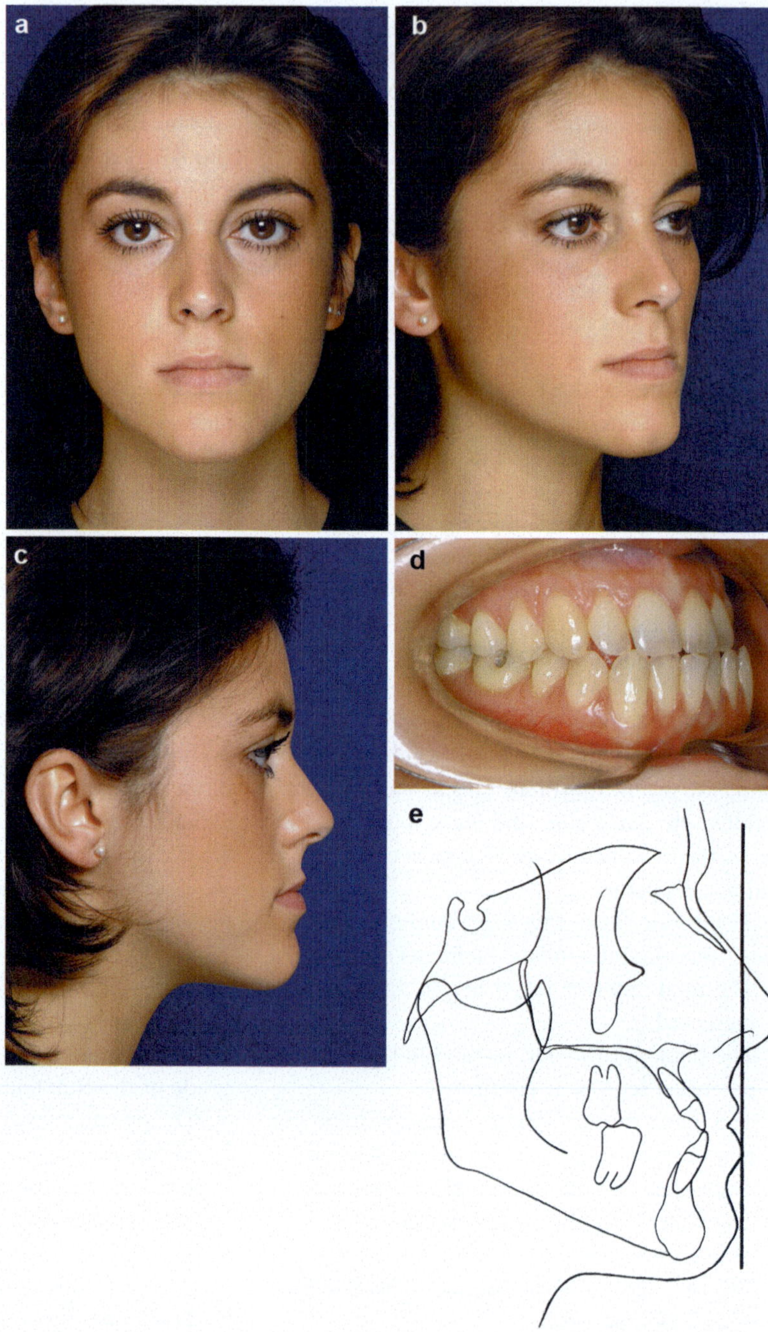

Fig. 9.3 A clinical case of class III dentofacial deformity. Frontal (**a**), oblique right (**b**), profile (**c**), intraoral right oblique views (**d**), and cephalometric tracing (**e**)

- The total chin–throat–neck outline length is reduced with an open cervicomental angle.
- The throat length is extremely short. The cephalometric tracing (Fig. 9.4d), obtained from the cephalograms in lateral view, shows the presence of overjet between the upper and lower incisors, as well as the molar class II relationship, and confirms the clockwise rotation of the mandible and the chin underprojection.

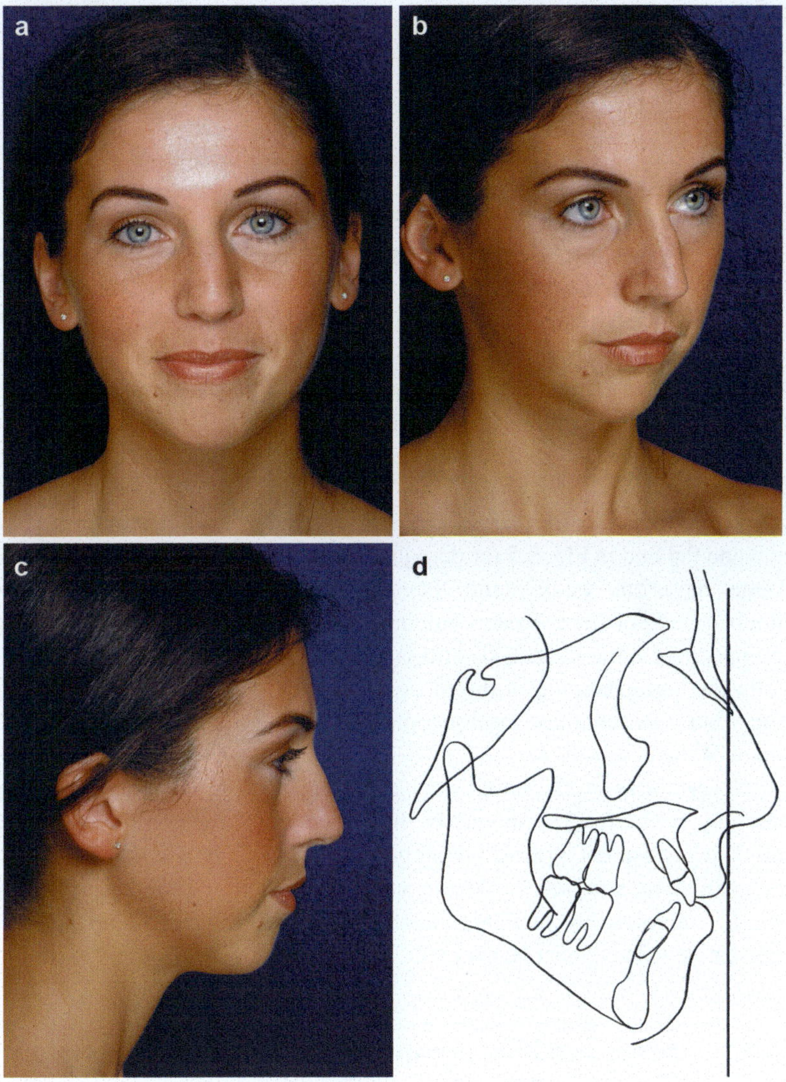

Fig. 9.4 A clinical case of class II dentofacial deformity. Frontal (**a**), oblique right (**b**), profile views (**c**), and cephalometric tracing (**d**)

9.1.5 Transverse Discrepancies and Asymmetry of the Jaws

An asymmetric arrangement of the dental arches is frequently associated with a corresponding facial asymmetry. The clinical case presented in Fig. 8.5 in the previous chapter is a clear example of that association. Analyzing the frontal and left views of the dental cast (Fig. 8.5a, b), we note these points:

- The mandibular midline is deviated on the left compared to that of the maxillary.
- Some teeth on the left side (colored in Fig. 8.5b) are in a reverse overbite relationship.
- The line connecting the two lower cuspids as well as the occlusal plane of the mandibular arch is counterclockwise rotated.

The facial frontal view (Fig. 8.5c) confirms that the facial asymmetry is coherent with the intraoral findings. In particular:

- The line connecting the two labial commissures is tilted counterclockwise.
- The chin is deviated to the left.

Figure 8.5c also shows some reference planes utilized in the assessment of the facial asymmetries, such as the lines connecting the medial canthus, the upper palpebral folds, or the apex of the eyebrows. Each of these lines must be checked in order to confirm their symmetry and therefore their reliability.

9.1.6 The Immense Number of Combinations of Different Types and Grades of the Basic Components of Facial Deformities

In a real clinical situation, there is almost never an isolated basic component of a facial deformity in a patient, and the grade of the deformity also varies greatly.

The real cases presented here in Figs. 9.1, 9.2, 9.3 and 9.4 and in Fig. 8.5 for demonstration purposes have one weak point: they are without doubt a mix of these basic components, so the preoperative clinical analysis still is not finished with the understanding of the most obvious element but must continue until a complete assessment of the case is done.

Nevertheless, in the initial steps of the analysis, any written notes should be based on the clinical assessment without taking precise metric or angular measurements. At this early stage, a rigid "computerized" method of analysis, with its normative values, must be avoided.

9.2 Direct and Photographic Clinical Analysis for Dentofacial Deformities

The biggest mistake we can make, when dealing with dentofacial deformities, is to limit our attention only to the jaw relationships. A severely retruded maxilla, for example, profoundly influences the aesthetics of the lower lids, zygomatic and orbital, nasal and paranasal, upper and lower lips, mandibular, and chin regions. For that reason, before continuing to read this chapter, I suggest that the reader should be familiar with the basic facial analysis (Chap. 5), the eyes and orbital analysis (Chap. 6), the nasal analysis (Chap. 7), and the lips, teeth, chin, and smile analysis (Chap. 8); furthermore, some points reported in the previous analysis checklists must be incorporated into the dentofacial analysis checklist.

When dealing with dentofacial deformities, during examination and photographic documentation, it is extremely important to obtain a relaxed lip position, a relaxed-rest mandibular position, and again the natural head position. How to obtain the natural head position is described in Chap. 3. In order to help the patient achieve the relaxed lip position, the examiner asks him to relax, strokes the lips gently, and takes multiple pictures on different occasions; an additional assessment of the lips is obtained with successive casual observations while the patient is unaware of being observed [2, 4].

Some authors [2, 13, 14] favor performing the direct and photographic analysis in centric relationship or centric occlusion, which means maintaining the two dental arches in contact, with the mandibular elevator muscles contracted. I disagree with this because normally a person is only in this position while swallowing, obtaining it for a fraction of a second. Maintaining it for a minute is a difficult task for patients because of the need for continuous muscle strain and the unnatural mandibular position.

Instead, for my basic aesthetic considerations, I want a relaxed position of the mandible in every case, doing a further facial examination in the close bite position only if a large difference in soft tissue arrangement exists between the two, as shown in Fig. 9.5.

As a general rule, in the clinical assessment of the total and regional vertical facial heights, it is possible to highlight more or less pronounced curves and more or less acute angles. In particular, the long face in profile and oblique views can be seen as an open accordion (Fig. 9.6a) with obtuse angles and flat curves, whereas a short face can resemble a closed accordion (Fig. 9.6b) with acute angles and pronounced curves.

Particular attention should be given to the cheekbone–nasal base–lip curve contour described by Arnett and Bergman [3]. In a subject with good facial proportions, it is composed of a convex, anteriorly facing, uninterrupted line that starts just anterior to the ear, follows the zygomatic arch, passing through the cheekbone

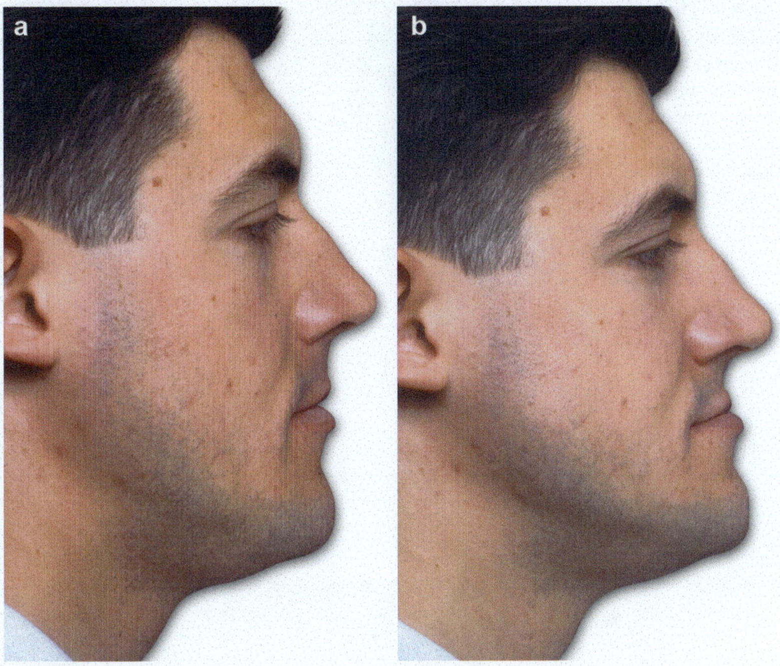

Fig. 9.5 Differences in facial soft tissue adjustment in the same subject in his habitual posture (**a**) and in the close bite mandibular position (**b**). The patient obtains the latter condition only during the act of swallowing

point, extending anterorinferiorly reaching the maxilla point, which constitutes its most anterior point, and then ending lateral to the commissure of the mouth (Fig. 9.7).

A maxillary retrusion is clinically related to a straight or concave cheekbone–nasal base–lip curve contour at maxilla point, a flat cheekbone point, and a clockwise rotation of the lower lid inclined in profile view, whereas the ogee profile on oblique view shows a flat outline at the level of the malar eminence (Fig. 9.8).

Utilizing the frontal and oblique views, further attention should be given to the triangular area situated between the nasal base at the alar crease junction and the upper end of the nasolabial sulcus, the paranasal triangle, evaluating its depth. Again, a maxillary hypoplasia is associated with a deep paranasal triangle (Fig. 9.9).

In order to visualize the relationship between the maxillary anteroposterior position, the nasal tip projection, and the chin projection better, I suggest drawing three angles over the life-size profile view photograph. The first is the angle obtained by connecting glabella, nasal tip, and soft tissue pogonion (G′-P-Pog′); the second is the angle obtained by connecting glabella, subnasale, and soft tissue pogonion (G′-Sn-Pog′), also called the angle of facial convexity; and the third is the angle obtained by connecting glabella, alar crease junction, and soft tissue pogonion (G′-ACJ-Pog′). Even if I do not measure these angles, simple observation of the drawing helps in finding and differentiating the anteroposterior relationships of the maxilla, chin, nasal tip, and anterior nasal spine, as shown in the clinical examples in Fig. 9.10.

The lip outline is evaluated considering the maxillary and mandibular sulcus contours, which should be two gentle concavities [3], as well as the anteroposterior relationship between the labrale superior and inferior, whose projection should differ minimally (Fig. 9.11).

The upper lip length should be considered in its absolute and relative values. It is the distance from subnasale and upper lip inferior, called "labial ledge" by Hoefflin [8], and should be between 19 and 22 mm [3]. Sometimes an apparently short upper lip can be confused with vertical maxillary excess, which also produces an increased upper incisors exposure, or a clockwise-rotated nasal tip, which "hides" the upper lip; in contrast, the counterclockwise-rotated nasal tip makes the upper lip appear longer (Fig. 9.12).

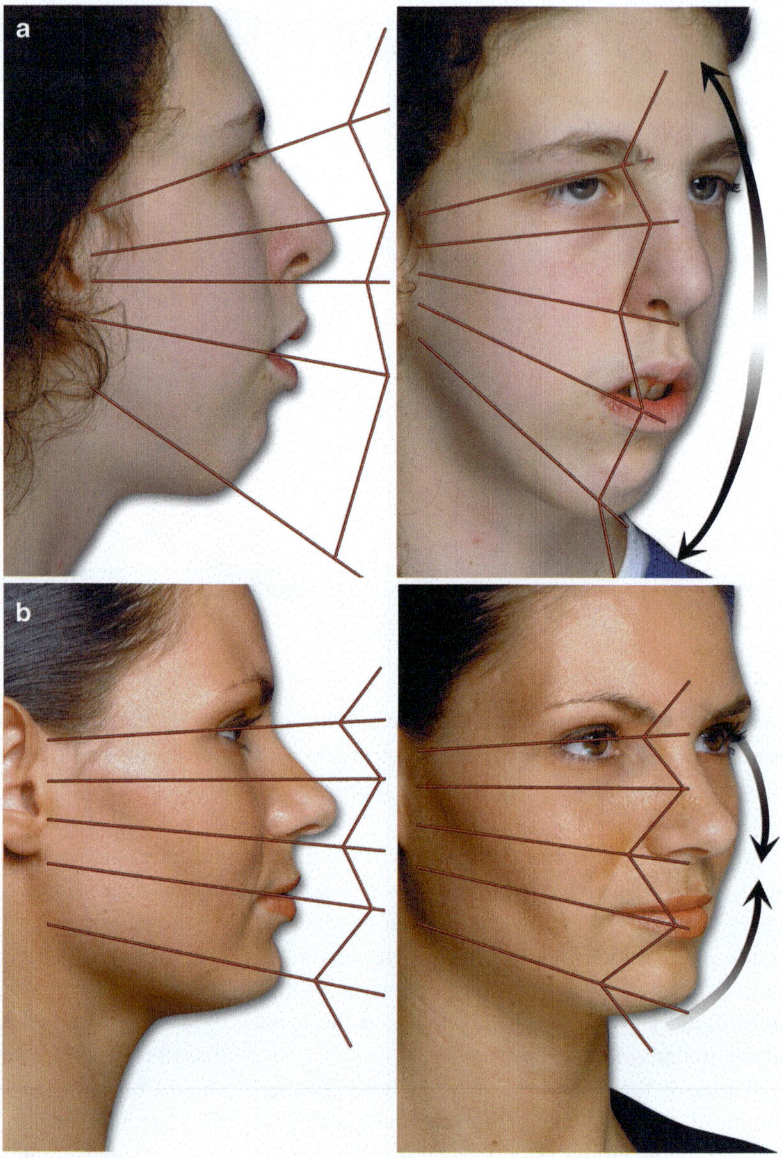

Fig. 9.6 The long face in profile and oblique views can be seen as an open accordion (**a**) with obtuse angles and flat curvatures, whereas the short face can resemble a closed accordion (**b**) with acute angles and pronounced curves

Another important step in the dentofacial deformities analysis is the assessment of the chin–throat–neck profile, as well as the mandibular border contour. The main points to consider are:

- Mandibular size. More than its absolute size, it is important to consider the relative dimensions and the supporting action offered to the overlying soft tissue, as well as the shape of the mandibular contour.
- Mandibular incline in profile view. Counterclockwise rotation of the mandible increases the chin projection, shortens the lower facial third height, and usually favorably affects the chin–throat–neck profile. In contrast, the mandibular clockwise rotation decreases the chin projection, increases the lower facial third height, and usually worsens the chin–throat–neck profile (Fig. 9.13).[6]
- Mandibular border definition from angle to chin. A thin soft tissue envelope and mandibular counterclockwise rotation produce a well-sculptured border, whereas a poor definition is

[6]See also the clinical cases in Fig. 5.17.

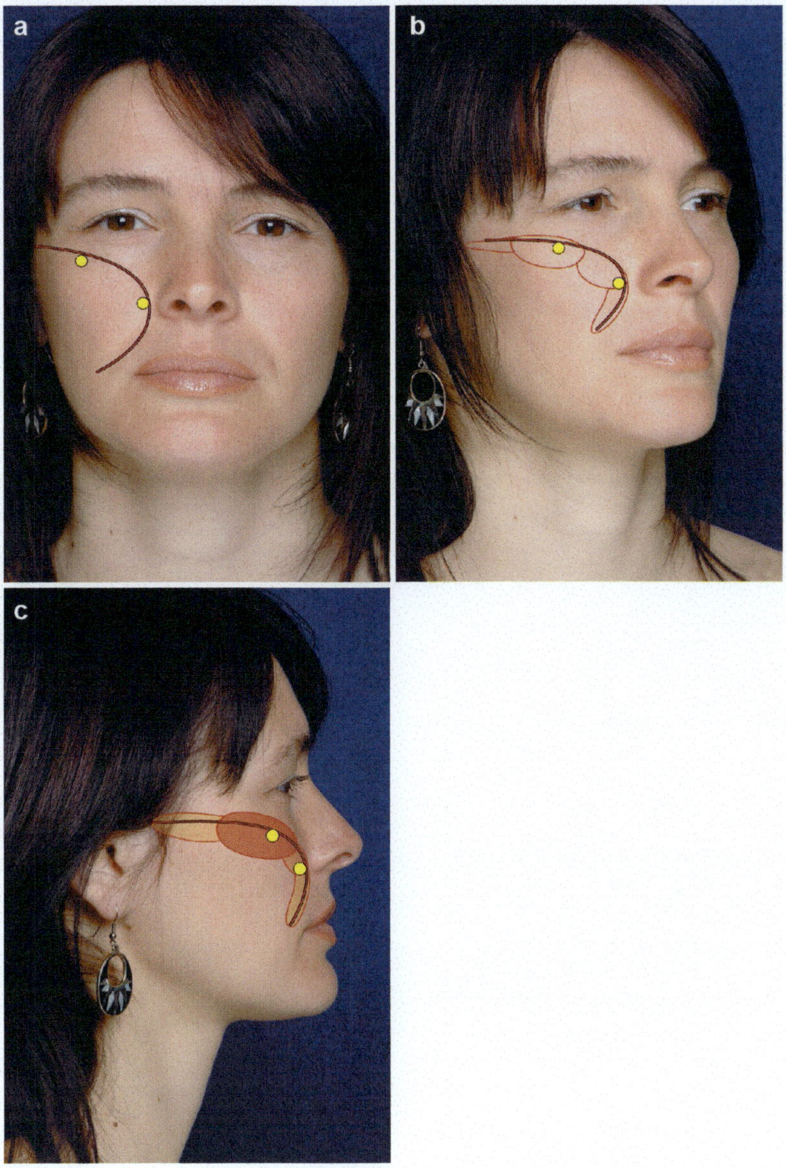

Fig. 9.7 The cheekbone–nasal base–lip curve contour described by Arnett and Bergman in frontal (**a**), oblique (**b**), and profile views (**c**) of a subject with good facial proportions. The cheekbone point, in a subject with good facial proportions, is the apex of osseous cheekbone that is located 20–25 mm inferior and 5–10 mm anterior to the outer canthus of the eye when viewed in profile and is 20–25 mm inferior and 5–10 mm lateral to the outer canthus of the eye when viewed frontally. A flat cheekbone point is often associated with malar deficiency and maxillary hypoplasia. The maxilla point is the most anterior point on the continuum of the cheekbone–nasal–lip contour described by Arnett and Bergman and is an indicator of maxillary anteroposterior position [3]

due to fat accumulation and mandibular clockwise rotation. The definitions of mandibular angle and posterior third of mandibular border are also variable, depending on the volume of the masseter muscle.

- Chin shape at rest and chin dynamics. As reported in Chap. 8, the assessment of the bony as well as the soft tissue components that determine the external chin shape is of paramount importance. The profile assumed by the subject when sustaining the lip seal with musculature contraction should also be noted.
- The throat length (NTP-Me′). This is the distance between neck–throat point (NTP) and soft tissue menton (Me′) on the lower facial outline (Fig. 9.14). The throat length is preferably assessed clinically to be short or long and not measured instrumentally [3].
- The throat incline. This is the angle formed between the throat outline and the horizontal plane passing through the soft tissue menton; a favorable incline is that which remains over or near the horizontal plane, whereas an excessively downwardly oriented incline is

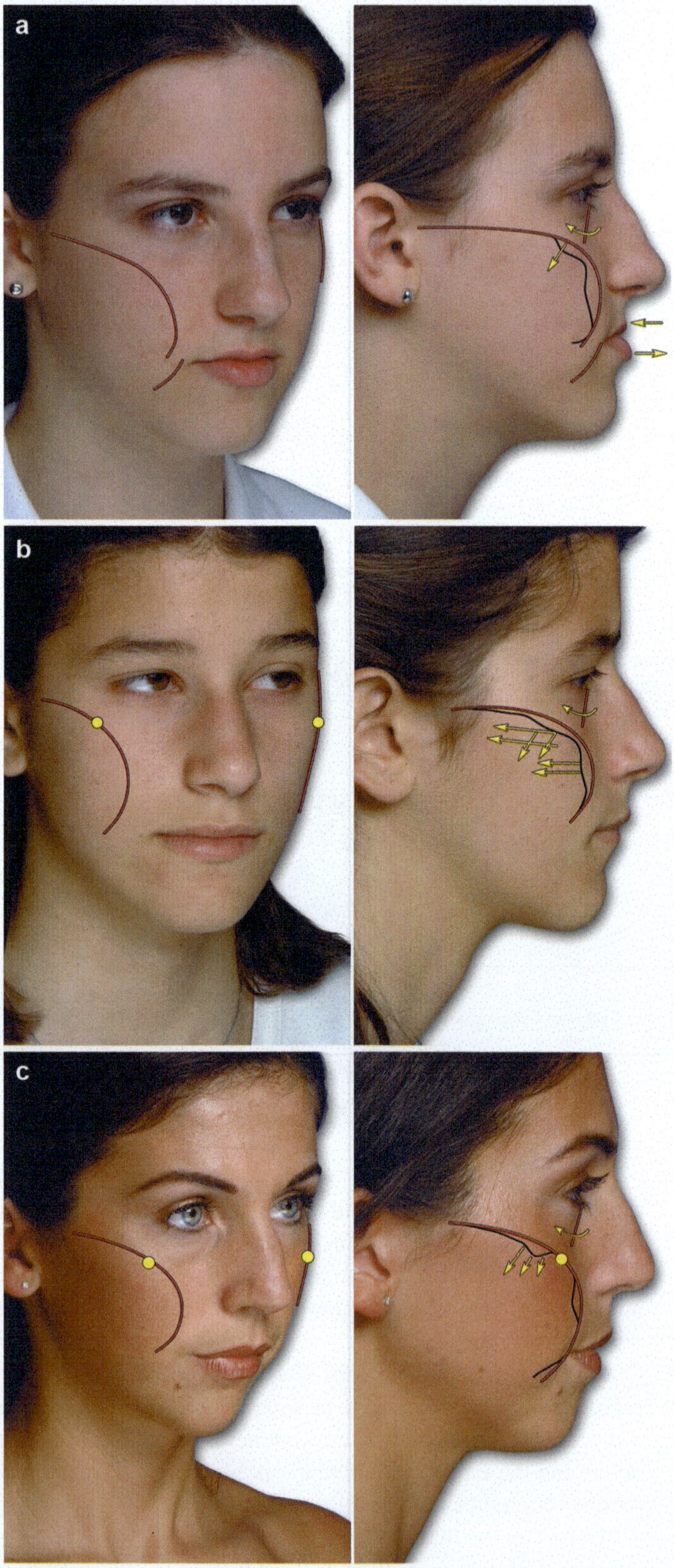

Fig. 9.8 Profile and oblique views of three subjects (**a**–**c**) with maxillary retrusion in which the cheekbone–nasal base–lip curve contour displays a flat cheekbone point, a posterior positioned maxillary point, and a clockwise rotation of the right lower lid incline in profile view, whereas the ogee profile on oblique view shows a flat outline at the level of the malar eminence

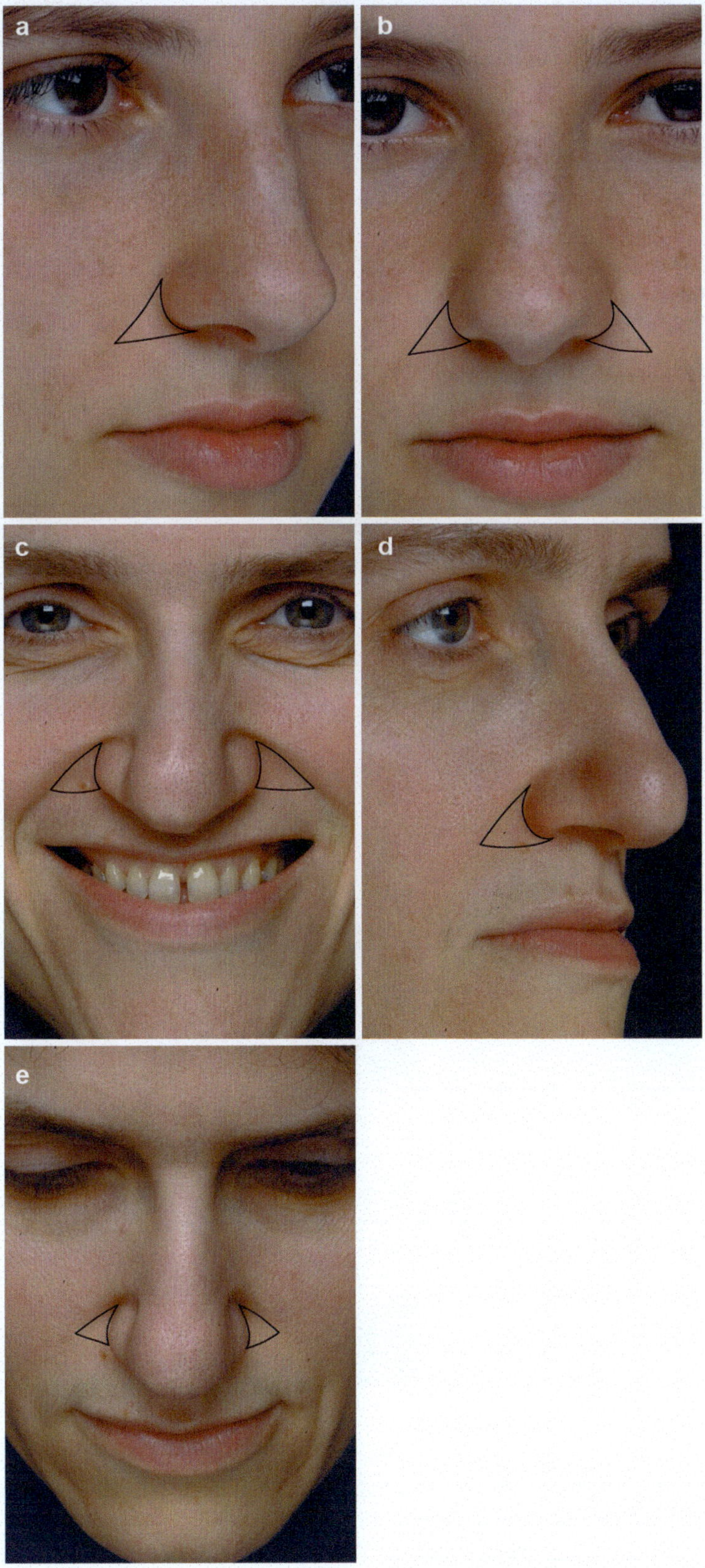

Fig. 9.9 Assessment of the paranasal triangle. In these two cases, the maxillary hypoplasia is associated with a deep paranasal triangle, the triangular area situated between the nasal base at the alar crease junction and the upper end of the nasolabial sulcus (**a**–**e**)

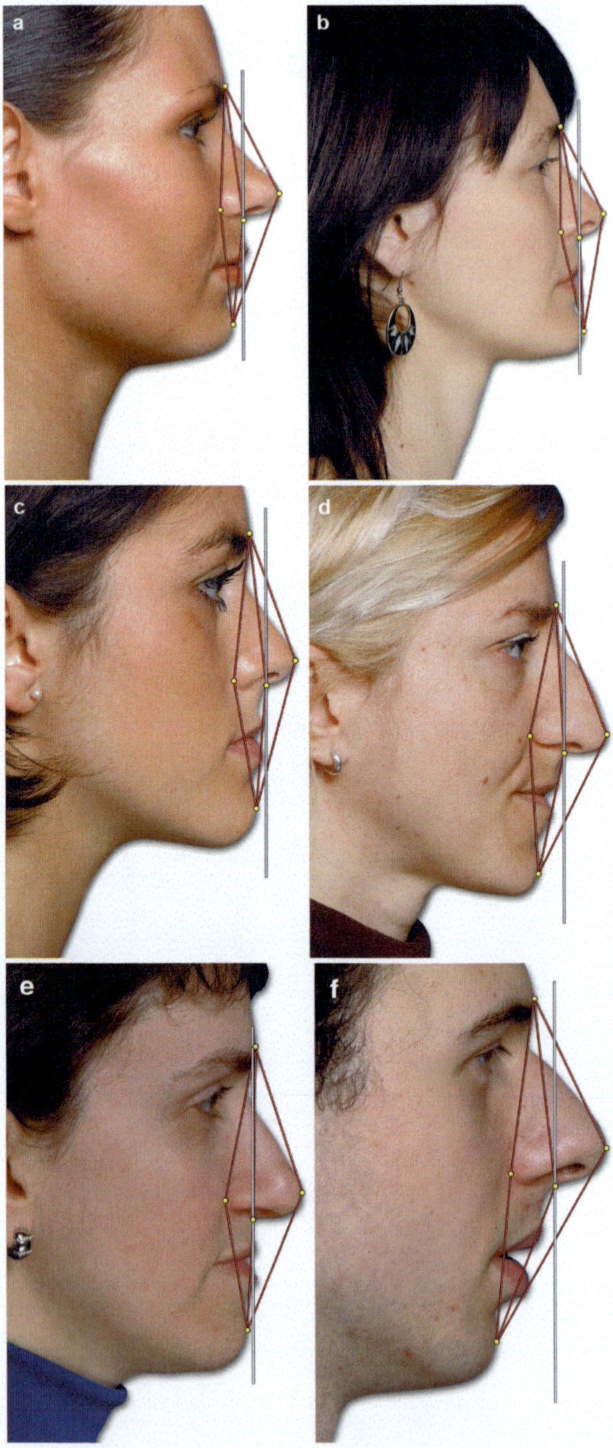

Fig. 9.10 In these profile views of six different cases, three angles are superimposed. The first is the angle obtained by connecting glabella, nasal tip, and soft tissue pogonion (G′-P-Pog′); the second is the angle obtained connecting glabella, subnasale, and soft tissue pogonion (G′-Sn-Pog′), also called the angle of facial convexity; and the third is the angle obtained connecting glabella, alar crease junction, and soft tissue pogonion (G′-ACJ-Pog′). A normal maxilla may be associated with a slight overprojected nasal tip (**a**) or an overprojected chin (**b**), whereas a hypoplasic nasal base and maxilla may be associated with a normal nasal tip and chin projection (**c**), an overprojected nasal tip (**d**), an underdeveloped nasal spine (**e**), and an overprojected nasal tip and a mandibular retrusion (**f**)

associated with poor aesthetics of the lower face. Again, it is not measured instrumentally but only clinically assessed (Fig. 9.14).

- Hyoid bone spatial position. The vertical and anteroposterior hyoid bone position greatly affects the throat length and incline and the submental–neck angle due to the need for a superoposteriorly positioned hyoid bone for favorable aesthetics. Palpation and lateral cephalograms help in differentiating a malpositioned hyoid

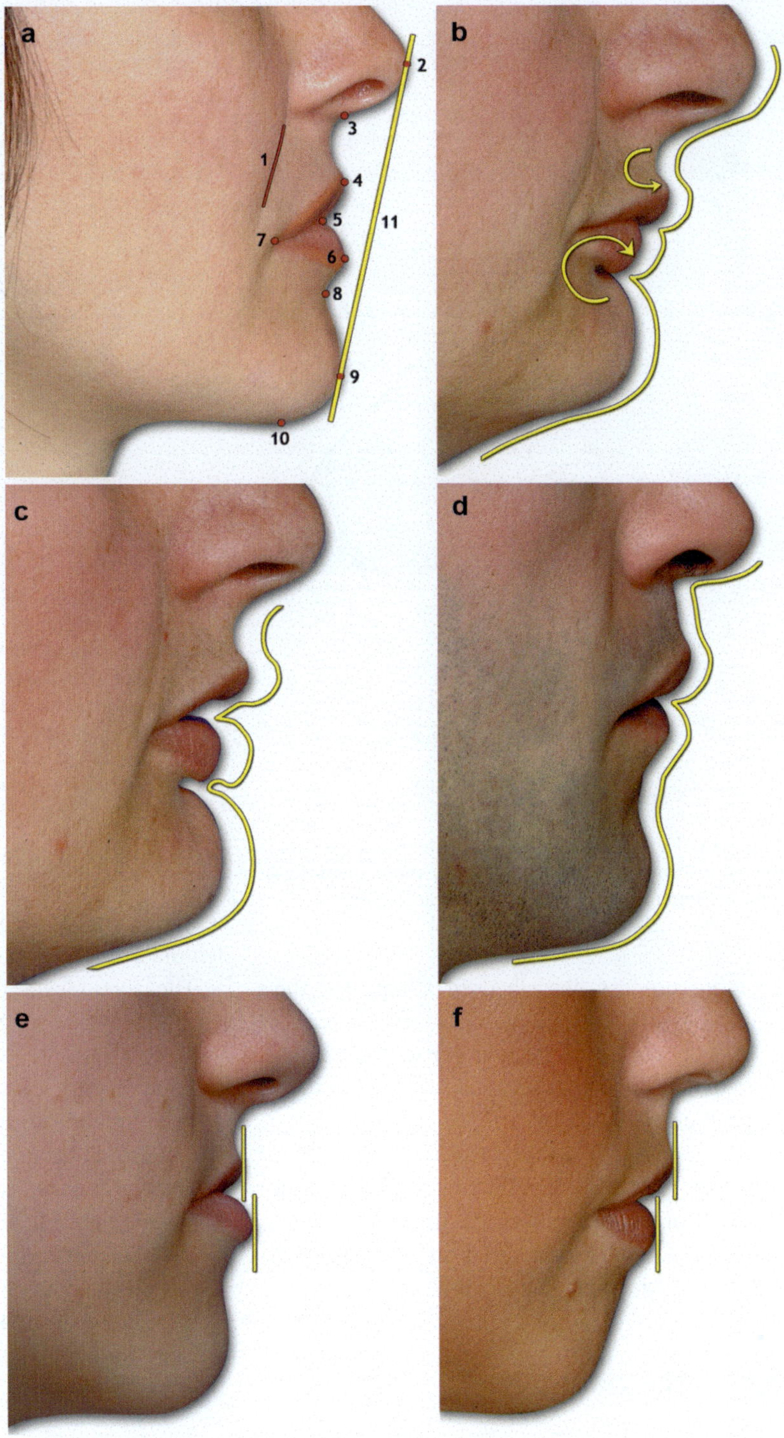

Fig. 9.11 The upper and lower lip outline should be two gentle curves with minimal differences in anteroposterior projection (reference points and Ricketts' lips projection reference E-line: *1* nasolabial sulcus, *2* nasal tip, *3* subnasale, *4* labrale superior, *5* stomion, *6* labrale inferior, *7* lip commissure, *8* labiomental sulcus, *9* soft tissue pogonion, *10* soft tissue menton, *11* Ricketts' E-line) (**a**). In a skeletal anterior vertical deficiency case, either in close bite (**b**) or in mandibular rest position (**c**), the lip outline contours present deep curves, whereas in anterior vertical excess, the lip outline contours present flat curves (**d**). In a skeletal class III discrepancy case, the labrale inferior is usually in front of the labrale superior (**e**) and vice versa for a skeletal class II discrepancy case (**f**)

bone from muscular bulging or true fat accumulation.

- Soft tissue thickness. The submental – throat–neck is one of the facial regions most prone to fat accumulation. Palpation helps in differentiating muscular bulging from true fat accumulation.
- Soft tissue redundancy and ptosis. Even if skin excess and platysma banding, as with many other problems, are associated with the

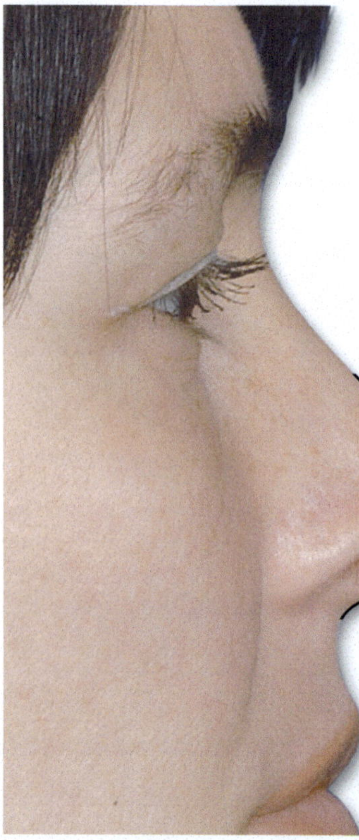

Fig. 9.12 The clockwise rotation of the nasal tip makes the upper lip appear shorter, whereas the counterclockwise rotation makes the upper lip appear longer

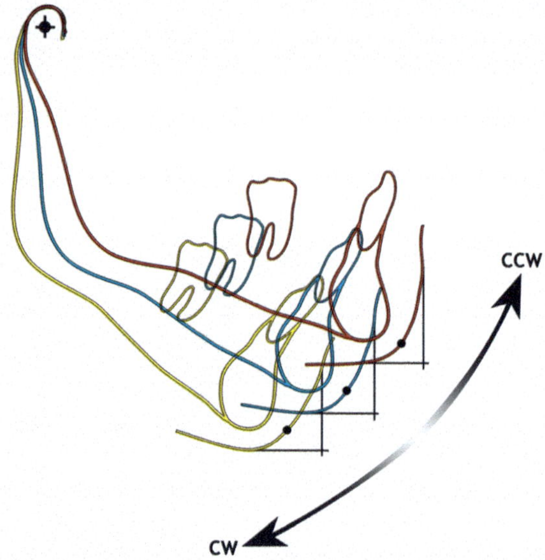

Fig. 9.13 The degree of mandibular incline is associated with many other features of the lower facial third. A mandibular clockwise (*CW*) rotation increases the chin projection, shortens the lower facial third height, and usually favorably affects the chin–throat–neck profile. In contrast, a mandibular counterclockwise (*CCW*) rotation decreases the chin projection, increases the lower facial third height, and usually worsens the chin–throat–neck profile

aging process described in Chap. 10, they must also be investigated and assessed in middle-aged subjects in order to differentiate between the various causes of the aesthetic problems.

In the case of an aesthetically poor chin–throat–neck profile, it is mandatory to separate the skeletal factors, such as the dimension, shape, and orientation, from the soft tissue factors related to the skin, platysma muscle, and fat.

9.3 The Youthful Neck

As for other facial regions, defining the ideal chin–neck features helps us to understand and analyze the clinical problems. Although the approach of Ellenbogen and Karlin [6], which utilizes five visual criteria in the assessment of the neck, and Dedo's classification of neck laxity [5] were devised for rhytidectomy patients, they are reported here because of the strong relationship between dentofacial deformities and neck problems.

The five visual criteria of Ellenbogen and Karlin [6] characterizing the ideal youthful neck are (Fig. 9.15):

1. The presence of a distinct mandibular border from mentum to angle with no jowl overhang
2. Subhyoid depression, which is a slight recess below the apex of the cervicomental angle[7]
3. Visible thyroid cartilage bulge
4. Visible anterior border of sternocleidomastoid muscle distinct in its entire length from the mastoid to sternum
5. Cervicomental angle between 105° and 120°

[7] I utilize the radius of curvature of the cervicomental angle for the second visual criteria. The ideal radius is rather small to give a well-defined cervicomental angle, whereas a long radius is related to an obtuse angle and poor aesthetics.

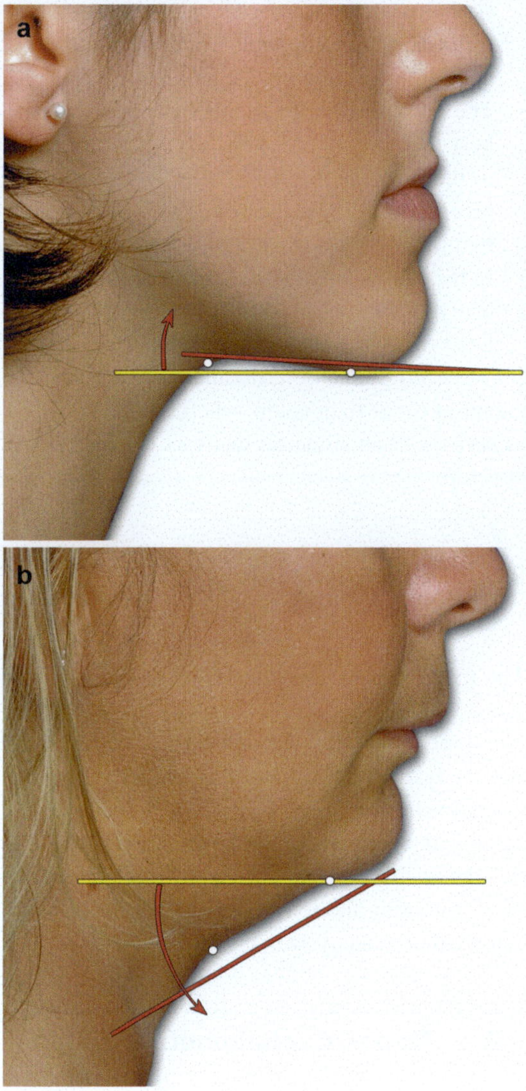

Fig. 9.14 Clinical evaluation of throat length and throat incline. A clinical case of long throat length and upwardly rotated throat incline (**a**) compared with the converse condition of a short throat length and downwardly rotated throat incline (**b**)

The classification of Dedo [5], which consists of six different classes, considers the different causes of neck aesthetic problems:

- Class I describes the case of no or minimal deformity still compatible with a youthful neck.
- Class II describes the case in which only skin laxity is present.
- Class III describes the case of excess of fat accumulation.

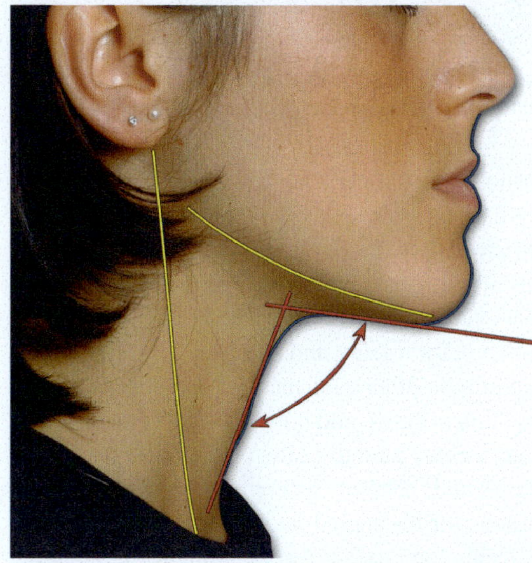

Fig. 9.15 A clinical case of a youthful neck. This shows a well-defined inferior mandibular border, cervicomental contour, and anterior border of the sternocleidomastoid muscle with a cervicomental angle of 103°

- Class IV refers to the presence of platysmal banding.
- Class V refers to the presence of microgenia (literally, this term identifies an underprojected chin) or retrognathia (literally, this term identifies a hypoplastic and retruded mandible).
- Class VI refers to the presence of a low-positioned hyoid bone.

It is obvious that more than one of Dedo's classes may be combined in the same clinical case.

9.4 Intraoral and Dental Cast Analysis

Intraoral and dental cast analysis is vital for the comprehension of dentofacial deformities and should be part of the background of all professionals dealing with facial aesthetics. In particular, the dental cast is the most utilized and easiest solid reproduction of a portion of the human body to obtain; it is also familiar to the patient himself, and, for these reasons, I utilize it extensively as a visual tool during the patient communication process.

The basic elements of dental analysis are illustrated in Chap. 8, to which the reader is referred.

9.5 Cephalometric Analysis

9.5.1 A Personal View on Radiographic Cephalometry

Orthodontics applied to jaw surgery was one of my earliest professional interests, and, as a consequence, over a couple of years, my library was full of books and articles on cephalometrics, and every day at least one new head film was in my viewbox for tracing and analysis. The head of the department often gave me the cephalograms from his clinical cases, and during 1989, I was in Milan every Friday attending the orthodontic section of the dental school, where the then chief was famous for his cephalometric analysis.

Cephalometrics is a demanding form of analysis, many points of reference are hidden in the depths of the face, and others are simply nonexistent (artificially constructed); it also requires anatomical, dental, and radiological knowledge, and it is a time-consuming activity. To control every step of the procedure, you need to know how to position the patient's head in the cephalostat; how to adjust the x-ray generator (time of exposure, milliampere, kV) in relationship to the skeletal structure, the film type, and the rare earth intensifying screen; and how to process the film. For these reasons, 10 years ago I decided to equip my office with the appliance for personally taking the cephalograms.

To complicate this field further, hundreds of different cephalometric analyses were published, giving the clinicians an immense number of different parameters and a correspondingly difficult technical language.

After 15 years of daily clinical experience, I am sure that I need less data from cephalometrics and more data from other sources in order to give better treatment to my patients. The evidence that cephalometric analysis is not decisive for planning orthodontic treatment was practically demonstrated in 1991 by Han and coworkers [7].

However, I still recommended that my young colleagues spend a regular part of their time studying and practicing it because:

- One of the largest group of specialists working with the face, the orthodontists, uses cephalometrics to classify, define, treat, and follow-up their clinical cases, and we all need to communicate with one another.
- The comparison of serial tracing is one of the best methods of studying what has happened to the facial profile and skeletal structure in a given clinical case, not only with orthodontic treatment but also with surgery.
- In the first years of practice, the other forms of analysis are not sufficiently developed to be utilized without an extra "cephalometric control."

We need cephalometric analysis early in our career in order to develop, whereas later we need to surpass cephalometric analysis to continue to develop.

9.5.2 Essential Radiographic Cephalometry

The most utilized cephalometric analyses contain a collection of parameters, which can be divided into three subgroups: dental, skeletal, and soft tissue analysis. The following paragraphs report a limited selection of the basic cephalometric measurements obtainable from the lateral cephalometric tracing; these are included with the main purpose of encouraging the reader to discover more about cephalometric analysis in his future practice.

9.6 Dental Cephalometric Analysis

The main scope of dental cephalometric analysis is to study the spatial position of the upper and lower central incisors. Every angle or distance measured must be correlated to the clinical findings reported in Chap. 8.

9.6.1 Interincisal Angle

The interincisal angle is drawn by passing a line through the incisal edge and the apex of the root of the maxillary and mandibular central incisors. Its normative value is 130°. In the case of a more acute value, one or both of the incisors are excessively labial (anteriorly) inclined, whereas in the

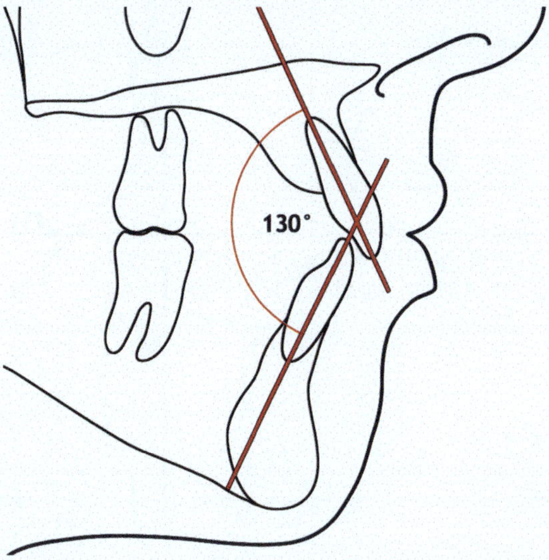

Fig. 9.16 Interincisal angle. Its normative value is 130°

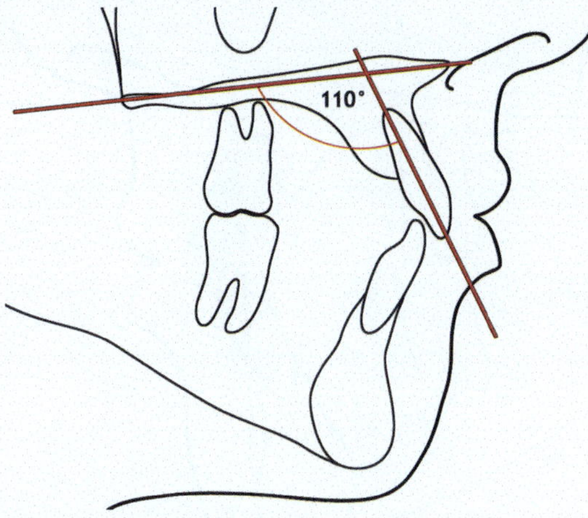

Fig. 9.17 Upper central incisors to maxillary plane angle. Its normative value is 110°

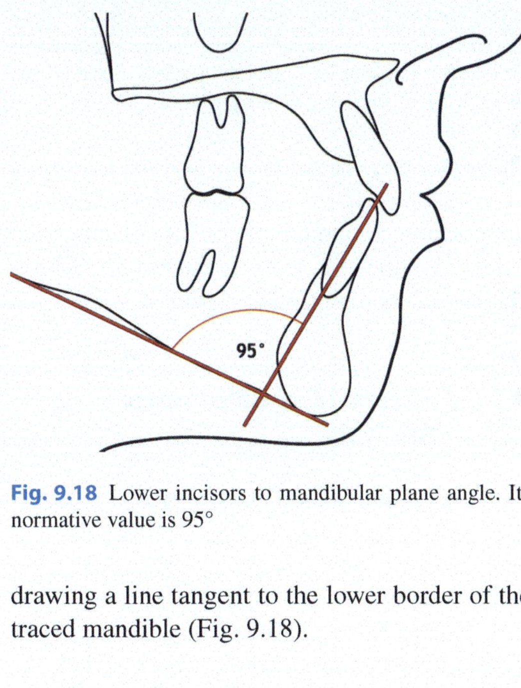

Fig. 9.18 Lower incisors to mandibular plane angle. Its normative value is 95°

case of a more obtuse value, one or both of the incisors are excessively lingual (posteriorly) inclined (Fig. 9.16). The measurement of the interincisal angle does not by itself clarify which set of incisors (the upper or the lower) is abnormally inclined.

9.6.2 Angle Between the Upper Central Incisors and the Maxillary Plane

The angle between the upper central incisors and the maxillary plane helps in analyzing the incline of the upper anterior teeth. Its normative value is 110°. The maxillary plane is constructed by passing a line through the anterior nasal spine and posterior nasal spine on the traced maxilla (Fig. 9.17).

9.6.3 Angle Between the Lower Incisors and the Mandibular Plane

The angle between the lower incisors and the mandibular plane helps in analyzing the incline of the lower anterior teeth. Its normative value is 95°. The mandibular plane can be constructed utilizing various methods, the simplest one is by drawing a line tangent to the lower border of the traced mandible (Fig. 9.18).

9.6.4 Protrusion of Maxillary Incisors

The protrusion (anteroposterior position) of the maxillary incisors is measured as the distance between the incisal edge of the maxillary central incisors and the line obtained passing through the A and pogonion points (A–pogonion line). Its mean normative value is 2.7 mm anterior to that reference line and ranges between 5.0 mm anterior and 1.0 mm posterior (Fig. 9.19).

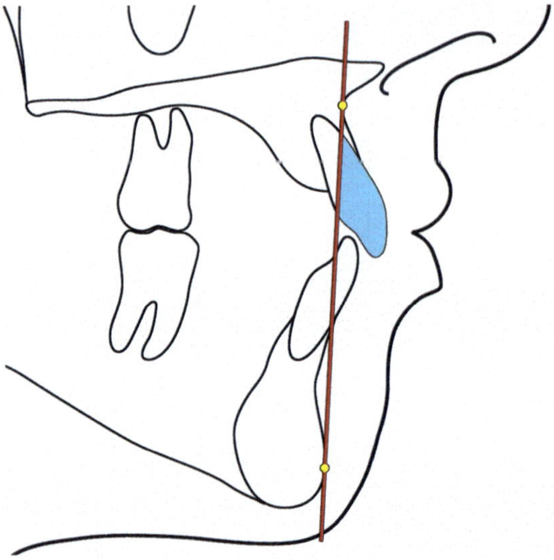

Fig. 9.19 Distance from the incisal edge of the upper central incisors to A-pogonion line. Its mean normative value is 2.7 mm anterior to that reference line and ranges between 5 mm anterior and mm posterior

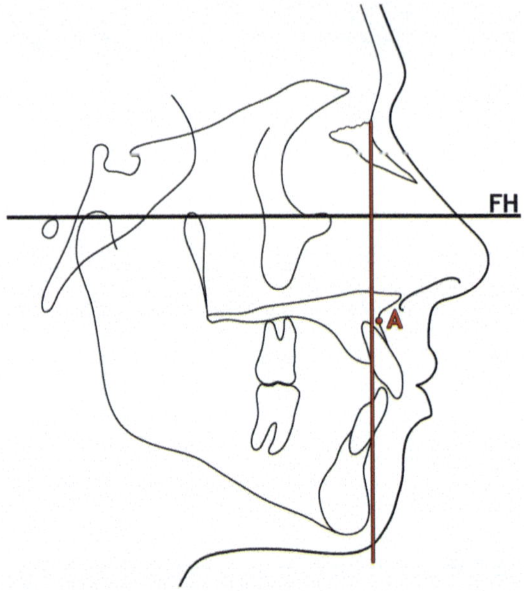

Fig. 9.20 McNamara's maxilla to cranial base anteroposterior assessment. The A point, in an ideal adult subject, should be 1 mm anterior to the reference line

This particular measurement is reliable only if the pogonion point is in its normal anteroposterior position; for example, in a case of a too posterior pogonion, this analysis can produce a false diagnosis of too protruding upper incisors.

9.7 Skeletal Cephalometric Analysis

The vertical and anteroposterior spatial relationship between the jaws and between the jaws and other skeletal structures can be studied in depth with cephalometry. The following parameters are part of a more complex modern analysis published by James McNamara in 1984 [10, 11].

9.7.1 Maxilla to Cranial Base Anteroposterior Assessment

This measurement utilizes a vertical reference line passing through the nasion. The A point, in an ideal adult subject, should be 1 mm anterior to the reference line (Fig. 9.20). As for the possibility of discrepancy between the clinical and cephalometric observation of the maxillary anteroposterior position, James McNamara suggests that "the clinical examination should take precedence. Treating a patient only in accordance with cephalometric norms must be avoided" [11].

9.7.2 Mandible to Cranial Base Anteroposterior Assessment

This measurement also utilizes a vertical reference line passing through the nasion. In an ideal adult subject, the pogonion should be comprised from 2 mm posterior to 4 mm anterior to the reference line (Fig. 9.21).

9.7.3 Mandible to Maxilla Assessment

To study the relationships between the mandible and maxilla, McNamara proposed the construction of a triangle (Fig. 9.22) consisting of the length of the mandible, measured as the distance from the condylion to the gnathion (Co–Gn); the length of midface, measured as the distance from the condylion to the A point (Co–A point); and the lower anterior facial height, measured as the distance between the anterior nasal spine and the menton (ANS–Me). Utilizing Table 9.1, it is

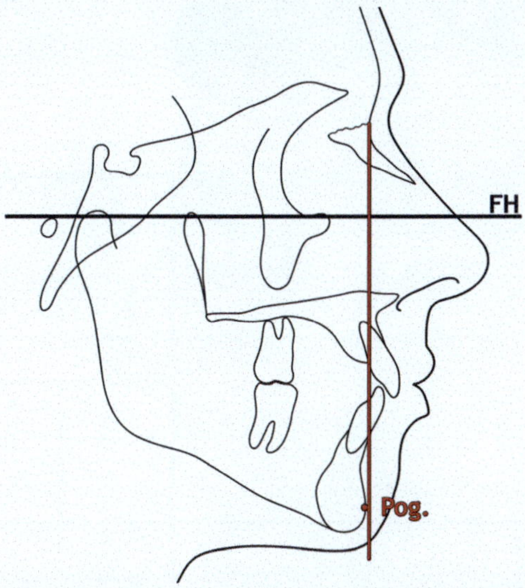

Fig. 9.21 McNamara's mandible to cranial base antero-posterior assessment. The point pogonion, in an ideal adult subject, should be comprised from 2 mm posterior to 4 mm anterior to the reference line

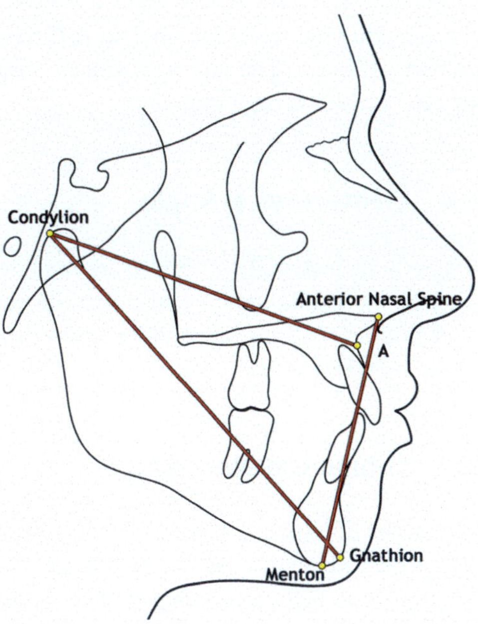

Fig. 9.22 McNamara's mandible to maxilla assessment. A triangle is constructed utilizing the length of the mandible, measured as the distance from the condylion to the gnathion (Co–Gn); the length of midface, measured as the distance from the condylion to A point (Co–A point); and the lower anterior facial height, measured as the distance between the anterior nasal spine and the menton (ANS–Me). The proportions between each of these three distances, in ideal subjects, are reported in Table 9.1

Table 9.1 McNamara's composite norms representing the relationship between the midfacial length, mandibular length, and lower anterior vertical height

Midfacial length (mm; Co–A point)	Mandibular length (mm; Co–Gn)	Lower anterior facial height (mm; ANS–Me)
80	97–100	57–58
81	99–102	57–58
82	101–104	58–59
83	103–106	57–58
84	104–107	59–60
85	105–108	60–62
86	107–110	60–62
87	109–112	61–63
88	111–114	61–63
89	112–115	62–64
90	113–116	63–64
91	115–118	63–64
92	117–120	64–65
93	119–122	65–66
94	121–124	66–67
95	122–125	67–69
96	124–127	67–69
97	126–129	68–70
98	128–131	68–70
99	129–132	69–71
100	130–133	70–74
101	132–135	71–75
102	134–137	76–76
103	136–139	73–77
104	137–140	74–78
105	138–141	75–79

Co–A point condylion to the A point, *Co–Gn* condylion to the gnathion, *ANS–Me* anterior nasal spine to the menton

possible to correlate, for any given midfacial length, the range of corresponding normal mandibular length and corresponding normal lower anterior facial height.

9.8 Soft Tissue Cephalometric Analysis

Many of the soft tissue cephalometric measurements can also be done on the life-size clinical photographs and directly on the subject, as anthropometric measurements. Each of the following examples of soft tissue analysis is presented utilizing a tracing and a photograph of two different subjects for comparison.

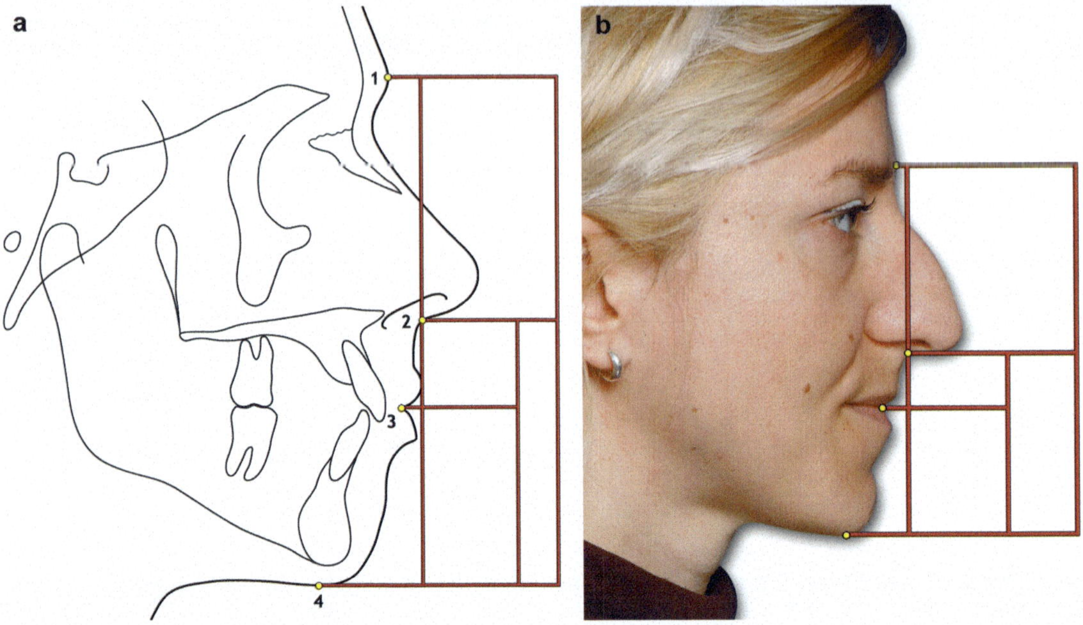

Fig. 9.23 Vertical proportion measured over a cephalometric tracing obtained from a lateral cephalometric radiograph (**a**) and over a profile view clinical photograph (**b**) of two different subjects

9.8.1 Vertical Proportions

The proportion of the upper and lower face can be evaluated dividing the vertical distance between the glabella and soft tissue menton at the subnasale point; the distance from glabella to subnasale should be equal to that from subnasale to soft tissue menton. The upper lip should be one-third of the subnasale to soft tissue menton vertical distance, whereas the lower lip should be about two-thirds (Fig. 9.23).

9.8.2 Nasofacial Angle

The nasofacial angle is formed by the intersection of the line drawn from glabella to soft tissue pogonion with a line drawn along the outline of the nasal dorsum. The average values range from 30° to 35° (Fig. 9.24).

9.8.3 Nasomental Angle

The nasomental angle is constructed by drawing a line along the outline of the nasal dorsum and a line connecting the tip of the nose to soft tissue pogonion (E-line). The average values range from 120° to 132° (Fig. 9.24).

9.8.4 Mentocervical Angle

The mentocervical angle is formed by the intersection of the E-line with a tangent to the submental outline. The average values range from 120° to 132° (Fig. 9.24).

9.8.5 Submental–Neck Angle

The submental–neck angle is formed by the tangents to the submental and neck outlines. The average value is 126° in men and 121° in women (Fig. 9.24).

9.8.6 Subnasal Vertical

A vertical line drawn through the subnasale can be used as a reference to assess the prominence of the upper and lower lip as well as the chin.

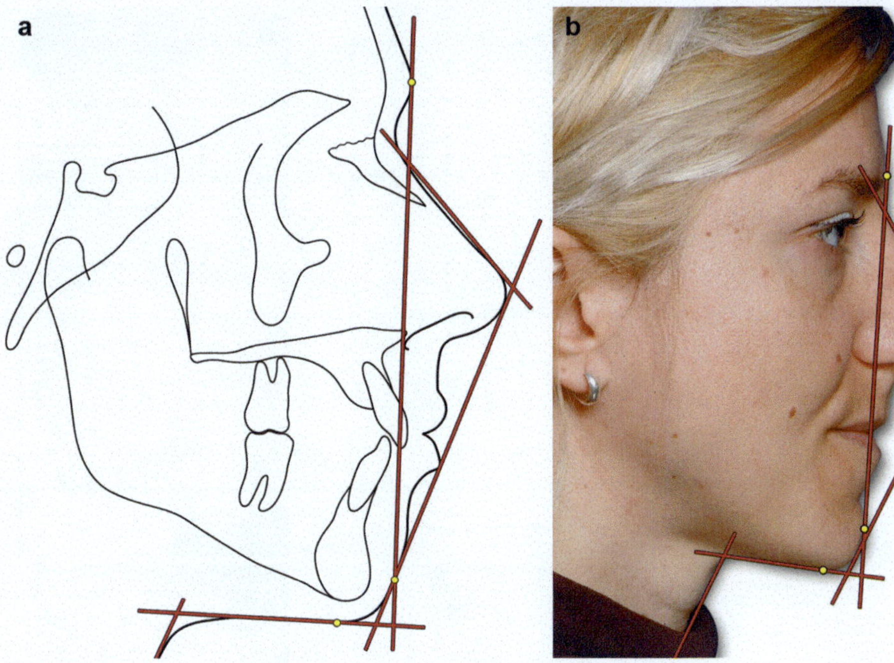

Fig. 9.24 Nasofacial, nasomental, mentocervical, and submental–neck angles measured over a cephalometric tracing obtained from a lateral cephalometric radiograph (**a**) and over a profile view clinical photograph (**b**) of two different subjects

Before selecting the subnasale as a reference, it is essential to obtain the natural head position and to exclude a regional deformity of the subnasal region itself, such as a prominent or recessive nasal spine, an overgrowth of the caudal septum, or any other condition leading to a malposition of the subnasale point.

The upper lip should be 1–2 mm in front of the subnasal vertical reference line, the lower lip should be on the line or 1 mm posterior to it, and the pogonion soft should be 1–4 mm posterior to it (Fig. 9.25).

9.8.7 Nasolabial Angle

The nasolabial angle is formed by the intersection of a columella tangent and an upper lip tangent. In an adult sample with an ideal occlusion and well-balanced face [11], the average value was 102°, with a standard deviation of 8° for both males and females. The angle can be further subdivided to assess the columella and the upper labial inclines independently utilizing a horizontal line passing through it (Fig. 9.26). Also, for this parameter, special effort should be made to detect any abnormal position of the subnasale point before judging the incline of the columella and the upper lip.

9.9 The Points, Lines, and Angles Difficult to Trace

Sometimes, one or more of the points, lines, or angles are difficult to identify and trace as a result of the subject's anatomical variability. In these cases, instead of mistakenly utilizing a cephalometric rule to obtain a linear or angular value, it is preferable to return to the direct clinical examination to assess a facial feature.

9.10 The Maxillomandibular Complex Concept

In many clinical cases, the findings obtained from the dental analysis are closely related to those obtained from the facial assessment. For example, a class II dental occlusion with a mandibular

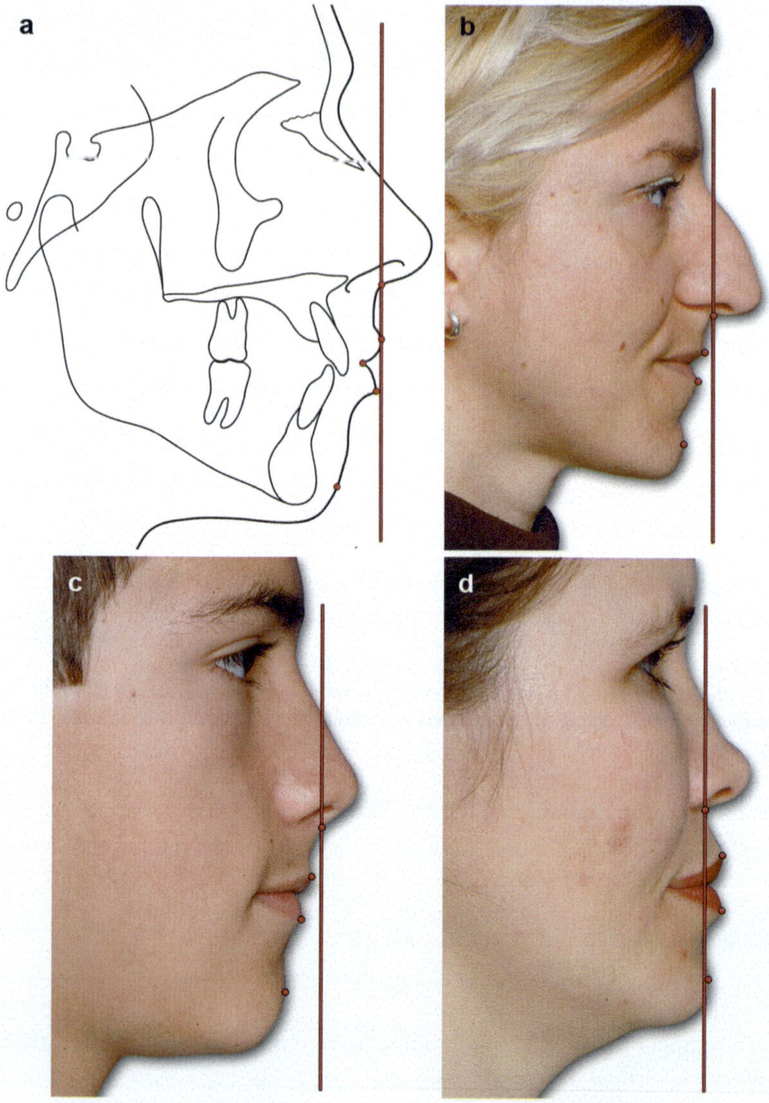

Fig. 9.25 Subnasal vertical reference line measured over a cephalometric tracing obtained from a lateral cephalometric radiograph (**a**) and over a profile view clinical photograph (**b**). A too anterior (**c**) or too posterior subnasale (**d**) needs to be detected in advance to avoid errors in the construction of the reference line

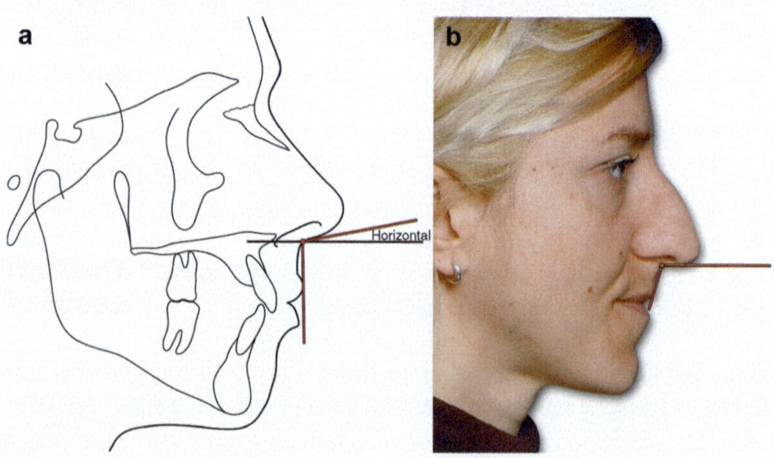

Fig. 9.26 The nasolabial angle is formed by the intersection of a columella tangent and an upper lip tangent. The angle can be further subdivided to assess the columella and the upper labial inclines independently utilizing a horizontal line passing through it (**a**). A clinical case of maxillary deficiency in which the whole nasolabial angle measures 103° but the columellar component is 0° and the upper lip component is 103° (**b**)

anteroposterior deficiency is usually correlated to a specific facial profile with a poor lower lip–chin–submental–neck contour, a recessive chin, and a relative overprojection of the nasal tip.

In other cases, a nearly perfect occlusion, either spontaneously developed or resulting from previous orthodontic treatment, is found in subjects with poor facial balance, subjects that at first sight can be quite similar to those with a dentofacial deformity. Unfortunately, a similar clinical scenario can also be seen after a surgical–orthodontic treatment in spite of correct dental occlusion having been achieved.

The concept of moving the maxillomandibular complex (MMC) backward or forward, upward or downward, and rotating clockwise or counterclockwise with jaw surgery is not new in the process of planning orthognathic surgery [12, 13] and should be extended in the future to every form of facial analysis as a basic tool.

Figure 9.27a shows the essential dental and skeletal components of the MMC obtained from a cephalometric tracing. The assessment of the spatial position of the MMC considers its anteroposterior, vertical, transverse, and the grade and point of rotation in clockwise or counterclockwise direction (Fig. 9.27b–e).

Figure 9.28 reports an example of a malpositioned MMC (the clinical case is presented in Fig. 9.1). Even if the dental occlusion is acceptable, due to previous orthodontic treatment carried out in his childhood, a developmental clockwise rotation of the MMC at the level of the anterior nasal spine is responsible for the flattening of the labiomental fold, the recessive soft tissue chin, the lack of definition of the mandibular border, and the poor chin–neck profile.

9.11 The Role of Dentofacial Deformities in Premature Aging Appearance

The shapes and volumes of dental, bony, and cartilaginous structures play a fundamental role in supporting the soft tissue envelope and greatly influence how the face ages. So, many of the "dentoskeletal" problems discussed in this chapter can be revisited as major determinants of the aging appearance of younger subjects. In particular, the conditions classified as midface retrusion, paranasal retrusion, mandibular retrusion and microgenia, upper and lower anterior teeth retrusion, and anterior vertical excess have the same effect, that of poorly supporting the soft tissue.

In Chap. 10, the intimate relationships of dentofacial deformities and a prematurely aged appearance are considered again in Sect. 10.1.

9.12 Dentofacial Analysis Checklist[8]

- Is the face symmetric?
  □ Yes
  □ No, because…
- Is the upper facial third symmetric?
  □ Yes
  □ No, because…
- Are the eye globes symmetric?
  □ Yes
  □ No, because…
- Is the middle facial third symmetric?
  □ Yes
  □ No, because…
- Is the lower facial third symmetric?
  □ Yes
  □ No, because…
- In the frontal view, the facial shape is:
  □ Wide
  □ Narrow
  □ Long
  □ Short
- Inferior scleral show:
  □ No
  □ Yes, right… mm. Left… mm
- Define the malar eminence:
  □ Hypoplastic
  □ Balanced
  □ Pronounced
- The total facial profile is:
  □ Straight
  □ Slightly concave
  □ Concave
  □ Slightly convex
  □ Convex

[8]Section 2 on Springer Extra Materials (extras.springer.com).

- Define the paranasal region (pyriform aperture):
  □ Correct
  □ Hypoplastic (retrusive)
- Are the lips symmetric?
  □ Yes
  □ No, because…
- Is the lip seal reached with muscular strain?
  □ Yes
  □ No
- Is the lip seal maintained when the perioral musculature is relaxed?
  □ Yes
  □ No
- In profile view, are there a series of gentle curves from the nasal tip to the soft tissue menton, without straight traits and a unique well-defined angle at the stomion?
  □ Yes
  □ No, because…
- The upper lip profile is:
  □ Normally projected
  □ Too anterior
  □ Too posterior
- Define the nasolabial angle:
  □ Ideal
  □ Too acute
  □ Too obtuse
- The lower lip profile is:
  □ Normally projected
  □ Too anterior
  □ Too posterior
- Define the maxillary incisors and gingival display when smiling:
  □ Absence of upper incisors display
  □ Poor upper incisors display
  □ Ideal upper incisors and gingival display (slightly above the gingival margin)
  □ Increased (esthetically acceptable gingival display)
  □ Excessive gingival display
- The anteroposterior projection of the upper frontal teeth is:
  □ Ideal (balanced with the facial profile)
  □ Too anterior
  □ Too posterior
- Is the bony chin symmetric?
  □ Yes
  □ No, because…
- Is the external chin shape symmetric?
  □ Yes
  □ No, because…
- Does the chin maintain its symmetry during smiling?
  □ Yes
  □ Dynamic asymmetry due to…
- In the frontal view, the chin shape is:
  □ Wide or narrow
  □ Vertically long
  □ Vertically short
- The chin profile is:
  □ Balanced
  □ Too protrusive
  □ Too recessive
- The soft tissue pogonion is:
  □ Too posterior to labrale inferior (Li)
  □ Slightly posterior (balanced) to Li
  □ Vertical to Li
  □ Anterior to Li
- Define the chin shape:
  □ Pointed
  □ Large
  □ Square
  □ Witch's chin (ptotic chin)
  □ Cleft chin
  □…
- The labiomental fold is:
  □ Balanced
  □ Deep
  □ Shallow
- The vertical lower lip/chin ratio is:
  □ Balanced
  □ Long lip and short chin
  □ Short lip and long chin
- Define the mandibular size relative to the whole face:
  □ Balanced
  □ Small
  □ Big
- Define the mandibular incline:
  □ Ideal
  □ Clockwise rotated
  □ Counterclockwise rotated
- Define the mandibular border definition from angle to chin:
  □ Ideal
  □ Poor

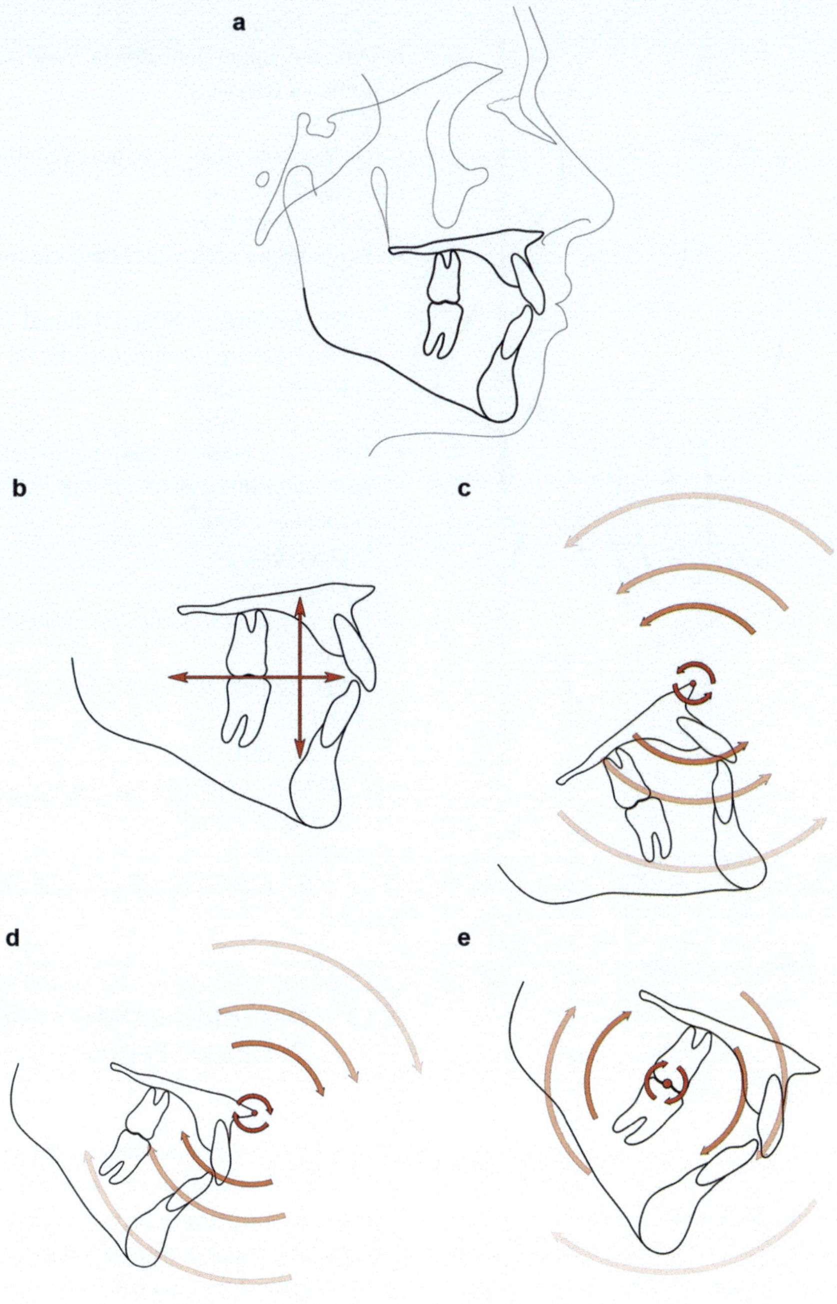

Fig. 9.27 The maxillomandibular (MMC) complex traced from a subject with good occlusal relationship (**a**). The assessment of spatial position of the MMC in profile view should consider its vertical and sagittal position (**b**), as well as its grade, point, and direction of rotation. A counterclockwise-rotated MMC on the anterior nasal spine produces a prominent soft tissue chin with little influence on the upper incisors (**c**), whereas the opposite rotation is responsible for a recessive chin again with little influence on the upper incisors (**d**). A clockwise-rotated MMC centered on the occlusal plane at the level of first molars produces the elongation of the lower third of the face as well as an advancement of the anterior nasal spine and a set back of the chin profile (**e**)

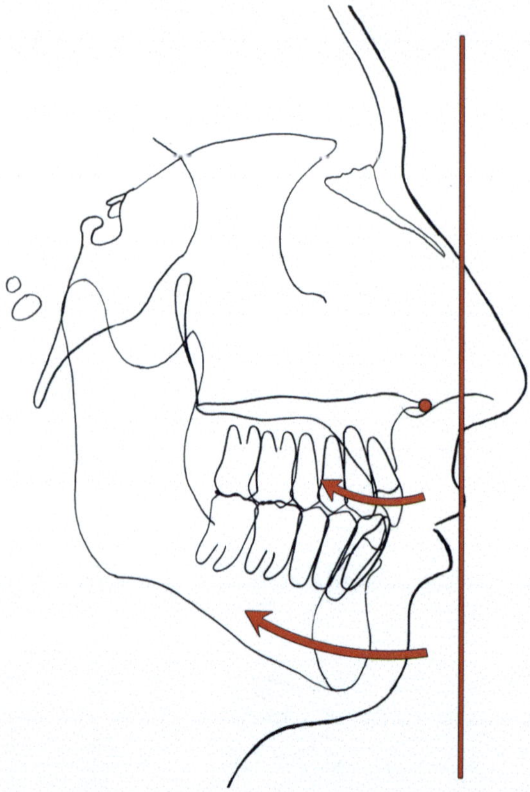

Fig. 9.28 The tracing of the MMC of the clinical case presented in Fig. 9.1. The clockwise rotation at the level of the anterior nasal spine of the MMC is responsible for the flattening of the labiomental fold, the recessive soft tissue chin, the lack of definition of the mandibular border, and the poor chin–neck profile

- Define the throat length:
  □ Ideal
  □ Too short
  □ Too long
- Define the throat incline:
  □ Ideal
  □ Excessively down oriented
- Define the cervicomental angle:
  □ Ideal
  □ Too acute
  □ Too obtuse
- Is the dental occlusion symmetric with the face?
  □ Yes
  □ No, because…
- Do the upper and lower dental midlines coincide with each other?
  □ Yes
  □ No, because…
- Are the upper incisors in front of the lower incisors (overjet)?
  □ Yes
  □ Yes, but they are horizontally separated (increased overjet)
  □ No (reverse overjet)
- Is the upper arch wider than the lower one?
  □ Yes
  □ No, because of bilateral dental crossbite
  □ No, because of unilateral dental crossbite
  □ Right crossbite
  □ Left crossbite
- Define the vertical relationship between upper and lower incisors (overbite):
  □ Ideal overbite
  □ Deep bite
  □ Open bite
- Define the soft tissue envelope thickness of the face:
  □ I Extremely thin (pathological)
  □ II Thin
  □ III Slightly thin
  □ IV Ideal thickness for age and sex
  □ V Slightly thick
  □ VI Thick
  □ VII Extremely thick (extremely obese patients)

9.13 Dentofacial Deformities: Preferred Terms[9]

- *Alar crease junction*. The most posterior point of the curved line formed by the alar crease as seen in profile view; it is utilized as a landmark for measuring tip projection.
- *Anterior nasal spine*. The most anterior point in the traced maxilla (tip of the nasal spine). It is a cephalometric reference point.
- *Cephalometric tracing*. The pencil drawing obtained by tracing from a cephalogram onto an acetate matte paper, the outline of some of the anatomical structures like teeth, facial and cranial bones, and soft tissue profile.

[9]Section 3 on Springer Extra Materials (extras.springer.com).

- *Cheekbone point*. In a subject with a balanced middle facial third, it is the apex of osseous cheekbone that is located 20–25 mm inferior and 5–10 mm anterior to the outer canthus of the eye when viewed in profile and is 20–25 mm inferior and 5–10 mm lateral to the outer canthus of the eye when viewed frontally [3]. A flat cheekbone point is often associated with malar deficiency and maxillary hypoplasia.
- *Chin deficiency*. Refers to a lack of anterior projection of the chin outline.
- *Chin pad*. The thick soft tissue overlying the bony chin.
- *Condylion*. The most posterosuperior point on the outline of the mandibular condyle seen on lateral cephalograms. It is a cephalometric reference point.
- *Crossbite*. When one or more of the maxillary teeth are lingually (internally) positioned relative to the respective mandibular teeth. The anterior crossbite is also called reverse overjet.
- *Dental classes*. The classification of the sagittal relationship between the dental arches. Class I: normal posteroanterior relationship between the two dental arches. Class II: too anterior upper dental arch and/or too posterior lower dental arch. Class III: too posterior upper dental arch and/or too anterior lower dental arch.
- *Dental crowding*. The absence of alignment between adjacent teeth. It is usually graded from mild to severe crowding.
- *E-line* (*esthetic line*). A reference line connecting the tip of the nose to the most anterior point of the chin contour (soft tissue pogonion).
- *Glabella* (*soft tissue glabella*). The most prominent anterior point in the midsagittal plane of the forehead [9]. It is influenced by pneumonization of the frontal sinus and varies widely in posteroanterior position.
- *Gnathion*. The most anteroinferior point on the outline of the mandibular symphysis seen on lateral cephalograms. It is a cephalometric reference point.
- *High/low mandibular plane angle*. The excessive clockwise (high) or counterclockwise (low) rotation of the mandibular plane. The high mandibular plane angle is correlated with the hyperdivergent facial pattern and the long face; the low mandibular plane angle is correlated with the hypodivergent facial pattern and the short face.
- *Hyper/hypodivergent facial pattern*. The increased (hyperdivergent) and decreased (hypodivergent) anterior facial height in relation to the posterior facial height (see also high/low mandibular plane angle).
- *Labiomental fold* (*mandibular sulcus contour*). The horizontal skin depression that separates the chin from the lower lip. It varies from a flat curve to a deep sulcus.
- *Labrale inferior*. A point indicating the mucocutaneous border of the upper lip. The most anterior point of the upper lip (usually). It is a cephalometric reference point.
- *Labrale superior*. The median point in the lower margin of the lower membranous lip.
- *Lip support*. The action of the anterior teeth and their surrounding alveolar bone in shaping the lips.
- *Dentoalveolar protrusion/retrusion*. The abnormal forward (protrusion) or backward (retrusion) position of the teeth and their alveolar bone in respect to the basal bone of the jaws. It can involve the maxillary and/or mandibular dental arches.
- *Malar eminence*. The point of maximal outer projection of the malar region.
- *Mandibular deficiency*. The hypoplasia of the whole mandible. It is the most common cause of class II dentofacial deformities.
- *Mandibular plane*. A cephalometric reference plane constructed by drawing a line tangent to the traced mandibular border.
- *Maxilla point*. The most anterior point on the continuum of the cheekbone–nasal–lip contour described by Arnett and Bergman [3]; it is an indicator of maxillary anteroposterior position.
- *Maxillary plane*. A cephalometric reference plane constructed by drawing a line passing through the anterior nasal spine and the posterior nasal spine on the traced maxilla.
- *Menton*. The lowest point on the symphyseal shadow of the mandible seen on lateral

cephalograms. It is a cephalometric reference point. Soft tissue menton – The lowest point on the contour of the soft tissue chin found by dropping a perpendicular line through the skeletal menton. It is a cephalometric reference point.

- *Microgenia*. This term refers to an under-projected chin independently from occlusal consideration.
- *Muscle strain*. The flattening of the chin outline due to muscular contraction produced to achieve lip seal. It is a frequent finding in many dentofacial deformities (dental and skeletal open bite, dental and skeletal class II).
- *Nasion*. The most anterior point on the frontonasal suture in the midsagittal plane. It is a cephalometric reference point. Soft tissue nasion – The point of greatest concavity in the midline between the forehead and the nose.
- *Neck–throat point*. The more posterior–superior point of the submental–neck outline.
- *Occlusal plane*. The line bisecting the overlapping cusp of the first molars and the incisal overlap.
- *Overbite*. The vertical overlap of the incisors obtained when the two dental arches occlude together. Deep bite – Excessive vertical overlap between upper and lower incisors. Open bite – In this condition, there is no overlap but a vertical separation.
- *Overjet*. The horizontal overlap of the upper incisors in front of the lower incisors. Normally, it is 2–3 mm due to the thickness of the edge of the upper incisors. Increased overjet is the excessive horizontal distance between the upper and lower incisors. Reverse overjet (anterior crossbite) – If the lower incisors are in front of the upper incisors.
- *Platysma bands* (*"turkey gobbler" effect*). The vertical skin bands, usually one for each side, of the aging submental and neck region. It is caused by platysma muscle attenuation, lengthening, and dehiscence, along with fat accumulation, skin excess and photodamage.
- *Pogonion*. The most anterior point of the bony chin contour. It is a cephalometric reference point. Soft tissue pogonion – The most prominent or anterior point of the chin contour. It is a cephalometric reference point.
- *Point A*. The most posterior midline point in the anterior concavity of the traced maxilla situated between the anterior nasal spine and the most inferior point on the alveolar bone overlying the maxillary incisors. It is a cephalometric reference point.
- *Posterior nasal spine*. The most posterior point of the palatine bone on the traced maxilla. It is a cephalometric reference point.
- *Pronasale*. The tip of the nose. The most prominent or anterior point of the nose.
- *Scleral show* (*inferior scleral show*). The presence of a strip of white sclera between the iris and the lower lid margin with the subject in natural head position and straight gaze. It may be a sign of exophthalmos, previous trauma, prior surgery, lower lid laxity, or dentofacial deformities with maxillary hypoplasia.
- *Skeletal classes*. The classification of sagittal relationship between maxilla and mandible. Class I: normal posteroanterior relationship between maxilla and mandible. Class II: too anterior maxilla and/or too posterior mandible. Class III: too posterior maxilla and/or too anterior mandible.
- *Subnasale*. The point at which the columella merges with the upper lip in the midsagittal plane [9]. It varies widely in relation to caudal septum prominence and nasal spine morphology.
- *Throat length*. The distance between the neck–throat point and the soft tissue menton on the lower facial outline. The throat length is preferably assessed clinically as short or long and not measured instrumentally [3].
- *Witch's chin deformity* (*ptotic chin*). The flattening and ptosis of the chin pad associated with the deepening of the submental crease. It can be age related or iatrogenic.

References

1. Ackerman JL (1998) An orthodontic viewpoint. In: Rosen HM (ed) Aesthetic perspective in jaw surgery. Springer, New York
2. Arnett GW, Bergman RT (1993) Facial keys to orthodontic diagnosis and treatment planning. Part I. Am J Orthod Dentofacial Orthop 103:299–312

The Aging Face

10

We have met the enemy...... and he is us!
– Walt Kelly (cited in [7])

Contents

The "process of aging" is the sum of factors acting on all the four main components involved in facial aesthetics:

- The soft tissue quality
- The soft tissue quantity
- The soft tissue dynamics
- The supporting bony, dental, and cartilaginous skeleton

The causes almost always start to act early on the facial tissue, but the consequences are manifest only over the long term. This reminds us of many of the great problems that humans are incapable of solving, such as wars, the hole in the ozone layer, the big financial crises, environmental pollution, and many others. In all cases, nobody recognizes himself as being guilty because our single action is so small and so distant in time and space that we have completely lost the connections when the problem arises in its full extent.

So, one of the difficult tasks in facial analysis is the early detection of the signs of aging in the younger patient, as well as the identification of the basic developmental deformities that worsen

F. Meneghini, P. Biondi, *Clinical Facial Analysis*,
DOI 10.1007/978-3-642-27228-8_10,

the final effects of aging. In other words, we must observe the young subjects now, also thinking in terms of future aging.

10.1 Structural Factors of Aging

When a young or middle-aged subject appears "aged," the presence of one or more structural factors of aging should be suspected, looked for, and assessed. For example, the association of two structural factors, one affecting the soft tissue, such as a vertically long upper lip, and another affecting the dental and skeletal framework, such as a vertical short maxilla, can produce an aged appearance affecting all the lower facial third. This negative combination also influences the act of smiling of the patient as a result of the reduced exposure of the upper anterior teeth (Fig. 10.1).[1]

Sometimes the structural factors of aging are not easily detected because of the compensation offered by the soft tissue envelope, which, in a young subject, has an important role of camouflage. A typical example is the effects of teeth extraction, performed in childhood for orthodontic needs, as in the clinical case of the young girl reported in Fig. 10.2. Before the orthodontic treatment, the main concern of her parents was the protruding anterior teeth; her dentist "solved" the problem by extracting an upper premolar on each side and retracting the upper incisors but left untreated (or misdiagnosed) the mandibular deficiency. When her case was documented, at the age of 26 years, the initial signs of aging on the upper lip were evident and will worsen in the future when the camouflage effects produced by the soft tissue envelope progressively disappear.

This case confirms the initial assertion that if our actions, i.e., the teeth extraction and orthodontic treatment, are so distant in time and space, we, and our patients too, lose the connections between cause and effect when the problem of aging arises in its full magnitude. To prevent the aesthetic problem of this dentofacial deformity as well as confronting the aging process, a different treatment should have been done when she was in her teens:

- Avoid the extraction of the upper premolars.
- Extract one inferior premolar on each side.
- Retract the inferior anterior teeth with orthodontics.
- Perform the surgical advancement of the mandible to correct the sagittal component of the malocclusion as well as the facial profile.

10.2 Soft Tissue Quality and Aging

Aging acts by changing the skin through two distinct basic processes: intrinsic and extrinsic. Intrinsic aging is inevitable, not beyond voluntary control, and reflects the genetic background of the subject. Extrinsic aging is mainly caused by sun exposure but also by smoking, excessive use of alcohol, and poor nutrition, so in some ways, it can be prevented [1] (see Sect. 13.14).

In clinical facial analysis, but also when communicating with the patient, it is imperative to differentiate between the quality of the skin, which consists of the skin color, texture, tone, elasticity, pigmented lesions, and the quantity and displacement of skin and other facial soft tissue (see also Sect. 5.5).

[1]The complete clinical facial photographic documentation of this case is available in Sect. 4 on Springer Extra Materials (extra.springer.com) (Clinical Case No. 8).

Fig. 10.1 In this 40-year-old woman, a structural vertically long upper lip is associated with a vertically short maxilla. Both are responsible for a prematurely aging appearance (**a**, **b**). A close analysis of the perioral region in profile view (**c**) permits us to point out some conclusions: (1) the skin portion of the upper lip is too long; (2) the upper lip is excessively clockwise rotated; (3) the upper vermillion portion of the upper lip is hidden to the observer; (4) the entire lip outline is poorly supported and lies too posterior with respect to the E-line (a reference line connecting the tip of the nose to the most anterior point of the chin contour). The prematurely aging appearance is confirmed during smiling as a result of her inability to obtain a normal display of the anterior upper teeth and gingiva (**d**, **e**)

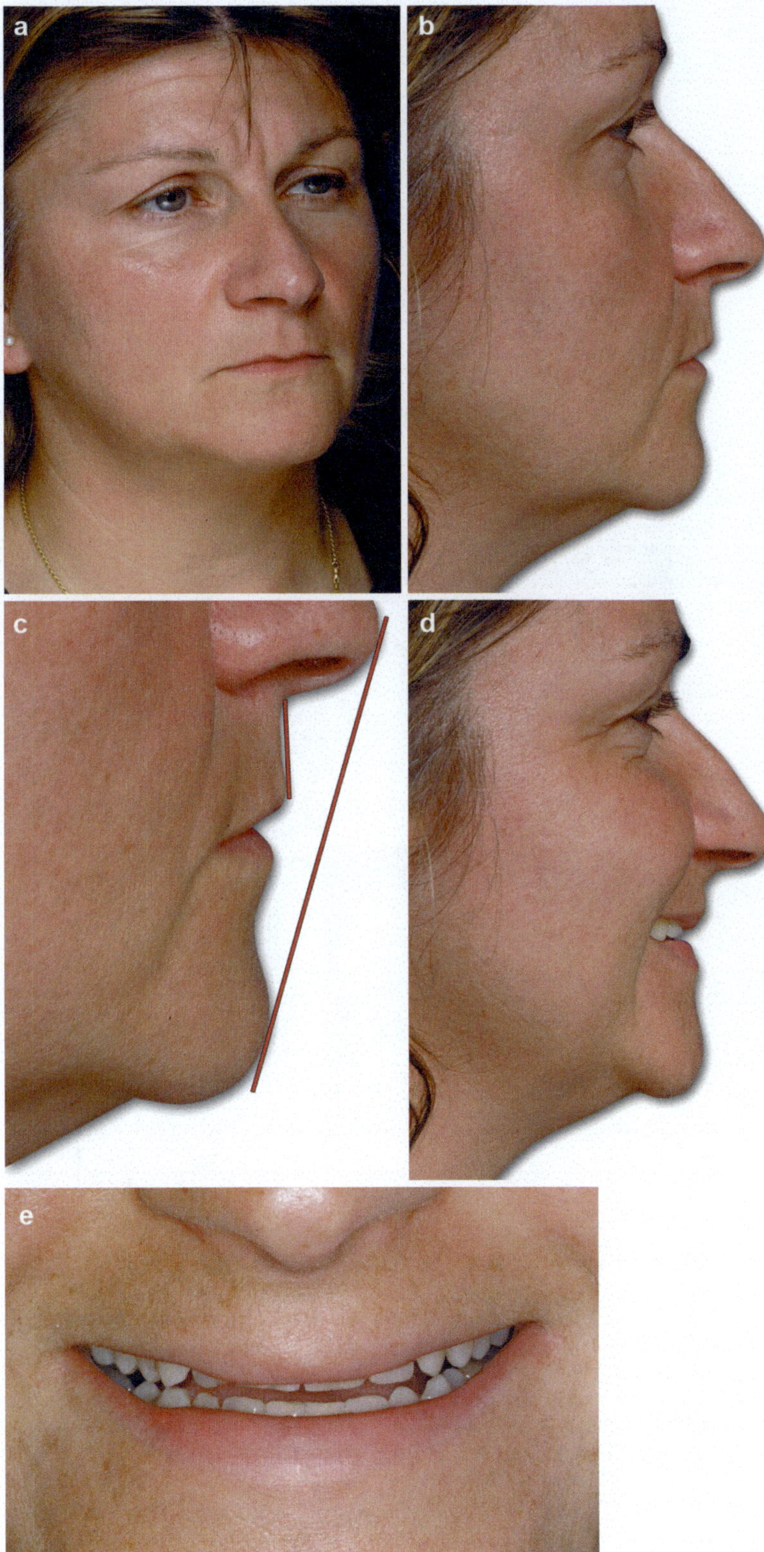
a
b
c
d
e

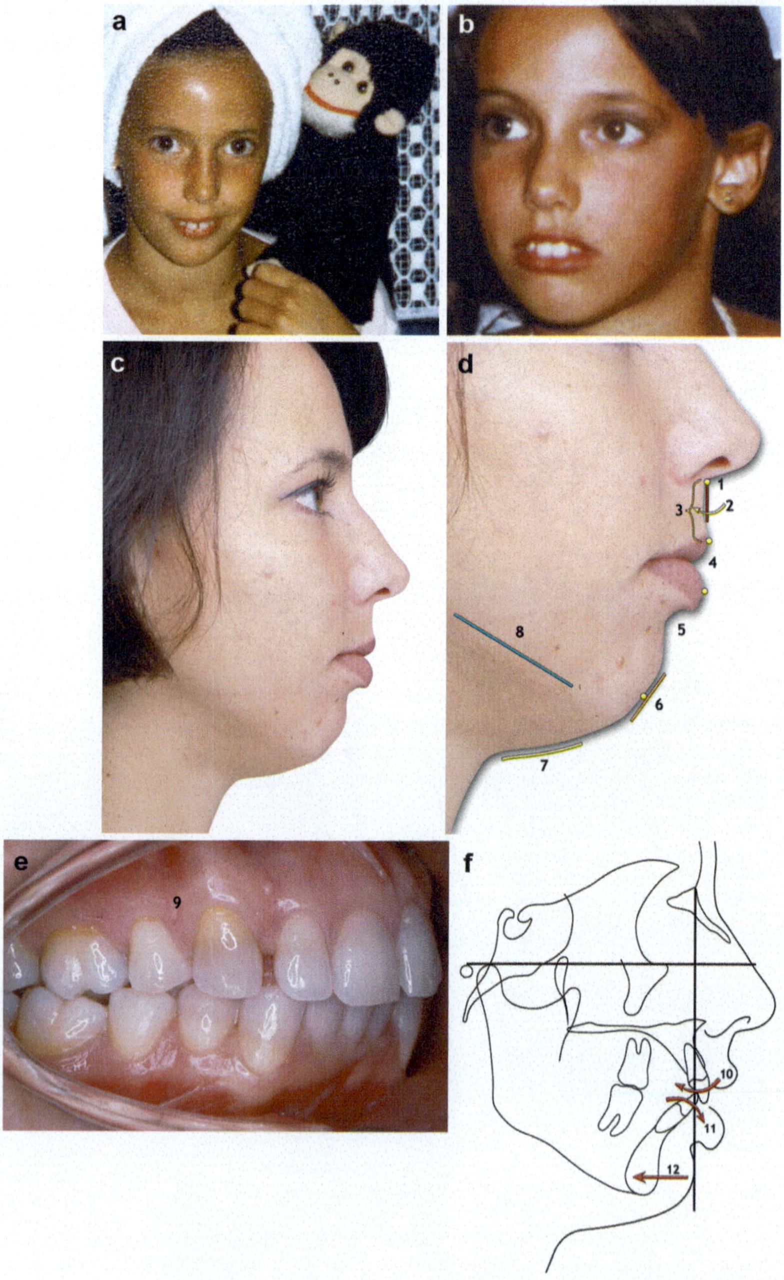

Fig. 10.2 In the two childhood photographs, taken from the personal album of the patient, clear protruding upper incisors were seen (**a**, **b**). When she was 26 years old, a complete facial analysis including the dental arches and cephalometric tracing (**c**–**f**) highlighted: *1* moderate vertical lengthening of the upper lip, *2* clockwise rotation of the upper lip outline, *3* flattening of the upper lip contour when the patient maintained the lip seal, *4* discrepancies between the vermillion exposure of the upper and lower lip, *5* excessive lower lip eversion, *6* flattening of the chin contour due to the muscular strain necessary to maintain the lip seal, *7* reduction of the throat length, *8* absence of definition of the mandibular border, *9* absence of one upper premolar on each side, *10* clockwise rotation of the upper incisors, *11* counterclockwise rotation of the lower incisors, and *12* a noticeable retrusion of the mandible

10.3 Soft Tissue Quantity and Aging

Aging also acts by reducing volumes, enlarging the surface, and displacing facial soft tissue. A process of atrophy (dermal atrophy, muscle atrophy, connective atrophy, fat atrophy) is responsible for volume reduction. A process of skin and connective tissue elongation, real or relative, is responsible for redundancy, "bag" formation, and ptosis. The interaction between the two previous processes also permits the displacing, in the vertical direction, of intraorbital, malar, facial, and neck fat. The same displacement can also affect the lacrimal and submandibular glands.

Some facial convexities become flat with aging, such as the cheeks and lips, and some flat areas bulge, such as the lower lid and submental.

10.4 Soft Tissue Dynamics and Aging

Muscular activity can produce evident skin creases and, at the same time, can hold up some skin areas, as happens with the eyebrow, giving the false impression that its position is correct. When analyzing the face, a special effort is made by the observer to envision the direction of underlying mimetic muscles and correlate it to external visible effects.

10.5 Skeletal Supporting Framework and Aging

A preexisting dentofacial deformity can aggravate and anticipate the aged look. If a patient looks older, check on the personal patient photographs searching for any preexisting aging signs and for the general features of the facial skeleton. The lack of support can be localized or extended over more subunits of the face, affecting the bone, cartilaginous, and dental framework.

10.6 Recognizing Aging in the Face

10.6.1 General Considerations

A comparison between youthful and aged faces reveals one or more of these changes:

- The general face form becomes longer and narrower. It can also shift from a triangular to a rectangular shape.
- Some subunits become empty and others become full.
- Some profile curves flatten.
- Some new curves appear.
- Some profile segments elongate.

10.7 Recognizing the Signs of Facial Aging

Some signs of aging are absent in a youthful face, such as the platysma bands, whereas others are already present in young subjects and their change, as when the nasolabial line transforms into the nasolabial groove and fold, underlines the progress of the aging.

Instead of discussing the theories of facial aging in depth (see Sect. 13.15), a list of the clinical signs of aging, from forehead to neck, is presented with some relevant specific considerations.

10.7.1 Forehead Transverse Furrows

The horizontal forehead furrows are usually two or three, continuous or centrally interrupted, lines. They are secondary to chronic frontalis muscle contraction produced as an effort to raise the descended eyebrows. As with any other mimetic wrinkle, line or furrow, the forehead transverse furrows are perpendicularly oriented to the underlying muscular fibers (Fig. 10.3).[2]

[2]The complete clinical facial photographic documentation of this case is available in Sect. 4 on Springer Extra Materials (extra.springer.com) (Clinical Case No. 9).

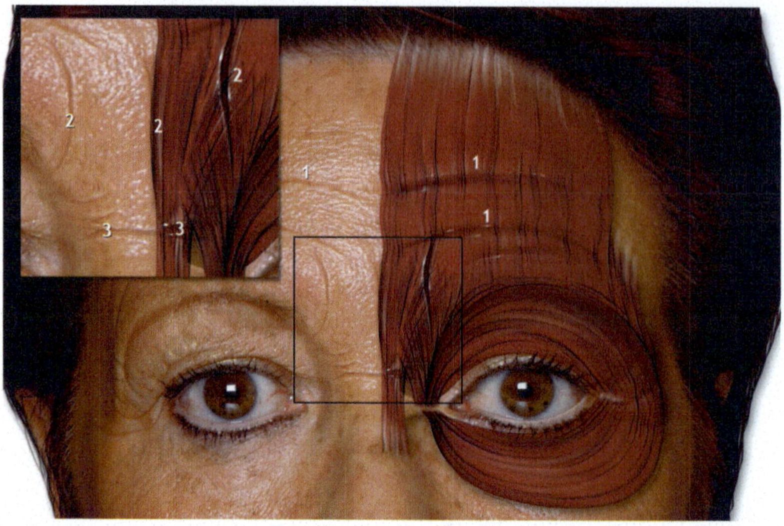

Fig. 10.3 Forehead and worry lines in a 65-year-old woman. These lines are all secondary to chronic muscular contraction of the frontalis muscle (*1* forehead lines), corrugator muscle (*2* paired vertical worry lines), and procerus muscle (*3* single horizontal worry line)

10.7.2 Frown Lines

The frown lines can be divided into vertical and horizontal. The vertical frown lines occupy the glabella, usually one for each side, and are perpendicular to the orientation of the fibers of the corrugator muscle, whereas the horizontal frown line is typically a single line occupying the radix of the nose and is perpendicular to the orientation of the fibers of the procerus muscle (Fig. 10.3). Each is considered to be a mimetic line.

10.7.3 Temporal Depression

The facial aging process can be seen in some areas as a progressive volume reduction of soft tissue, producing the effect called skeletonization, whereas in others, the soft tissue progressively increases or is made redundant, producing the opposite effect of hiding the skeletal and muscular contour. The temporal region usually undergoes a gradual loss of volume, producing a depression that is responsible for highlighting its skeletal boundaries: the zygomatic arch, the lateral orbital rim, and the temporal crest (Fig. 10.4).

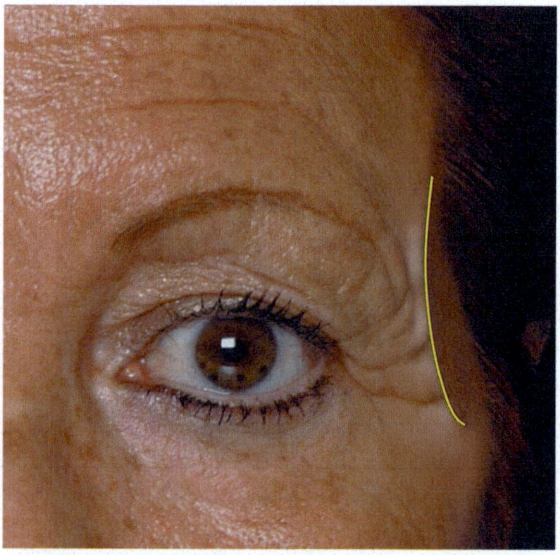

Fig. 10.4 Low-grade temporal depression in a 65-year-old woman. The skeletal boundaries of the temporal region are highlighted

10.7.4 Eyebrow Ptosis

Detecting eyebrow ptosis is not so easy because of the contraction of the frontalis muscle, which produces some degree of "balancing" elevation, as well as confusing the brow ptosis as a unique problem of hooded upper eyelid skin (Fig. 10.5a).

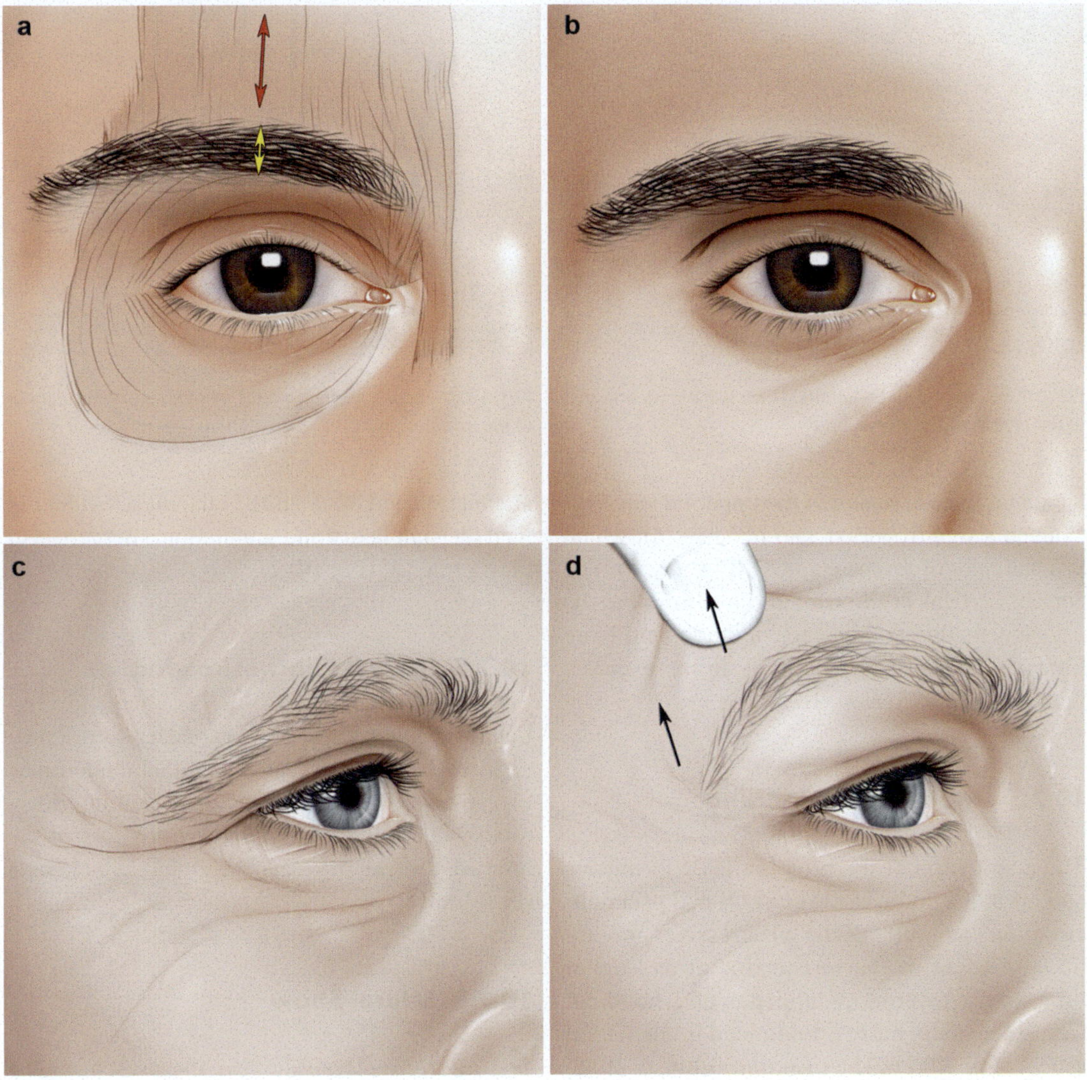

Fig. 10.5 The vertical position of the eyebrow is dynamically related to the activity of the frontalis muscle (**a**). A horizontal shadow at the level of the upper eyelid gives the illusion that the eyebrow is more ptotic than it really is (**b**). A lateral extension over the eyelid and onto the lateral periorbital region of the upper lid crease, or Connell's sign, is a hallmark of forehead ptosis (**c**). The correct vertical position of the eyebrow can be envisioned during the consultation, utilizing Flower's maneuver, by holding up the eyebrow with a fingertip (**d**)

The eyebrow, as with many other facial structures, is a moving target! So, after the correction of a ptotic upper marginal lid, the frontalis muscle contraction reduces with a downward repositioning of the eyebrow, which is now clearly ptotic to the examiner and patient.

Another problem lies in the illusional effect produced by a deep upper palpebral fold and/or prominent upper orbital margin. The resulting horizontal shadow makes the eyebrow "more ptotic" even if it is in the same vertical position. The loss of upper palpebral volume, either to a progressive involution or secondary to aggressive surgical treatment, creates a skeletonized orbit that is also responsible for this shadow (Fig. 10.5b).

In eyebrow analysis, it is important to detect a lateral extension over the eyelid and onto the

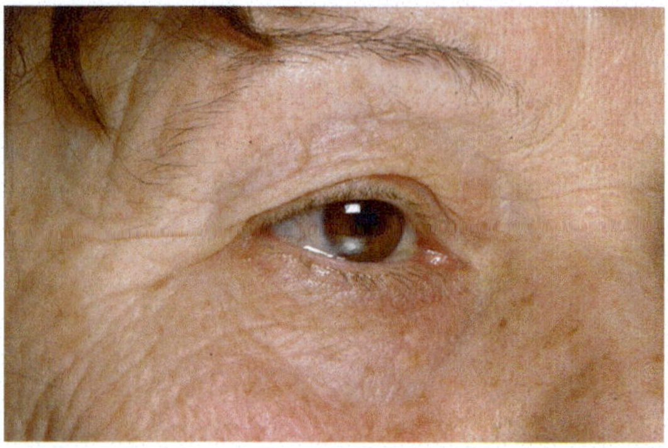

Fig. 10.6 Upper eyelid hooding, which is more pronounced in the lateral aspect of the orbit

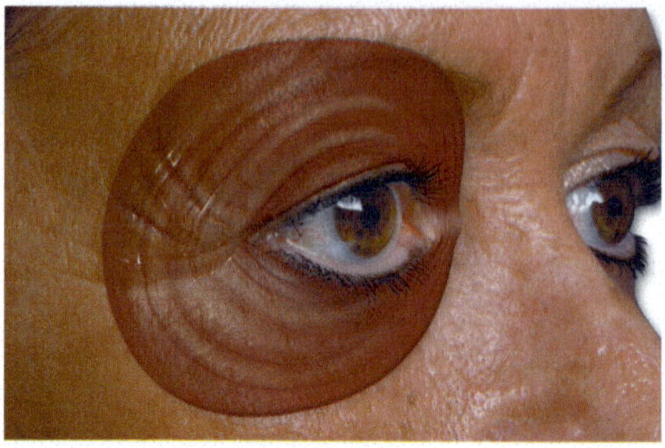

Fig. 10.7 Crow's feet and eyelid wrinkles and their relation to the orientation of the orbicularis oculi muscle

lateral periorbital region of the upper lid crease or Connell's sign (reported also in Chap. 6), which is a hallmark of forehead ptosis (Fig. 10.5c). The correct vertical position of the eyebrow can be envisioned during the consultation, utilizing Flower's maneuver, by holding up the eyebrow with a fingertip [5] (Fig. 10.5d).

10.7.5 Upper Eyelid Hooding

The attenuation of the orbicularis oculi muscle and orbital septum, the orbital fat pad pseudoherniation, as well as the progressive gravitational descent of the forehead skin and upper lid laxity, can produce upper eyelid hooding, which is usually more pronounced in the lateral aspect (Fig. 10.6). The eventual fullness in the medial aspect is due more to orbital fat pad pseudoherniation than skin excess. The redundancy of the skin, or dermatochalasis, can be assessed by pinching the excess of eyelid skin with a forceps until the eyelashes begin to evert (see Fig. 6.7).

10.7.6 Crow's Feet and Eyelid Wrinkles

Crow's feet and eyelid wrinkles are fine wrinkles or lines developing on the lower lid and the lateral aspect of the orbital region perpendicular to the fibers of the underlying orbicularis oculi muscle. In the evolution toward more evident lines, the attenuation and elongation of the muscle fibers as well the skin laxity and gravitational descent also play a role [3] (Fig. 10.7).

10.7.7 Lateral Canthal Bowing

Lateral canthal bowing is secondary to the progressive laxity of the lateral canthal tendon (see Fig. 6.6f). The visible effect is an inferiorly rotated lateral lid commissure with a loss of the upward lateral tilt of the intercanthal axis (Fig. 10.8).

10.7.8 Scleral Show

The inferior scleral show is the presence of a strip of white sclera between the iris and the lower lid margin with the subject in natural head position and straight gaze (Fig. 10.9). As a sign of aging, it is caused by the progressive laxity of the canthal tendons and the tarsus of the lower lid.

10.7.9 Baggy Lower Eyelid

The baggy lower eyelid is secondary to the combination of attenuation and lengthening of the skin, the orbicularis oculi muscle, the canthal tendons, and the orbital septum with pseudoherniation of orbital fat (Fig. 10.10). Orbital fat

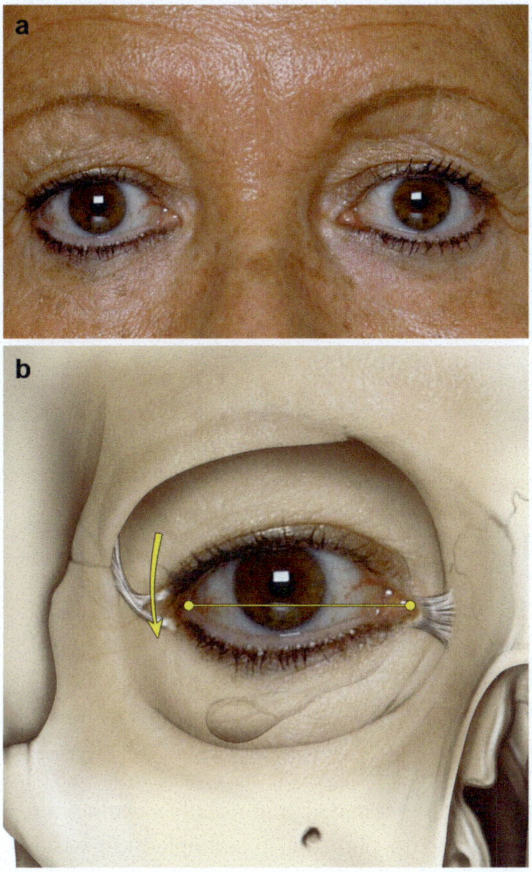

Fig. 10.8 Moderate lateral canthal bowing with a near horizontal intercanthal axis (**a**, **b**)

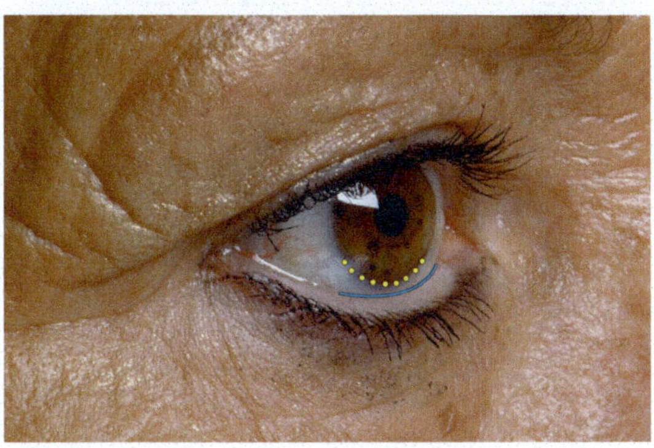

Fig. 10.9 Low grade of inferior scleral show caused by the progressive laxity of the canthal tendons and the tarsus of the lower lid

pseudoherniation can be pointed out and documented with the eye view looking-up picture (see Fig. 6.9b).

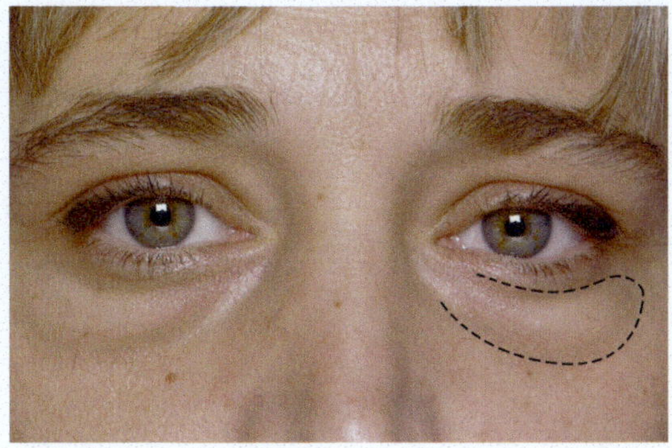

Fig. 10.10 A case of baggy lower eyelids in a middle-aged subject

10.7.10 Tear Trough Deformity (Palpebrojugal Fold) and Palpebral Malar Groove

A tear trough deformity (palpebrojugal fold) is a depression that develops along the medial part of the inferior orbital rim, which makes the region skeletonized. It is related to loss of fat secondary to aging or aggressive surgical lipectomy, but it can also be present in young untreated subjects. The eventual demarcation between the lower lid and the malar area, as a lateral continuation of the palpebrojugal fold, is the palpebral malar groove (Fig. 10.11).

10.7.11 Malar Bags (Festoons, "Cheek Bags")

Malar bags or festoons can be differentiated from the baggy lower eyelid because they occur below the level of the inferior orbital rim (Fig. 10.12). They are caused by attenuation of the orbicularis oculi muscle and overlying skin as well as by ptosis of the suborbicularis oculi fat pad [3].

10.7.12 Nasolabial Fold

This is the landmark that separates the lip from the cheek. Loss of cheek support results in antero-inferior descent of subcutaneous fat with inferior accumulation of tissue, deepening the fold, and

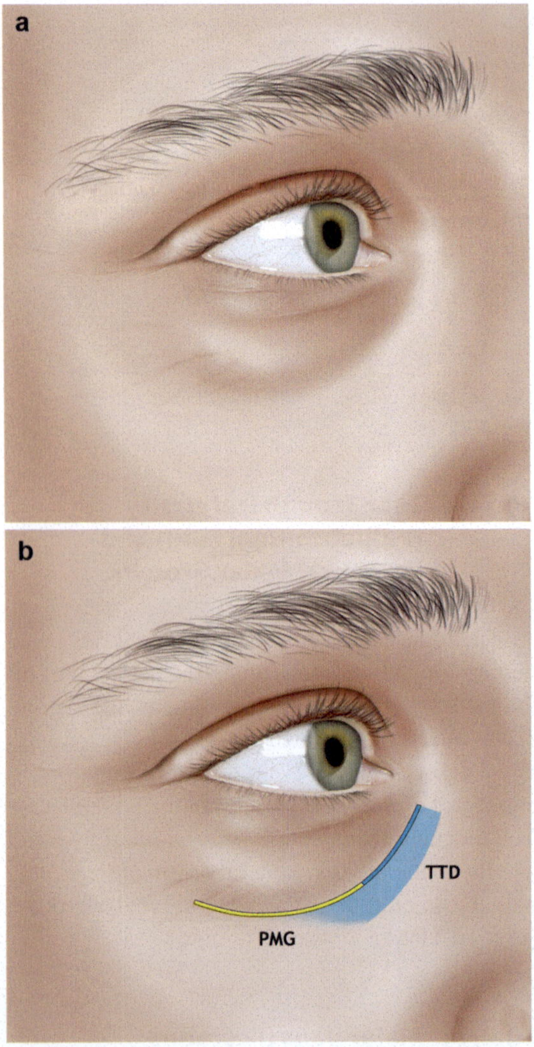

Fig. 10.11 Tear trough deformity (palpebrojugal fold) and palpebral malar groove (**a**). The spatial location of tear trough deformity (*TTD*, palpebrojugal fold) is depicted in *light blue*, whereas the palpebral malar groove (*PMG*) is depicted in *yellow* (**b**)

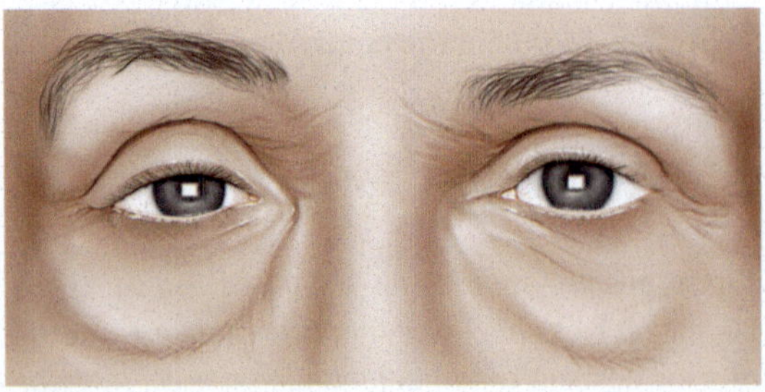

Fig. 10.12 Malar bags or festoons

superior loss of tissue. The fat cannot continue its descent because of the presence, at the level of the nasolabial line, of a dense fascia-to-dermis adherence; this leads to the formation of a deep nasolabial groove and a heavy nasolabial fold more or less associated with a skeletonized appearance of the cheekbone [3] (Fig. 10.13).

10.7.13 Preauricular Lines

These vertically oriented lines, usually two or three, develop in the preauricular region, in front of the tragus and the lobule (Fig. 10.13b).

10.7.14 Lip Lines

The upper and lower radial lip lines are mimetic wrinkles that are more pronounced as they reach the vermillion (Fig. 10.13). They are caused by the association between repeated muscular contracture, dermal atrophy, and attenuation and lengthening of the orbicularis oris muscle. This horizontally oriented line usually develops over the upper lip philtrum as a single skin wrinkle (Fig. 10.13).

10.7.15 Horizontal Upper Lip Line

This horizontally oriented line usually develops over the upper lip philtrum as a single skin wrinkle (Fig. 10.13).

10.7.16 Vertical Lengthening of the Upper Lip and Ptosis of the Lip Commissures

The vertical length of the skin portion of the upper lip increases during the entire lifetime with a progressive augmentation of the skin/vermillion ratio. Also the thickness and the anterior projection in profile view are prone to diminish with a reduction in volume of the red portion of the lip (red lip involution). An accompanying sign is the ptosis of the two commissures (Fig. 10.13).

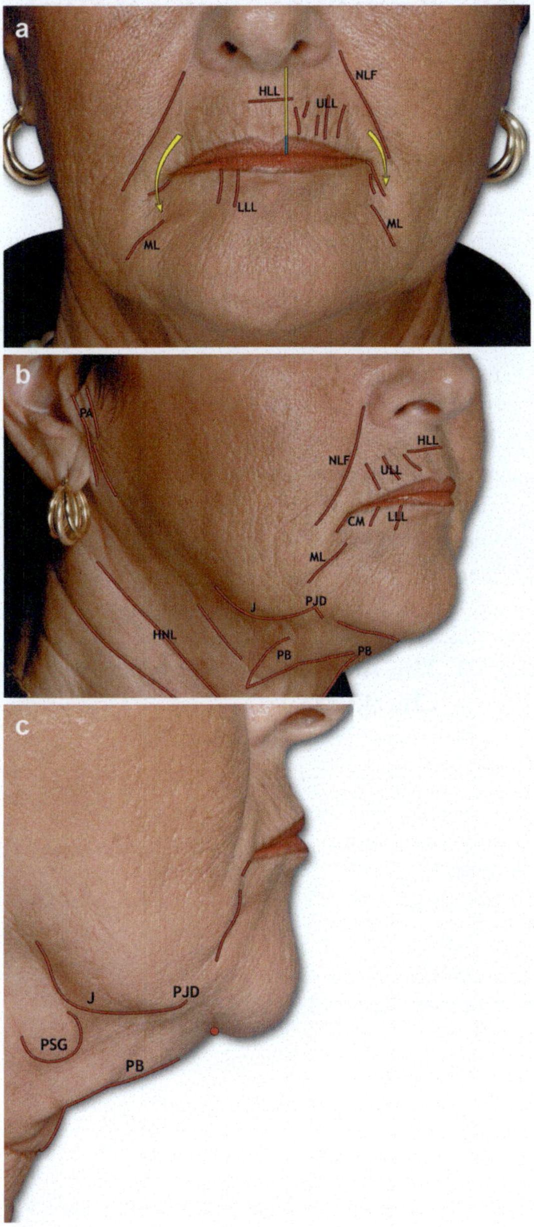

Fig. 10.13 Aging signs affecting the lower third of the face in frontal (**a**), oblique (**b**), and profile views (**c**). *NLF* nasolabial fold, *PA* preauricular lines, *HLL* horizontal upper lip line, *ULL* upper lip lines, *LLL* lower lip lines, *CM* corner of the mouth lines, *ML* marionette lines, *J* jowls bulge, *PJD* prejowl depression, *PB* platysma bands, *HNL* horizontal neck lines, *PSG* ptotic submandibular gland bulge. The upper lip skin/vermillion ratio is increased due to the lengthening of the skin portion and reduction of the vermillion portion

10.7.17 Corner of the Mouth Lines (Commissural Lines) and "Marionette" Lines

The corner of the mouth lines are short, vertically oriented, bilateral, sometimes very deep lines that depart from the oral commissure, whereas the marionette lines are longer, vertical lines that laterally circumscribe the chin (Fig. 10.13).

10.7.18 Jowls and Prejowl Depression

The "jowls" is an accumulation of subcutaneous fat along and inferior to the mandibular border. Its anterior limits, the prejowl depression, are defined by the presence of the mandibular retaining ligaments, which prevent any further anterior migration of fat [3] (Fig. 10.13).

10.7.19 Witch's Chin Deformity (Ptotic Chin)

The witch's chin deformity or ptotic chin is the flattening and ptosis of the chin pad associated with the deepening of the submental crease. It can be age-related or secondary to previous surgery (Fig. 10.13).

10.7.20 Platysma Bands and Loss of Cervicomental Angle

Platysma bands are vertical, large skin bands, one for each side, rising from the submental area and extending inferiorly, altering the cervicomental profile (Fig. 10.13). Muscular attenuation, lengthening, and dehiscence, along with fat accumulation and neck skin relaxation, cause these bands.

10.7.21 Horizontal Neck Lines

The horizontal semicircular neck lines occupy the anterior neck skin and are perpendicular to the underlying fibers of platysma muscle (Fig. 10.13). Their presence, in the form of fine lines, precedes the other signs of neck aging.

10.7.22 Ptotic Submandibular Gland

The ptosis of the inferior pole of the submandibular gland produces a bulge on the submandibular region, 1 or 2 cm inferior to the mandibular border (Fig. 10.13). The glandular origin of the bulge is confirmed with palpation.

10.8 Recognizing Nasal Aging

With aging, the nose undergoes many important changes that should not be ignored during clinical examination. Furthermore, in adult or older subjects, the probability of finding signs of a previous nasal trauma or surgery is high.

The nasal skin soft tissue envelope loses elasticity and becomes attenuated, permitting a gravitational descent of the tip. The cartilaginous framework reduces some of its tensile strength, and the ligamentous structures that maintain the lower lateral cartilages together and suspended to the upper lateral ones become less efficacious [2, 6]. Some of the visible and palpable effects of nasal aging are:

- The presence of the horizontal frown line occupying the radix perpendicular to the orientation of the fibers of procerus muscle
- Skin atrophy except for the tip area, which can undergo an increased sebaceous activity, augmenting its thickness
- The clockwise rotation of the tip, which becomes ptotic and underprojected
- Ptosis of the columella with a reduction in the nasolabial angle and a relative deepening of the subnasal point
- Increased prominence of the dorsal hump as a secondary effect of progressive skeletonization of the nose and loss of tip projection

The external signs are associated with many internal changes that are responsible for a progressive reduction of the function of the nose, such as warming, humidifying, and cleaning the ambient air on inspiration. These changes must not be underevaluated in the preoperative phase.

10.9 Recognizing Aging in the Oral Frame

Many visible effects of aging in the lower third of the face are concentrated in the oral frame:

- The reduction of exposed vermillion is accompanied by the disappearance of the lip white rolls.
- The progressive elongation of the upper lip obscures the upper anterior teeth both in repose and while smiling.
- The progressive lower lip descends, increasing the exposure of the lower anterior teeth both in repose and while smiling.
- The teeth morphology changes due to abrasion of the incisors and canine margin and gingival retraction (the resulting length of anterior visible teeth depends on the combination of marginal abrasion and gingival retraction).

10.10 The Aging Face Analysis Checklist[3]

- In the frontal view, the facial shape is:
  □ Triangular
  □ Rectangular
  □ Wide
  □ Narrow
  □ Long
  □ Short
- Does the face look old?
  □ No
  □ Yes, because…
- Does the face look skeletonized?
  □ No
  □ Yes, because…
- Define the facial supporting skeletal framework:
  □ Ideal for sex and age
  □ Altered, because…
- Define the facial fat distribution:
  □ Ideal for sex and age
  □ Altered, because…
- Define the facial skin redundancy:
  □ Absent
  □ Moderate
  □ Marked

[3]Section 2 on Springer Extra Materials (extra.springer.com)

- The hairline is:
  □ Normally positioned
  □ Too high
  □ Too low
- The forehead profile is:
  □ Flat
  □ Round
  □ Presence of inferior concavity (clear definite orbital bar)
- The supraorbital bar is:
  □ Normally shaped
  □ Protruding
  □ Recessive
- Forehead transverse lines:
  □ Just visible
  □ Moderate
  □ Marked
- Vertical frown lines (glabellar lines):
  □ Absent
  □ Moderate
  □ Marked
- Horizontal frown line (nasal radix line):
  □ Absent
  □ Moderate
  □ Marked
- Temporal depression:
  □ Absent
  □ Moderate
  □ Marked
- Does the orbital region look aged?
  □ No
  □ Yes, because…
- Define the eyebrow vertical position (eyebrow ptosis?):
  □ Ideal for sex and age
  □ Altered, because…
- Define the symmetry of the eyebrows:
  □ Present
  □ Absent due to…
- Define the symmetry of the eye globes:
  □ Present
  □ Absent due to…
- Define the symmetry of the eyelids:
  □ Present
  □ Absent due to…
- Define the upper lid crease position:
  □ Ideal
  □ Too high
  □ Too low
- Define the upper lid margin position:
  □ Ideal
  □ Too high
  □ Too low
- Define the lower lid margin position:
  □ Ideal
  □ Too high
  □ Too low
- Define the lateral canthus position:
  □ Ideal
  □ Altered, because…
- Upper eyelid dermatochalasis (upper eyelid hooding):
  □ Absent
  □ Moderate
  □ Marked
  □ Limiting the superotemporal visual field (pathological)
- Upper eyelid ptosis:
  □ Right,…
  □ Left,…
- Upper lid herniated orbital fat:
  □ No
  □ Right
  □ Left
- Prolapsed lacrimal gland:
  □ No
  □ Right
  □ Left
- Skeletal lower lid support:
  □ Poor
  □ Acceptable
  □ Ideal
- Define the malar eminence:
  □ Hypoplastic
  □ Balanced
  □ Pronounced
- Lower eyelid laxity:
  □ No
  □ Right
  □ Left
- Baggy lower eyelid:
  □ Absent
  □ Moderate
  □ Marked
- Lower lid herniated orbital fat:
  □ No
  □ Right
  □ Left

- Lateral canthal bowing:
  □ Absent
  □ Moderate
  □ Marked
- Scleral show:
  □ No
  □ Yes, right… mm, left… mm
- Hypertrophic orbicularis oculi muscle (tarsal portion):
  □ Right,…
  □ Left,…
- Crow's feet and eyelid wrinkles:
  □ Absent
  □ Moderate
  □ Marked
- Tear trough deformity (palpebrojugal fold):
  □ Absent
  □ Moderate
  □ Marked
- Palpebral malar fold:
  □ Absent
  □ Moderate
  □ Marked
- Malar bags (festoons, cheek bags):
  □ No
  □ Right
  □ Left
- Eye globe proptosis (exophthalmos):
  □ Right,…
  □ Left,…
- Eye globe enophthalmos:
  □ Right,…
  □ Left,…
- Does the nose look aged?
  □ No
  □ Yes, because…
- Does the nose look skeletonized?
  □ No
  □ Yes
- Is there loss of tip projection?
  □ No
  □ Yes
- Is there columellar ptosis?
  □ No
  □ Yes
- Preauricular lines:
  □ Absent
  □ Moderate
  □ Marked
- Nasolabial fold:
  □ Ideal for sex and age
  □ Increased
  □ Heavy
- Does the mouth look aged?
  □ No
  □ Yes, because…
- Vertical length of the upper lip:
  □ Short
  □ Ideal for sex and age
  □ Slightly augmented
  □ Augmented
- Upper lip skin/vermillion ratio:
  □ Ideal for sex and age
  □ Increased
- The upper lip profile is:
  □ Normally projected
  □ Too anterior
  □ Too posterior
- The lower lip profile is:
  □ Normally projected
  □ Too anterior
  □ Too posterior
- Upper lip lines:
  □ Absent
  □ Moderate
  □ Marked
- Horizontal upper lip line:
  □ Absent
  □ Moderate
  □ Marked
- Lower lip lines:
  □ Absent
  □ Moderate
  □ Marked
- Ptosis of the lip commissures:
  □ Absent
  □ Moderate
  □ Marked
- Corner of the mouth lines:
  □ Absent
  □ Moderate
  □ Marked
- Marionette lines:
  □ Absent
  □ Moderate
  □ Marked
- "Jowls":
  □ Absent
  □ Moderate
  □ Marked

- Witch's chin deformity (ptotic chin):
  □ Absent
  □ Moderate
  □ Marked
- Does the neck look aged?
  □ No
  □ Yes, because…
- Horizontal neck lines:
  □ Minimal
  □ Moderate
  □ Marked
- Platysma bands:
  □ Absent
  □ Moderate
  □ Marked
- Ptotic submandibular gland:
  □ Absent
  □ Moderate
  □ Marked R L
- Define the mandibular border definition from angle to chin:
  □ Ideal
  □ Poor
- Define the throat length:
  □ Ideal
  □ Too short
  □ Too long
- Define the throat incline:
  □ Ideal
  □ Excessively down oriented
- Define the cervicomental angle:
  □ Ideal
  □ Too acute
  □ Too obtuse

10.11 The Aging Face: Preferred Terms[4]

10.11.1 Wrinkles, Mimetic Lines, Mimetic Furrows, and Folds

The superficial age-related changes in the skin can be classified as follows (Fig. 10.14): [4]

- *Wrinkles* (fine superficial lines). They are associated with textural changes of the skin surface.

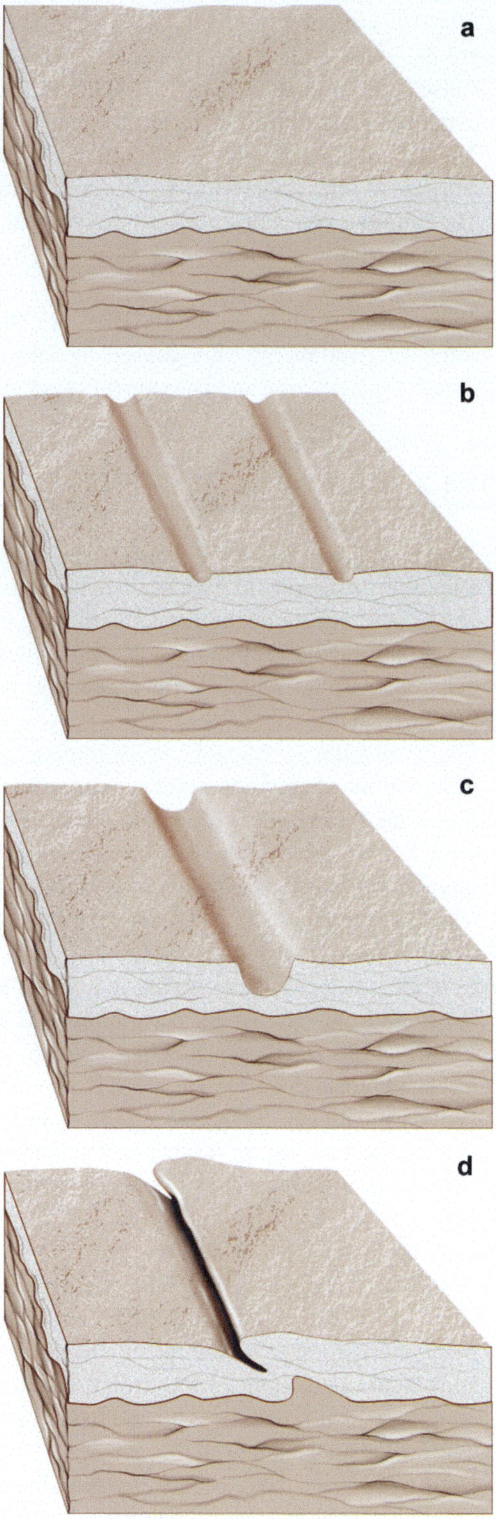

Fig. 10.14 Wrinkles (**a**), mimetic lines (**b**) and furrows (**c**), and skin Folds (**d**)

[4]Section 3 on Springer Extra Materials (extra.springer.com)

- *Mimetic wrinkles* (lines and furrows). They are the visible effect of deep dermal creasing caused by repeated facial movement and expression combined with dermal elastosis. These lines are perpendicularly oriented with respect to the underlying muscular fibers. The mimetic wrinkles can be divided into lines (partial thickness) and furrows (full thickness).
- *Skin folds* (overlapping skin). They are the result of overlapping skin caused by laxity, loss of tone, gravity, and consequent sagging.

10.11.2 Other Terms

- *Baggy eyelid* (*inferior lid bags*). The bulge affecting the lower lid area secondary to the combination of attenuation and lengthening of the skin, orbicularis oculi muscle, canthal tendons, and orbital septum with pseudoherniation of orbital fat.
- *Blepharochalasis*. Should be differentiated from dermatochalasis. It is an uncommon condition characterized by episodic edema and erythema of the eyelids. Blepharochalasis is more common in young women and may result in premature relaxation and laxity of the eyelid skin with wrinkling and hooding.
- *Connell's sign*. A lateral extension over the eyelid and onto the lateral periorbital region. The Connell's sign is considered a hallmark of forehead ptosis [5].
- *Crow's feet and eyelid wrinkles*. Fine wrinkles or lines developing on the lower lid and the lateral aspect of the orbital region perpendicular to the fibers of the underlying orbicularis oculi muscle.
- *Eyelid bags* (*baggy eyelid*). The visible bags of the lower eyelid caused by the processes of pseudoherniation of orbital fat and the attenuation and lengthening of the orbital septum, orbicularis oculi muscle, skin, and lower canthus (see also "Festoons").
- *Dermatochalasis*. Excess of eyelid skin that is usually more prevalent in the upper eyelids. It is a frequent condition in middle-aged subjects and a common one in the elderly.
- *Festoons* (*or cheek bags, malar bags*). Ptosis of the suborbicularis oculi fat. Malar bags should be differentiated from eyelid bags because they occur below the inferior orbital rim.
- *Forehead transverse furrows* (*worry lines*). The long horizontal mimetic furrows developing on the forehead perpendicular to the fibers of the underlying frontalis muscle.
- *Glabellar creases* (*frown lines, vertical glabellar lines*). The mainly vertical oriented mimetic skin lines developing on the glabella perpendicular to the fibers of the underlying corrugator muscle.
- *Herniated orbital fat* (*pseudoherniated orbital fat*). The anterior displacement of the fat located under the orbital septum. It should be examined with the patient in the upright sitting or standing position. The orbital fat pads are classically divided into two upper compartments (medial and central) and three lower compartments (medial, central, and lateral).
- *Horizontal upper lip lines* (*transverse upper lip lines*). One or two horizontal lines located centrally over the philtrum of the upper lip.
- *Intercanthal axis*. The imaginary line connecting the medial and lateral canthus.
- *Jowls*. A visible accumulation of subcutaneous fat along and inferior to the mandibular border. Its anterior limits, the prejowl depression, are defined by the presence of the mandibular retaining ligaments, which prevent any further anterior migration of fat.
- *Labial commissure*. The point of lateral confluence of the lips. During the act of smiling, it consists of the inner and the outer commissure.
- *Lagophthalmos*. Incomplete eyelid closure.
- *Lateral canthal bowing*. Secondary to the progressive laxity of the lateral canthal tendon. The visible effect is an inferiorly rotated lateral lid commissure with a loss of the upward lateral tilt of the intercanthal axis [3].
- *Lid tone* (*eyelid laxity*). The ability of the lids to maintain spontaneously and recover (recapture) quickly their normal position against the globe. The presence of horizontal lid laxity should be assessed by performing the snap test and the lid distraction test.

The lid should not be pulled more than 7 mm away from the globe (distraction test) and should snap back into its normal position immediately (snap test).

- *Lip white rolls*. The linear white skin relief placed around the vermillion border of both lips. It flattens and sometimes totally disappears with aging.
- *Lip lines*. The upper and lower radial lip lines. They are mimetic wrinkles, which are more pronounced as they reach the vermillion.
- *Marionette and commissural lines* (*corner of the mouth line*). Vertically oriented lines, which develop directly from the oral commissure (commissural line) or above and laterally to it (marionette line).
- *Nasolabial fold and nasolabial groove* (*nasolabial line*). The landmark that separates the lip from the cheek. Loss of cheek support results in anteroinferior descent of subcutaneous fat with accumulation of inferior tissue, deepening the fold, and loss of superior tissue. The fat cannot continue its descent because of the presence of a dense fascia-to-dermis adherence at the level of the nasolabial line; the various final effects are the formation of a deep nasolabial groove and a heavy nasolabial fold.
- *Palpebral malar groove*. The eventual demarcation between the lower lid and the malar area.
- *Platysma bands* ("*turkey gobbler*" *effect*). The vertical skin bands, usually one for each side, of the aged submental and neck region. They are caused by platysma muscle attenuation, lengthening, and dehiscence, along with fat accumulation and skin excess and photodamage.
- *Preauricular lines*. Vertically oriented lines, usually two or three, which develop in the preauricular region, in front of the tragus and the lobule.
- *Prolapsed lacrimal gland*. A prolapsed lacrimal gland can produce an excessive fullness of the upper eyelid in the temporal third (there is no orbital fat in the upper temporal angle of the orbit).
- *Red lip involutions*. The progressive reduction of exposed vermillion as well as its volume, combined with the augmentation of the vertical length of the upper lip skin.
- *Scleral show* (*inferior scleral show*). The presence of a strip of white sclera between the iris and the lower lid margin with the subject in natural head position and straight gaze. It may be a sign of exophthalmos, previous trauma, prior surgery, lower lid laxity, or dentofacial deformities with maxillary hypoplasia.
- *Submandibular gland ptosis*. The visible bulge produced by the inferior pole of the submandibular gland in the submandibular triangle.
- *Tear trough deformity* (*palpebrojugal fold*). A depression that develops along the medial part of the inferior orbital rim, which makes the region skeletonized. It is related to loss of fat secondary to aging or aggressive surgical lipectomy, but it can also be present in young untreated subjects.
- *Temporal atrophy*. The progressive loss of soft tissue volume that affects the temporal region and makes its skeletal boundaries more visible.
- *Transverse nasal line*. The horizontal single frown line occupying the radix perpendicular to the orientation of the fibers of procerus muscle.
- *Witch's chin deformity* (*ptotic chin*). The flattening and the ptosis of the chin pad associated with the deepening of the submental crease. It can be age-related or iatrogenic.
- *Worry lines*. See Sect. 10.7.1.

References

1. Baumann L (2002) Cosmetic dermatology. Principle and practice. McGraw Hill, New York
2. Lam SM, Williams EF (2004) Rejuvenation of the aging nose. In: Williams EF, Lam SM (eds) Comprehensive facial rejuvenation. Lippincott Williams & Wilkins, Philadelphia
3. LaTrenta G (2004) Atlas of aesthetic face and neck surgery. Saunders, Philadelphia
4. Lemperle G, Holmes RE, Coven SR, Lemperle SM (2001) A classification of facial wrinkles. Plast Reconstr Surg 108:1735–1750
5. Marten TJ, Knize DM (2001) Forehead aesthetics and preoperative assessment of the foreheadplasty patient.

In: Knize DM (ed) The forehead and temporal fossa. Anatomy and technique. Lippincott Williams & Wilkins, Philadelphia, pp 91–99
6. Rohrich RJ, Hollier LH, Gunter JP (2002) The aging nose. In: Gunter JP, Rohrich RJ, Adams WP (eds) Dallas rhinoplasty. Nasal surgery by the master. Quality Medical Publishing, St. Louis
7. Senge PM (1990) The fifth discipline: the art and science of the learning organization. Doubleday Dell, New York

11 Continuing Facial Analysis Utilizing Four Images by Man Ray

Contents

This chapter is based on three portraits and one self-portrait by one of the most influential and inventive artists of the last century: Man Ray. He had a special sensitivity with regard to the positioning and lighting of subjects for photographic portraits and developed, probably unconsciously, a personal approach to highlighting facial features.

The works of art by Man Ray reproduced in this chapter are the property of the Marconi Foundation in Milan. The authors wish to thank Giorgio Marconi for his substantial contribution to our project.

11.1 Man Ray's Unconventional Oblique Views

Being an artist, Man Ray was completely free from the standards and fixed conventions reported in this text when he created his portraits. An example of this is the way in which we kept the camera at the same height as the subject or the way in which we aligned them with their heads in a natural position. However, when studying Man Ray's prolific photographic work, it is evident that some details of his approach are also immovable, repetitive, and conventional:

- The shoulders are only just inside the picture frame.
- A vast, uniform, and neutral background surrounds the entire head.

F. Meneghini, P. Biondi, *Clinical Facial Analysis*,
DOI 10.1007/978-3-642-27228-8_11, © Springer-Verlag Berlin Heidelberg 2012

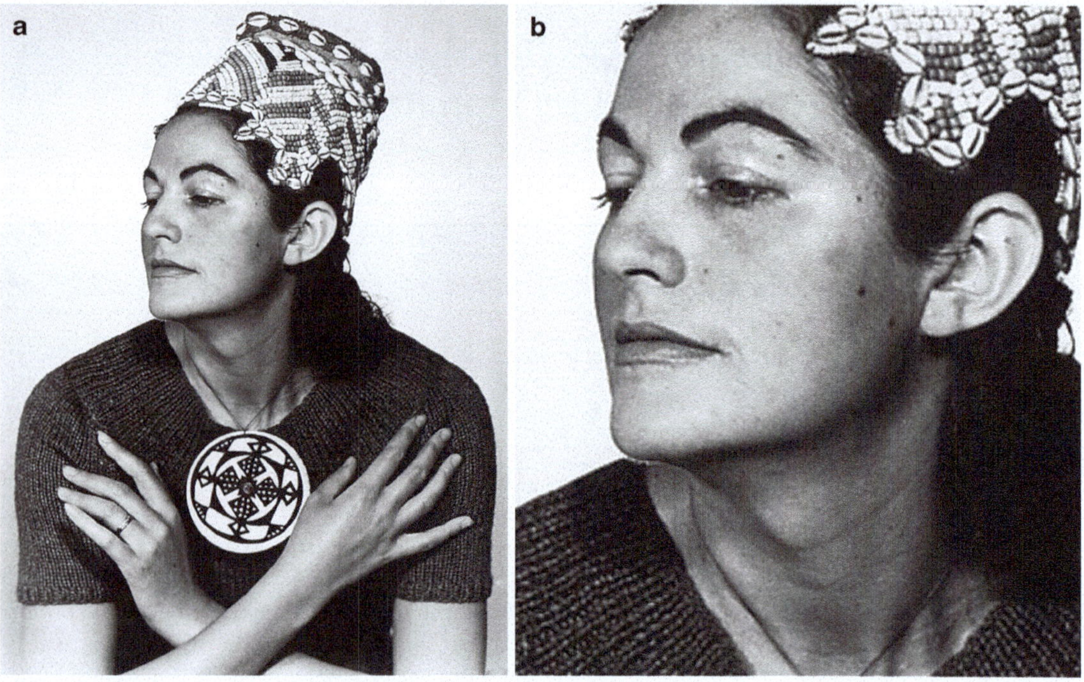

Fig. 11.1 (**a**, **b**) Man Ray: Mode au Congo (1937). Three quarter view with the head tilted slightly upward in order to advance the chin and stretch the neck skin. In this case, the frame best shows the projection and proportion of the right cheekbone-cheek-chin silhouette

- Three quarter views are mostly utilized, preferring those that highlight the nose or cheekbones best.
- The head is turned slightly upward to advance the chin and pull tight the skin of the neck.

Man Ray's portraits depict some facial features very well – particularly the nose, cheekbones, lips, and chin. This is also the result of the distance of the camera from the subject, giving us a better idea of the person depicted in terms of personality, behavior, and attitude.

A clear example of this is shown in Figs. 11.1, 11.2, and 11.3 which were all selected from the series "Mode au Congo" of 1937. That year, Harper's Bazaar asked Man Ray for a set of fashion photos for which the artist was granted the freedom by the editor to personally select hats or headdresses utilizing unusual styles and material.

Perhaps a broader documentation of the patient, including some photos taken at an increased distance by the physician/photographer, would also give the patient a more independent and, thus, a more spontaneous role in exhibiting and expressing himself. This could be considered in the near future, taking into account the difficulties imposed by an unconventional approach.

11.2 Man Ray's Asymmetrical Face

Figure 11.4 is a self-portrait which clearly illustrates the awareness of Man Ray of his asymmetrical face. The original idea lies in the fact that Man Ray selected as a reference the deformed, deviated lower third of his nose instead of more stable, symmetrical facial features such as his eye globes or the glabella.

The photo taken in 1930 was realized by crossing two thin black lines, one horizontal and one vertical, between the lower third and the middle

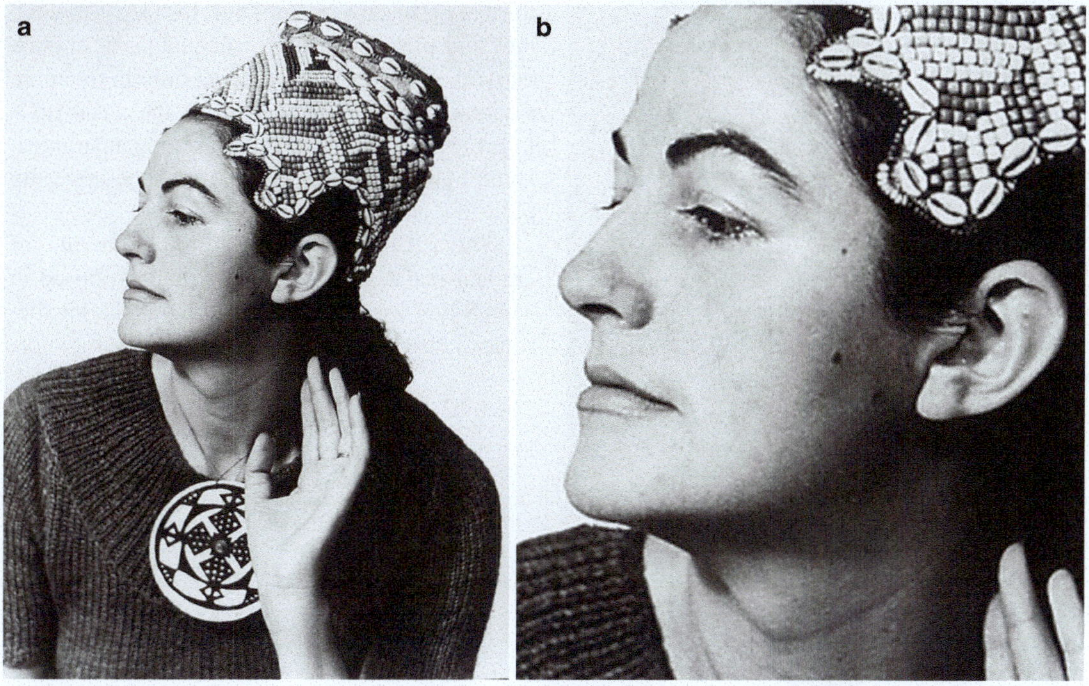

Fig. 11.2 (**a**, **b**) Man Ray: Mode au Congo (1937). Three quarter view with the head tilted slightly upward in order to advance the chin and stretch the neck skin. In this case, the frame shows the nasal features off best

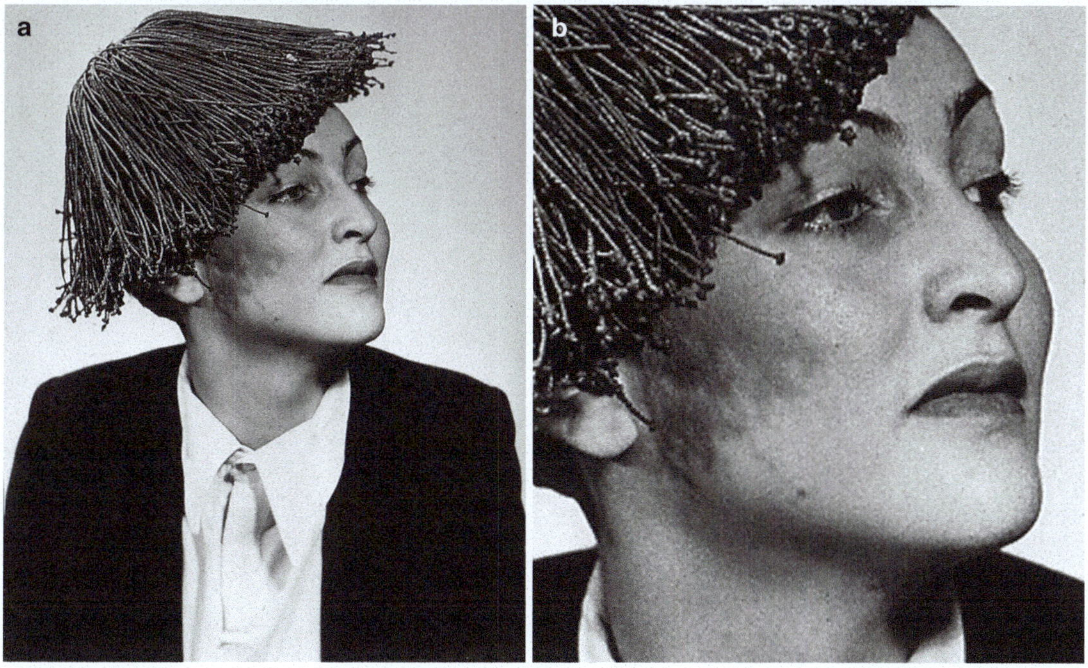

Fig. 11.3 (**a**, **b**) Man Ray: Mode au Congo (1937). Three quarter view with the head tilted slightly upward in order to advance the chin and stretch the neck skin. As in Fig. 11.1a, b, this frame shows the projection and proportion of the left cheekbone–cheek–chin silhouette off best

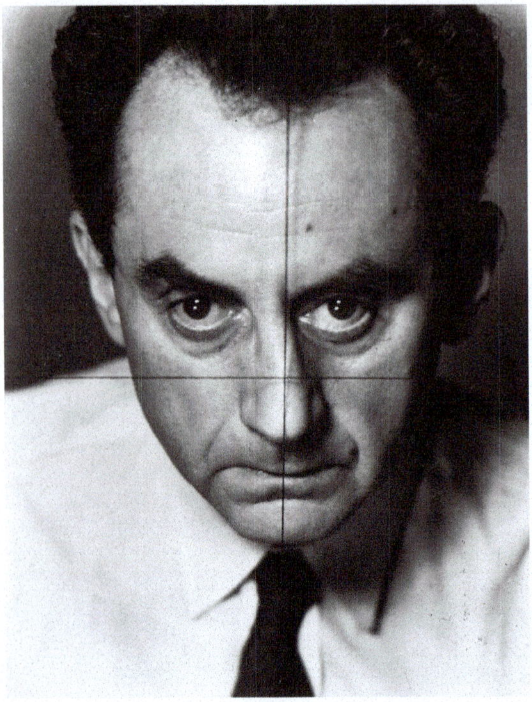

Fig. 11.4 Man Ray: self portrait (1930). The reference lines cross over the deformity of the deviated nose instead of the symmetrical features of the face

third of his nasal dorsum. Thus, his face is divided into four principal, clearly unequal parts, and the vertical reference line, centered only in the more asymmetrical part of the face – the nasal tip – fails to touch any of the other existing anatomical medial points such as the glabella, the upper lip philtrum, and the chin.

With a "Copernican" revolution of the rules of clinical facial analysis, the method proposed in Man Ray's self-portrait greatly helps the inexperienced observer to appreciate facial asymmetry.

Continuing Facial Analysis

12

The important thing is not to stop questioning
– Albert Einstein

Contents

Following the "spiral of analysis" requires continuous effort in many phases of our practice. When you have an individually tailored and patient-accepted treatment plan for the following day's surgery, these continuous efforts are directed toward the checking activity. Again, the most important advice is not to stop analyzing and questioning.

12.1 Meet the Patient the Day Before the Operation

One of my favorite moments in the preoperative phase is the meeting the day before. Even if all the preoperative steps are concluded and the informed consent documentation is signed, I like to go over the goals of the procedure together with my patient only a few hours before the surgery. The other main points of the meeting the day before are:

- Verify all the medical records. Do they contain evidence of first-visit patient education? Do they contain evidence of the procedure you will later perform? Do they include a complete history and physical examination? Do they include a complete and itemized patient priority list? Are the preoperative analysis and planning sheets ready for tomorrow?
- If the patient is a smoker, verify that she has stopped smoking before the procedure.
- Verify that she has not taken aspirin in the previous 2 weeks.

F. Meneghini, P. Biondi, *Clinical Facial Analysis*,
DOI 10.1007/978-3-642-27228-8_12,

- Verify that you have the opportunity to meet the patient's wishes with the treatment plan!

I believe it is absurd and dangerous to operate on a patient without a recent and conclusive preoperative meeting.

12.2 Continuing Facial Analysis in the Operating Room

12.2.1 The Basic Preoperative Documents Are Hanging up in the Operating Room

For any major facial surgery procedure, I hang the following documents up on the nearest wall of the operating room:

- The step-by-step operative surgical sequence planned.
- The printed photographs containing the notes written during the previous consultation together with conventional radiographs, CT scans, etc.
- The itemized list of goals for the procedure. At any time during the procedure, I can stand up, take two or three steps, and verify, on the documents, that my surgery fits the treatment plan.

12.2.2 Problems Related to General Anesthesia and Patient Positioning During Facial Surgery

> But, suddenly, they were like a car that loses its headlights while speeding down a mountain road on a dark night.
>
> – Champy and Nohria [1]

Looking at the patient's face a moment before the surgical incisions, you can note several important problems:

- It is probably the first time that you have seen this patient in the supine position.
- The head positioning is technically limited to avoid the risk of cervical trauma and to assure a stable and safe body position on the operating table.
- Your viable points of view are quite different from those utilized during the consultation.
- Gravity acts on mobile structures, the mandible and the soft tissue, with a vector oriented from the tip of the nose toward the ear instead of the usual cephalocaudal axis.
- The effects of gravity on the soft tissue are not counteracted by muscular tone due to the effects of general anesthesia.
- The drapes partially hide the face and, due to their weight, stretch and deform the facial skin.
- The intense operative light illuminates a restricted area and produces hard and unnatural shadows.
- Around the operative field, the light brightness decreases, creating a visual contrast.
- The endotracheal tube and the surgical tape utilized to fix it deform and hide some areas of the face.
- Orthognathic surgery and other facial procedures require a particular head position, such as the extended one, which contributes to an unnatural way of visualizing.
- The disinfecting solution partially erases your preoperative skin drawings.
- The infiltration of the soft tissue with local anesthetic solution produces a localized swelling.

These 12 intraoperative problems, which are only partially avoidable, require that during every step of the surgical procedure, the surgeon can see and compare his actions to the preoperative photographic and planning documentation. Again, keeping a well-prepared preoperative work in the operating theater is fundamental for facial surgery.

12.3 The Intraoperative and Postoperative Procedure Documentation

Taking intraoperative photographs or small video sequences of the main surgical steps should be common practice in the operating theater, at least for the most demanding procedures, and in every case, something of particular interest is found.

The surgeon should describe the surgical steps in detail immediately following surgery, not delegating the task to others. Making drawings during the operation, or filling in specific graphical templates, can be useful in the postoperative

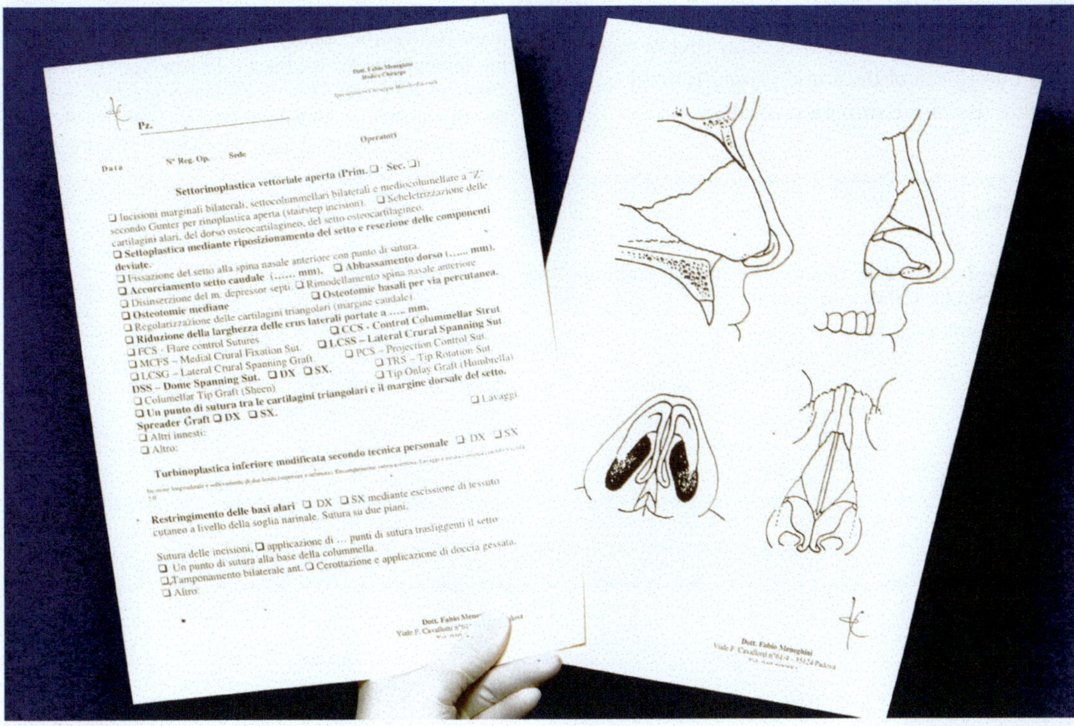

Fig. 12.1 Open rhinoplasty description worksheet. On one side, the surgeon fills in the form and reports any steps or adjunctive procedures performed. On the other side, he draws and adds notes over a modified version of the "Gunter diagram," enhancing the amount and value of the information recorded

analysis to enhance the value of the work performed in the operating theater.

For each of my open rhinoplasty cases, for example, I have adapted a modified version of the "Gunter diagram" (Fig. 12.1) printed onto a worksheet with a form reporting the most utilized steps of the procedure [2, 3].

12.4 The Continuing Facial Analysis in the Early Postoperative Phase

The final result is not the unique result!

When treating the face, the most visible – important – anatomical region of a person, we are also responsible for the postoperative discomfort of our patients, the postoperative external aspect, the time needed to return home, the time needed to return to work, and the time needed to restart physical activity. Close monitoring of the healing phase, sometimes with accurate photographic documentation, offers particular extra value to the surgeon, such as:

- The possibility of judging the immediate and early effects of the treatment on the patient
- The chance to reassure the patient about the unavoidable small problems of the postoperative phase
- The opportunity to check that the patient correctly follows the postoperative therapy
- A further opportunity to vary the postoperative therapy, if necessary
- A further way to maintain direct – uninterrupted – communication with the patient

12.5 The Continuing Facial Analysis in the Late Postoperative Phase

The initial clinical facial analysis material should not become a freeze-frame of an old case. It is the starting point of a dynamic process in which we must find as many cause-and-effect relationships as possible.

For any major surgical procedure, the routine postoperative photographs are taken at least

3 months and 1 year postoperatively. The new photographic set is taken only after reviewing the initial one to select the same projections in order to obtain the best comparative values.

References

1. Champy J, Nohria N (2000) The arc of ambition. Perseus Books, Cambridge, p 113
2. Gunter JP (1989) A graphic record of intraoperative maneuvers in rhinoplasty: the missing link for evaluating rhinoplasty results. Plast Reconstr Surg 84:204
3. Tebbetts JB (1998) Practice management documents for rhinoplasty – appendix D. In: Tebbetts JB (ed) Primary rhinoplasty. A new approach to the logic and techniques. Mosby, St. Louis

Aesthetic Facial Surgery: First Consultation Notes, Essential Medical History, and Clinical Diary

13

Contents

In 2005, the senior author (FM) conceived and produced a new pliable case sheet for aesthetic facial surgery patients named *Aesthetic Facial Surgery*: *First Consultation Notes*, *Essential Medical History* & *Clinical Diary* (*AFS Folder*) (Fig. 13.1a, b). One thousand copies of the *AFS Case Sheet* were printed, and these were utilized for every new patient who was seeking aesthetic facial surgical procedures.

The objectives of this simple, cheap instrument are numerous and as follows:

- To help surgeons establish the best line of communication
- To facilitate cooperation between patient and physician
- To organize a "basic" standard patient interview
- To record, in the most straightforward way, the patient's initial requests
- To help surgeons select patients and decide if a person is an ideal candidate for aesthetic facial surgery
- To help the surgeon to plan surgery and communicate objectives and drawbacks
- To help surgeons to describe the exact position and length of every planned facial surgical scar
- To gather preoperative medical reports, x-rays, clinical facial photographs, etc., into the two envelopes
- To document stages of consent with precise notes and drawings which have been developed by the patient and physicians as a team

F. Meneghini, P. Biondi, *Clinical Facial Analysis*,
DOI 10.1007/978-3-642-27228-8_13, © Springer-Verlag Berlin Heidelberg 2012

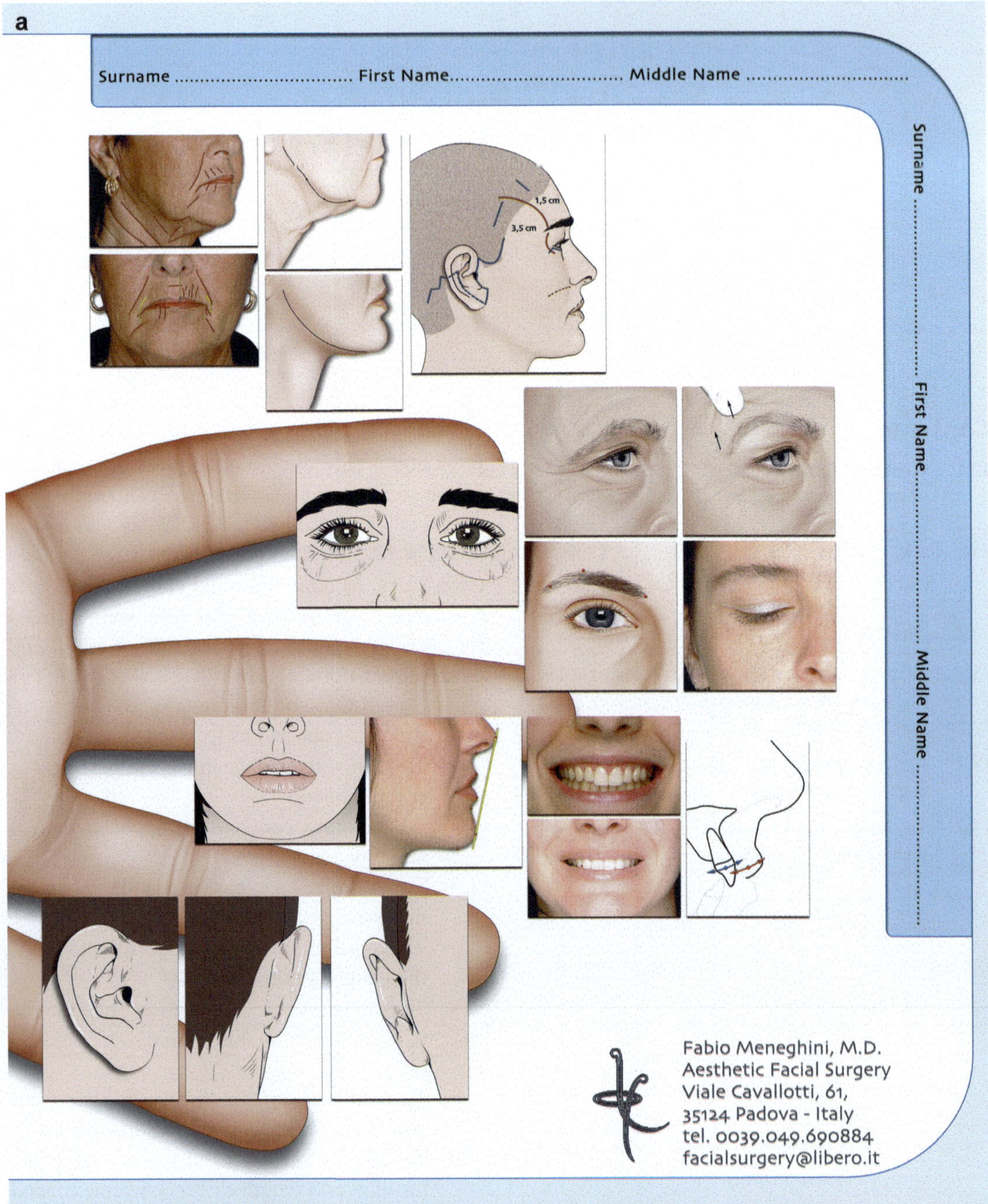

Fig. 13.1 *Aesthetic facial surgery: first consultation notes, essential medical history, and clinical diary* (**a**) Front cover, (**b**) Back cover, (**c**) Internal pages

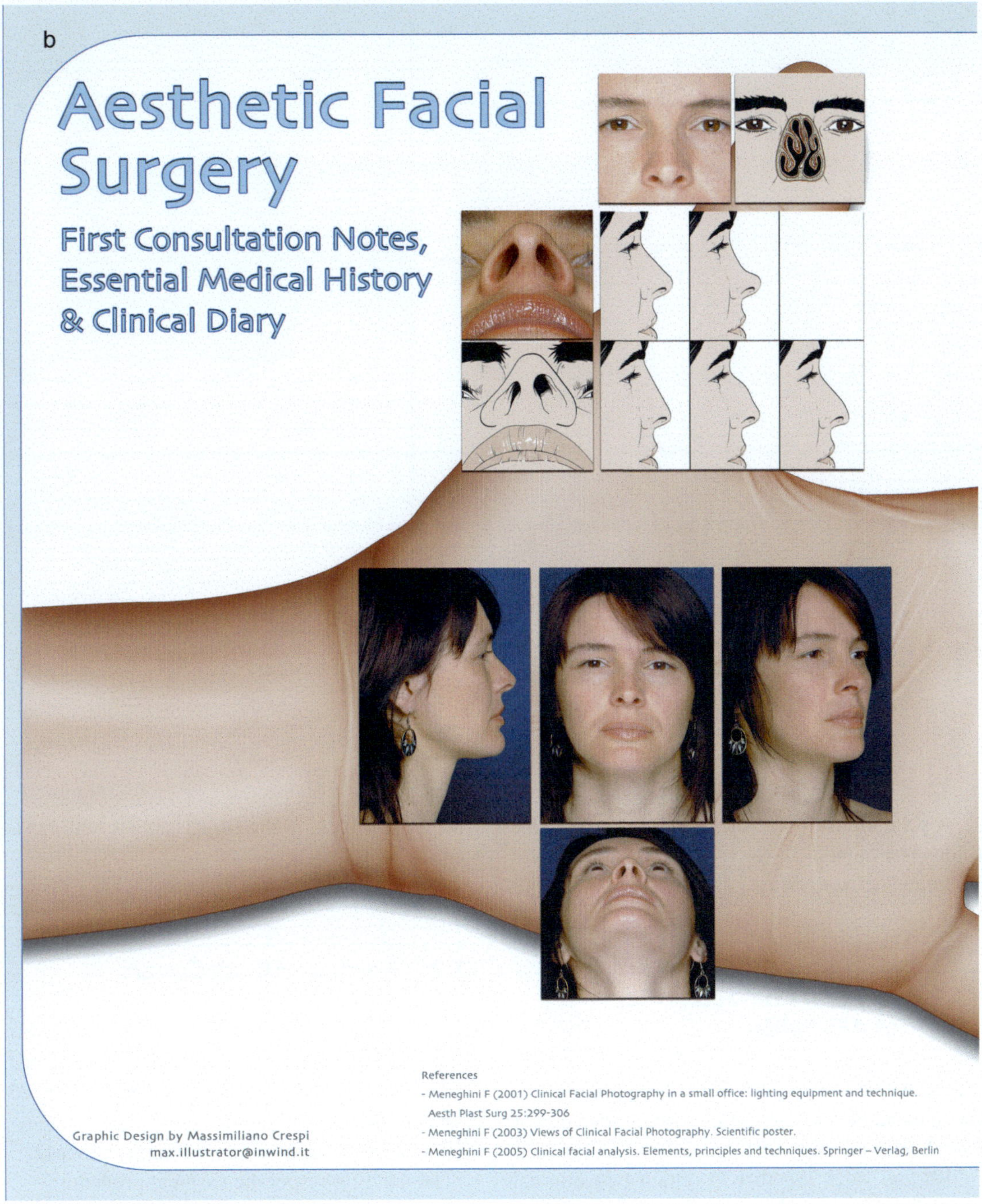

Fig. 13.1 (continued)

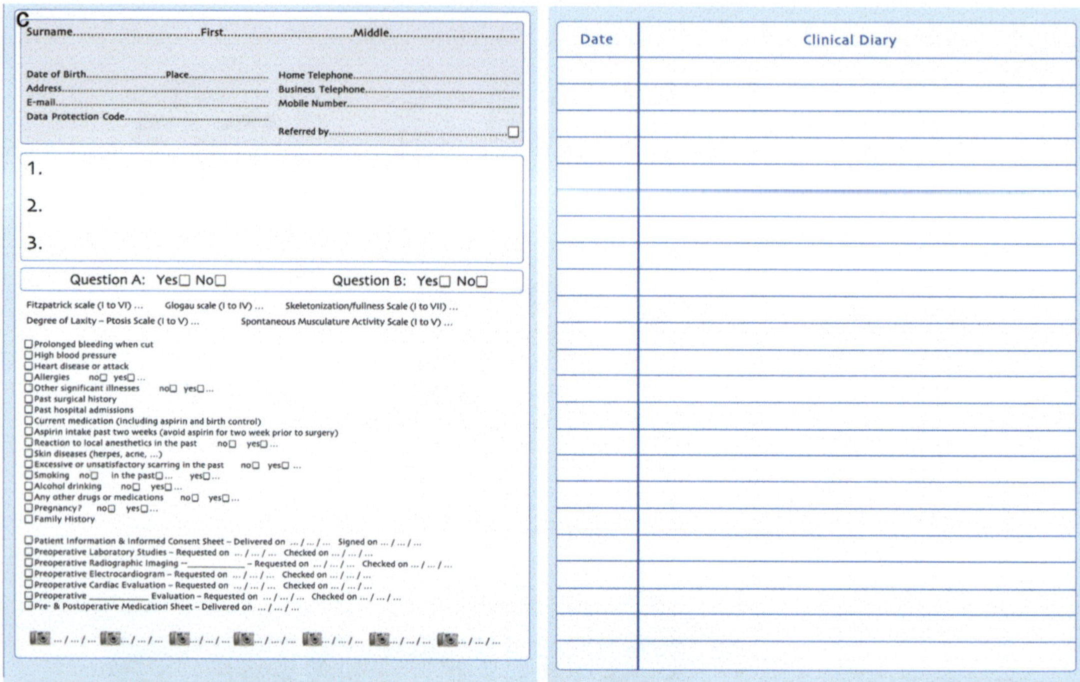
C
Surname................................First..................................Middle..................................

Date of Birth.........................Place.........................
Address..
E-mail...
Data Protection Code..
Home Telephone..
Business Telephone..
Mobile Number...
Referred by...☐

1.

2.

3.

Question A: Yes☐ No☐ Question B: Yes☐ No☐

Fitzpatrick scale (I to VI) ... Glogau scale (I to IV) ... Skeletonization/fullness Scale (I to VII) ...
Degree of Laxity – Ptosis Scale (I to V) ... Spontaneous Musculature Activity Scale (I to V) ...

☐Prolonged bleeding when cut
☐High blood pressure
☐Heart disease or attack
☐Allergies no☐ yes☐ ...
☐Other significant illnesses no☐ yes☐ ...
☐Past surgical history
☐Past hospital admissions
☐Current medication (including aspirin and birth control)
☐Aspirin intake past two weeks (avoid aspirin for two week prior to surgery)
☐Reaction to local anesthetics in the past no☐ yes☐ ...
☐Skin diseases (herpes, acne, ...)
☐Excessive or unsatisfactory scarring in the past no☐ yes☐ ...
☐Smoking no☐ in the past☐ ... yes☐ ...
☐Alcohol drinking no☐ yes☐ ...
☐Any other drugs or medications no☐ yes☐ ...
☐Pregnancy? no☐ yes☐ ...
☐Family History

☐Patient Information & Informed Consent Sheet – Delivered on ... / ... / ... Signed on ... / ... / ...
☐Preoperative Laboratory Studies – Requested on ... / ... / ... Checked on ... / ... / ...
☐Preoperative Radiographic Imaging –____________ – Requested on ... / ... / ... Checked on ... / ... / ...
☐Preoperative Electrocardiogram – Requested on ... / ... / ... Checked on ... / ... / ...
☐Preoperative Cardiac Evaluation – Requested on ... / ... / ... Checked on ... / ... / ...
☐Preoperative ____________ Evaluation – Requested on ... / ... / ... Checked on ... / ... / ...
☐Pre- & Postoperative Medication Sheet – Delivered on ... / ... / ...

... / ... / ... ... / ... / ... ... / ... / ... ... / ... / ... ... / ... / ... ... / ... / ... ... / ... / ...

Date	Clinical Diary

Fig. 13.1 (continued)

A printable full-size electronic copy of AFS folder is available in Sect. 5 on Springer Extra Materials (extras.springer.com).

13.1 General Characteristics of *AFS Folder*

The case *AFS Folder* is made of strong, matt cardboard to enable drawing and writing with a pen or pencil on both sides with ease. The cardboard is folded and stuck together to obtain two internal large envelopes which are very handy for gathering the patient's clinical reports, such as photographs, CD-ROMs, DVDs, x-rays, preoperative blood tests, and other materials (Fig. 13.2).

The front cover contains two distinct boxes in which the patient's surname, first name, and middle name are recorded along the horizontal and vertical margins (Fig. 13.3) and which allows for storage of folders in the filing cabinet both horizontally and vertically.

13.2 Front and Back Covers

The main objective of the two covers of the *AFS Case Sheet* is that of offering, with a single large "map," some helpful images that can be utilized to inform the patient about:

- His facial deformities and/or aging process
- The need for a specific surgical procedure
- The placement of surgical incisions and resulting scars
- Any other detailed or in-depth information or explanations utilizing images rather than verbal explanations

This "map" contains many images divided into small specific groups relating to the nasal, orbital, ear, chin-neck, and perioral area. Some

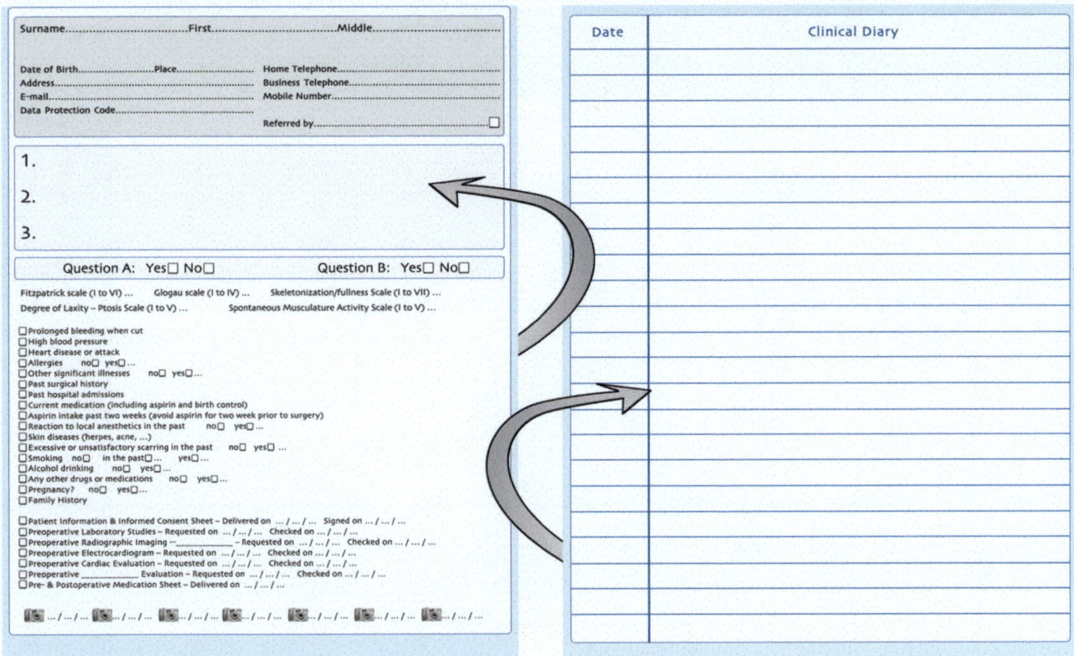

Fig. 13.2 The two large envelopes are obtained by folding and sticking the cardboard together

frontal images and a drawing with facelift skin surgical incisions are also inserted.

13.2.1 Frontal, Oblique, Profile, and Basal Full Face View

These images are central in the cover "map" of the *AFS Case Sheet* (Fig. 13.4): they are very useful when discussing facial features, proportion, and symmetry with the patient. Planned surgery can be illustrated by drawing the skin incision line and the area in which the effects of the surgery are expected to be directly onto the images. For example, when introducing the procedure of subchin liposuction, the profile view helps me to point out where fat will be reduced, while the frontal view gives me the opportunity to illustrate the position and extension of the incision line with precision (Fig. 13.5).

13.2.2 Nasal Area Images

The three images in the nasal area regard both aesthetic and functional problems. In Fig. 13.6, five nasal profiles are depicted to help the patient to compare a well-balanced, proportioned profile (the upper left-hand image) with the other four which are clearly deformed in one specific way. Figure 13.7 illustrates a coronal section of the anterior face in which one can see a deviated septum and the different dimensions between the right and left inferior turbinate; it is difficult to describe what a deviated septum or hypertrophic inferior turbinate is without the aid of a specific image. Figure 13.8 shows a basal nasal view of a normal, symmetrical nose (upper image), and a right nostril collapse restricting the airway (lower drawing); the basal nasal view is useful in explaining the exact position of the surgical incision to the patient in case of "open approach rhinoplasty" (Fig. 13.9).

13.2.3 Facial Aging and Facelift Incision Line Area

With a patient requesting facial rejuvenation procedures, the surgeon should discuss signs of aging, objectives of the treatment, and surgical scar positions. Figure 13.10 helps define signs

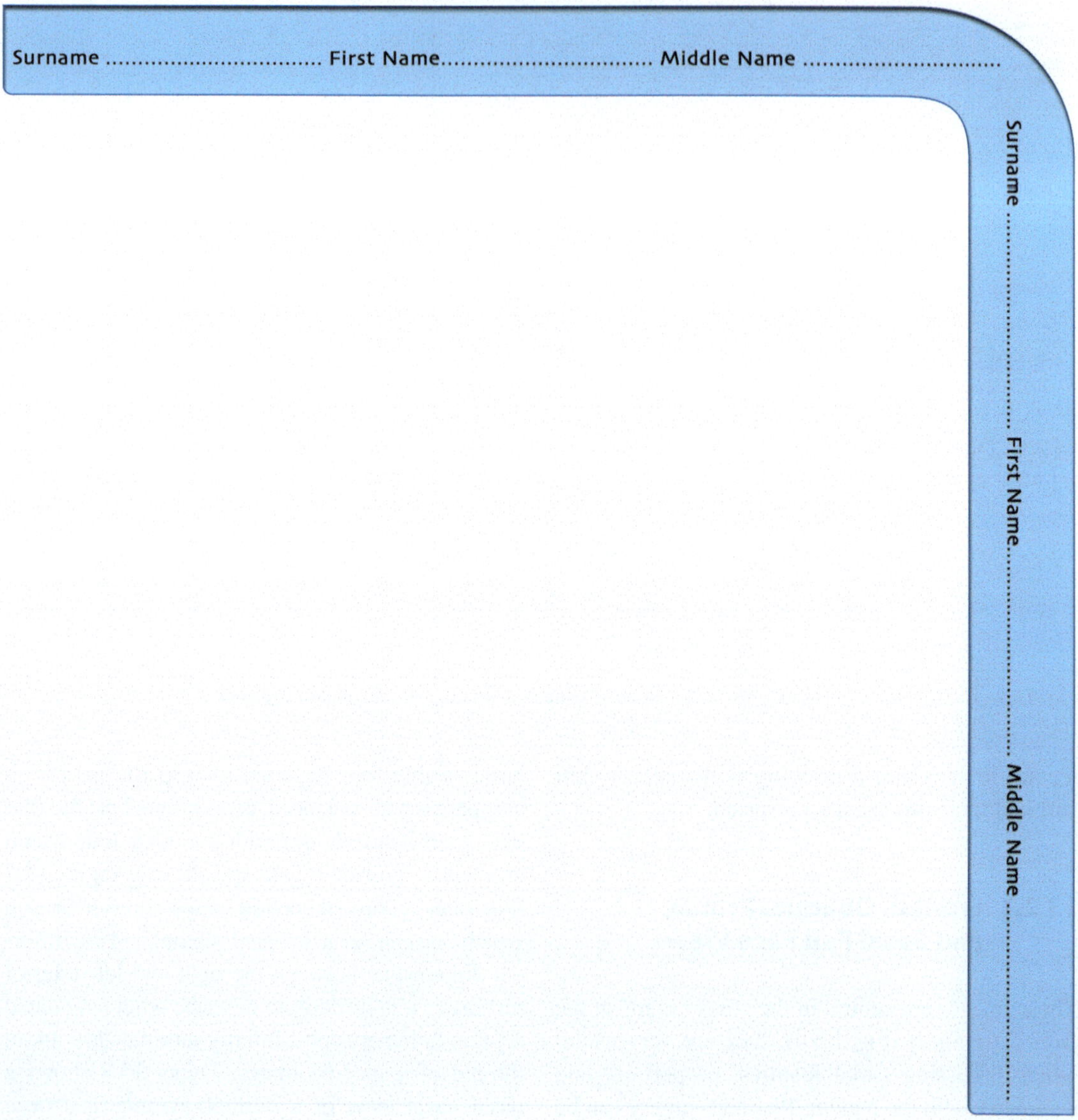

Fig. 13.3 The upper right-hand corner of the front cover with two boxes, one vertical and one horizontal, for writing the patient's surname, first name, and middle name

of aging in the lower third of the face, for example, deep folds from the nose to the mouth, vertical and horizontal upper lip lines, the increase of the skin height of the upper lip associated with the reduction of the vermillion height, vertical lower lip lines, marionette lines, and chin ptosis. Figure 13.11 compares the juvenile and aged chin/neck with the appearance of platysma bands, submandibular gland ptosis, loss of mandibular border definition, and witch's chin deformity (chin ptosis, flattening of lip-to-chin fold, and deepening of the subchin crease). Figure 13.12 shows main skin incisions and intraoral incision utilized by the authors in facelift procedures. The skin incisions are potentially a location for postoperative visible scars and should be clearly explained to the patient prior to surgery.

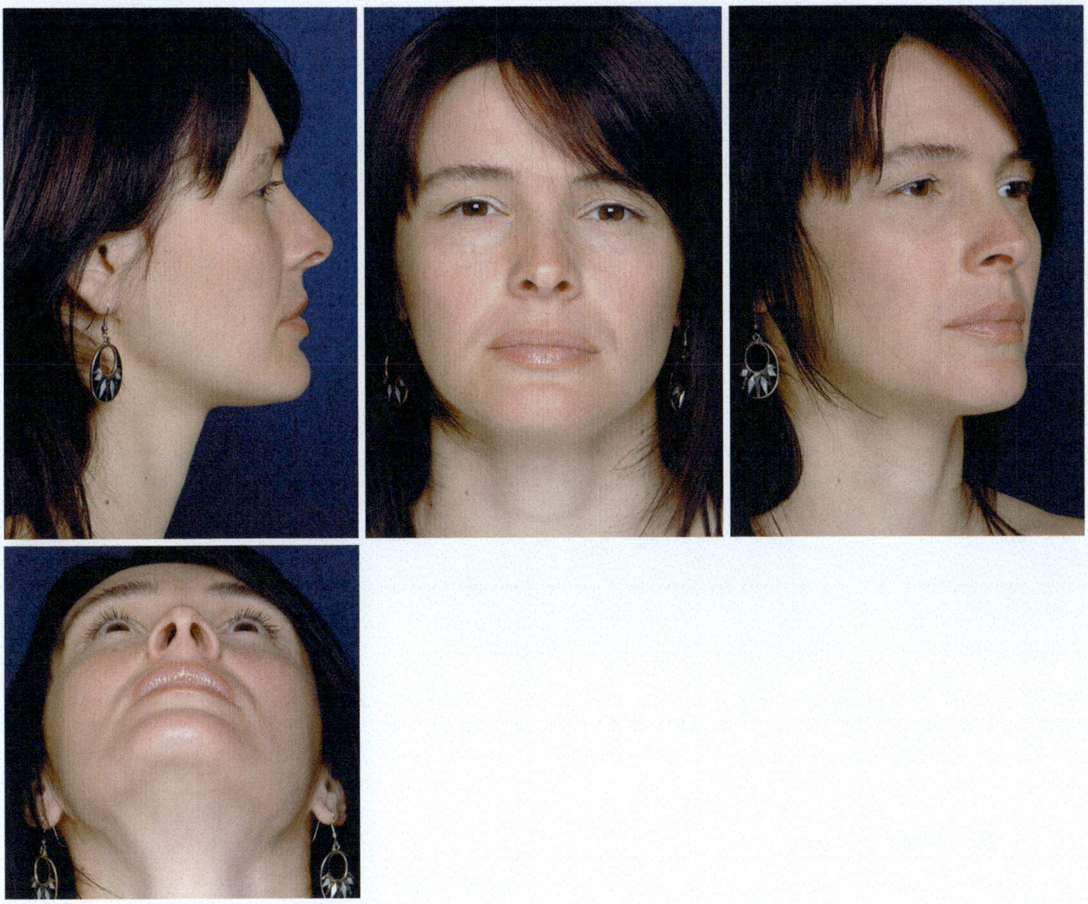

Fig. 13.4 Frontal, oblique, profile, and basal full face views

13.2.4 Eyebrow and Eyelid Area Images

The five images in this group concern the upper third of the face, or in other words the eyebrow and eyelid. Figure 13.13 shows the ptosis of the lateral portion of the eyebrow (above left), the need to elevate the lateral brow in order to correct or ameliorate the Connell sign – lateral extension of the upper lid crease onto the temporal region – (above right), and the normal shape and orientation of a female eyebrow (bottom left-hand image). The bottom right-hand image of Fig. 13.13, that is, a right eye view looking downward, is very helpful in the case of an upper blepharoplasty when the surgeon illustrates where the incision line is expected to be (Fig. 13.14).

In Fig. 13.15, the drawing helps to understand the baggy lower lid and shows the patient the lower lid subciliar incision (Fig. 13.16).

13.2.5 Lip and Smile Area Images

The fifth group of images on the cover of the *AFS Case Sheet* deals with the lips, the smile, the ratio between the upper incisors, and the upper lip (Figs. 13.17 and 13.18). These are utilized when communicating the objectives of jaw surgery, chin surgery, lip augmentation procedures, and other procedures involving the lower third of the face. In case of upper lip lifting, the location and amount of skin excision can be shown to the patient as in Fig. 13.19.

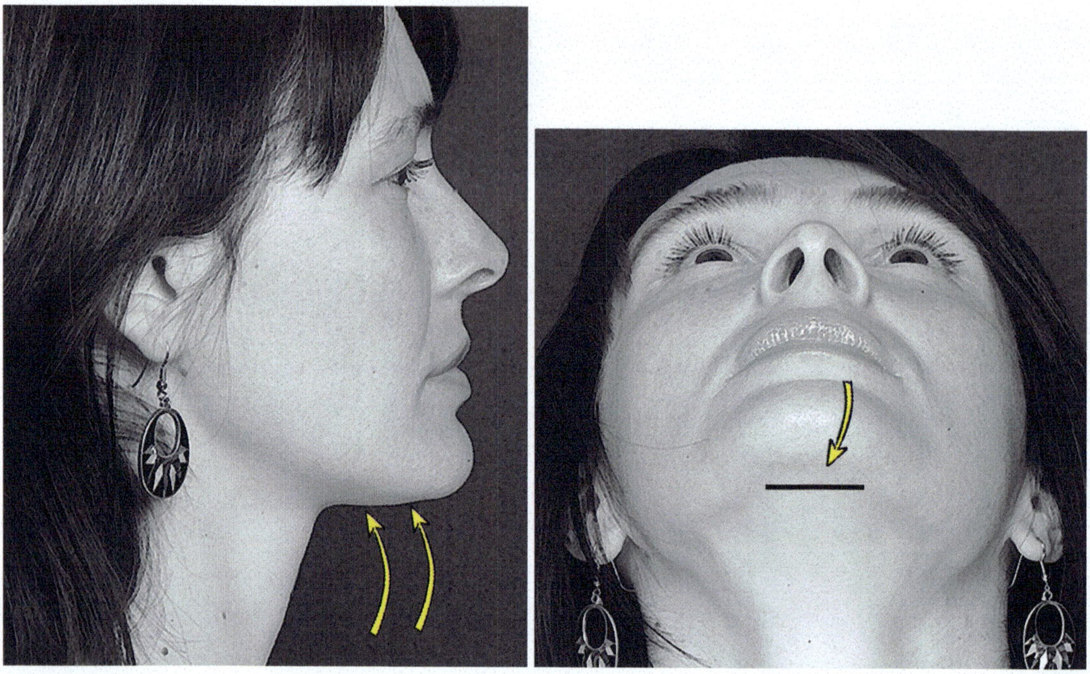

Fig. 13.5 In the case of subchin liposuction, the *arrows* drawn over the profile view indicate the anatomical area treated with the procedure, while the *black line* drawn on the basal view illustrates the skin incision line and resulting surgical scar

13.2.6 Ear Area Images

The three projections (lateral, rear, and frontal) of a normal right ear contribute toward the possibility of a better patient/surgeon relationship in case of aesthetic and reconstructive surgery of the external earlobe (Fig. 13.20): as mentioned above, the figures are helpful in describing the position and extent of the incision line as well as the objectives of the surgery proposed to the new patient.

13.3 Left-Hand Side of Inside Page of the *AFS Folder*

The left-hand side of the page should be completed fully and in detail at the first consultation.

Detailed data are filled in by the secretarial staff in the box with a pale gray background at the top of the page (Fig. 13.21). Special attention should be paid to the person (colleague, previous patient, friend, etc.) who has referred the new patient and, after the first visit has taken place, the doctor should always call to thank him. As a reminder that the call has been made, the little box in the lower right-hand corner of the box should be ticked (Fig. 13.22).

The other areas of the inside page on the left-hand side must be completed by the doctor himself in the presence of the patient during the consultation in order to illustrate his personal dedication to the patient's requests and problems.

We have dedicated the central box numbered 1, 2, 3 to the *Initial Patient Priority List* (Fig. 13.23). This was conceived in order to record the patient's principal requests, written down in simple terms (avoiding technical or medical terms) and which have been communicated by the patient himself in order of importance. The aim is to guarantee that everything that is important to him is also important, fully understood, and recorded by the doctor as one of the first actions at the consultation.

Figure 13.24 reports some typical statements made by a patient seeking nasal surgery. In this

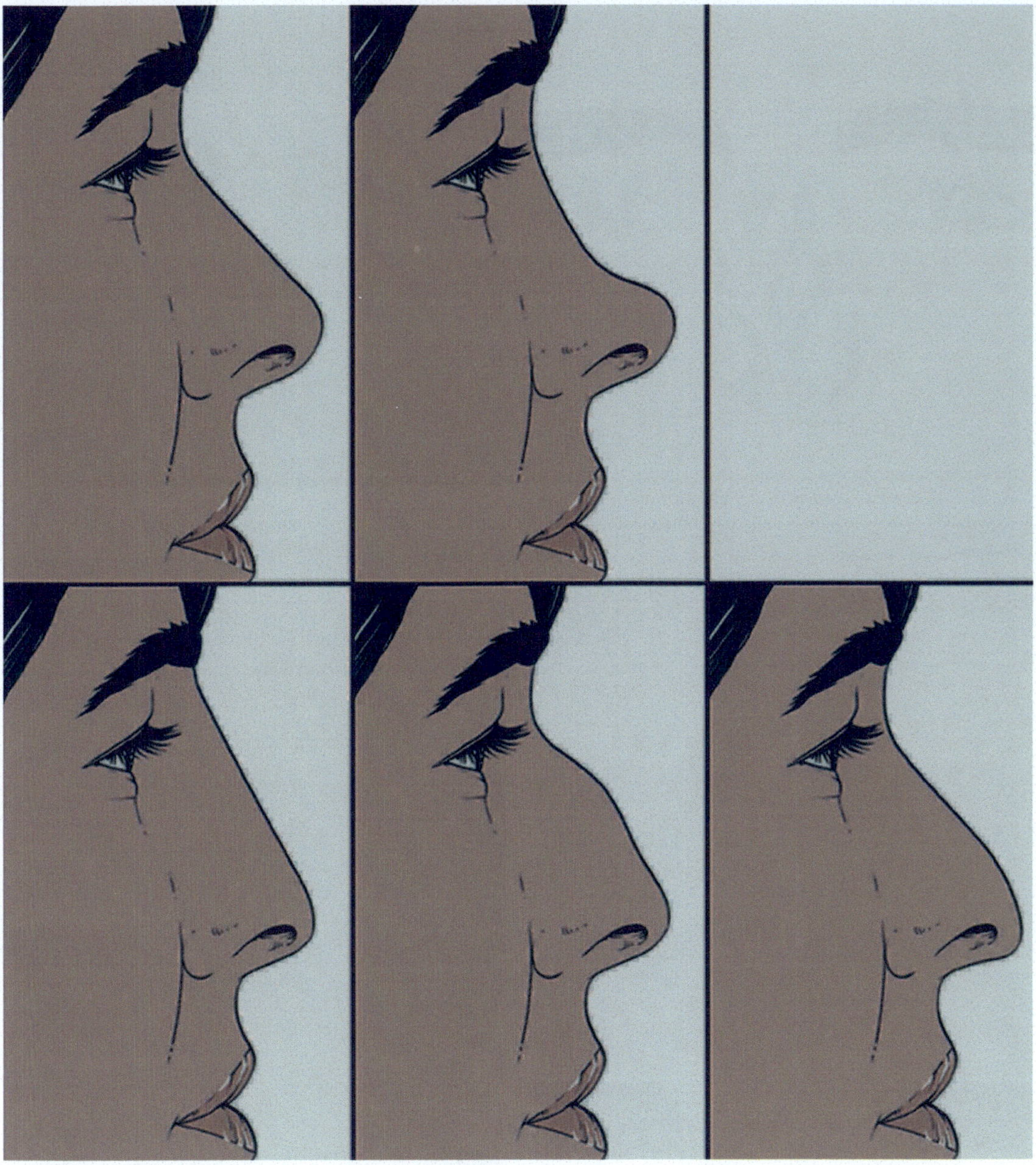

Fig. 13.6 Five nasal profiles. The upper left-hand image represents a well-balanced and aesthetically proportioned nasal profile

case, he is principally concerned with the aesthetics of his nasal dorsum (1. *big, ugly nasal hump*) than nasal function (2. *difficult nasal breathing, especially left-hand side*) and lower nasal symmetry (3. *nasal tip deviated to the left*). When, later in the preoperative stage, the objective of the treatment should be discussed and shared with the patient, this *Initial Patient Priority List* will be recalled, confirmed, or modified, taking nasal function into great consideration.[1]

During the first and successive preoperative consultations, the doctor should ask himself *questions A* and *B* (Fig. 13.25).

[1] Also see Sect. 16.8.

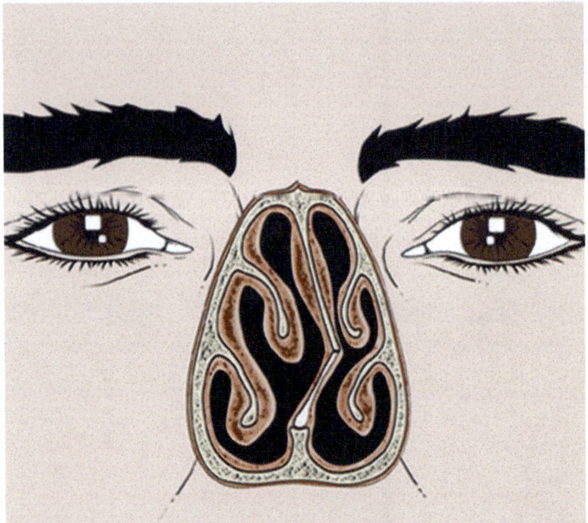

Fig. 13.7 A coronal section of the anterior nose showing a deviated nasal septum and asymmetrical inferior turbinates

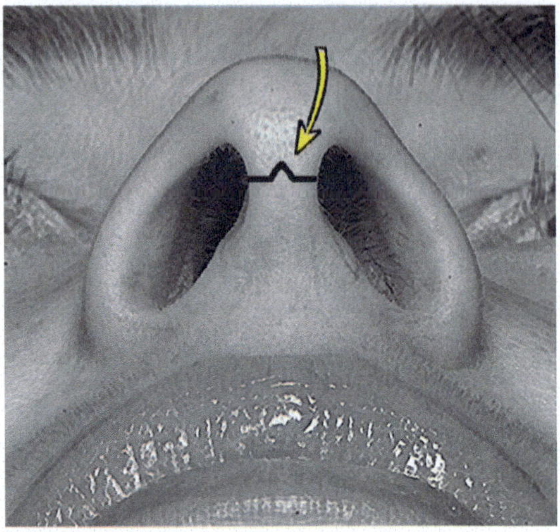

Fig. 13.9 Examples of surgical incision line performed in the case of "open approach rhinoplasty"

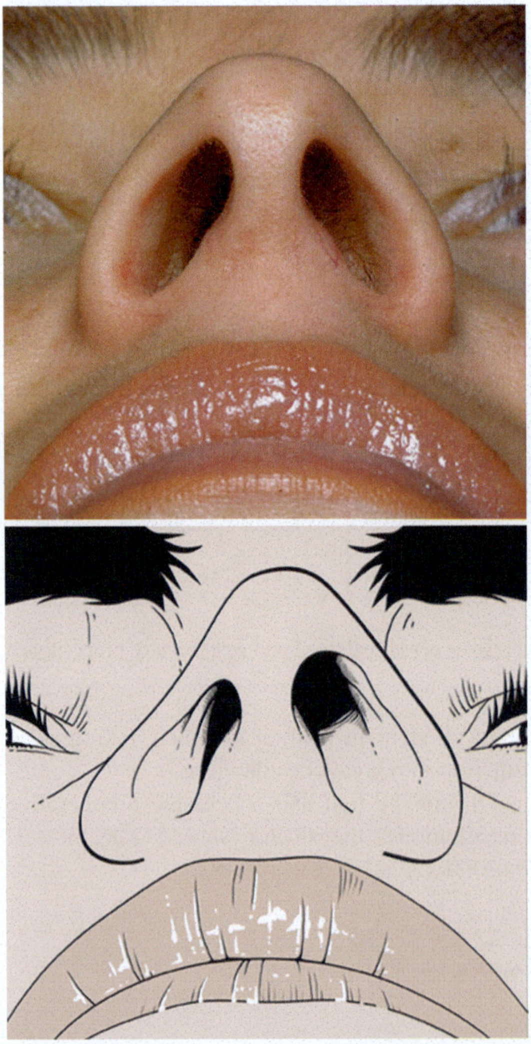

Fig. 13.8 *Above*: symmetrical, well-proportioned nasal base. *Below*: asymmetric nasal base with right nostril collapse restricting the airway

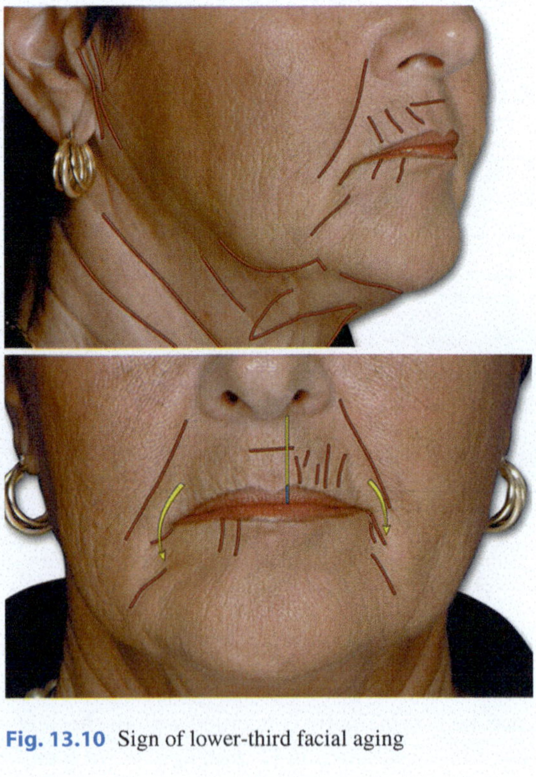

Fig. 13.10 Sign of lower-third facial aging

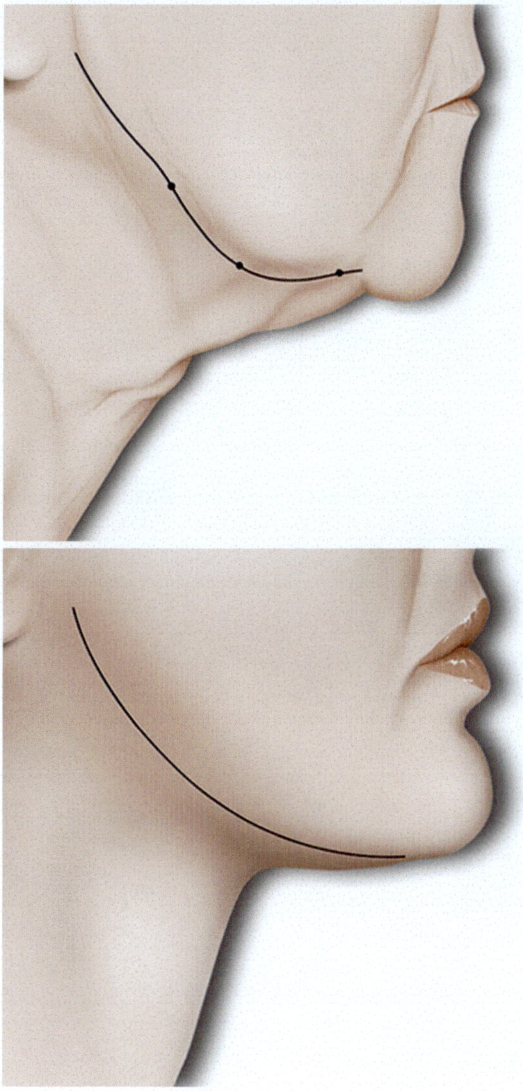

Fig. 13.11 *Above*: signs of chin-neck aging with interrupted jawline. *Bottom*: youthful chin-neck with uninterrupted jawline

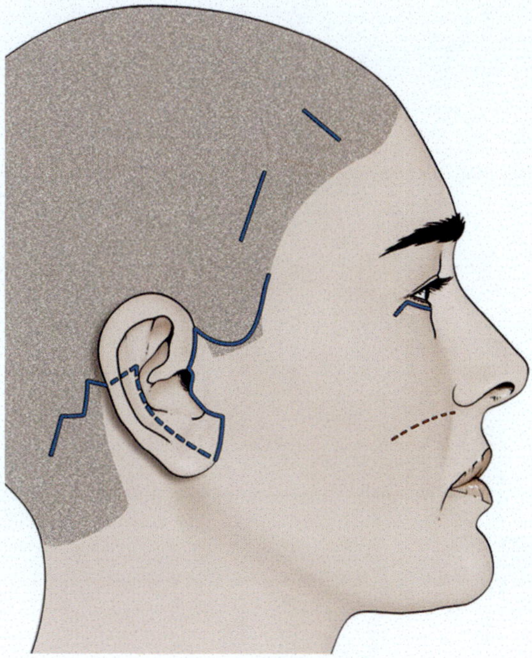

Fig. 13.12 Principal skin incisions and intraoral incision for facelift procedures

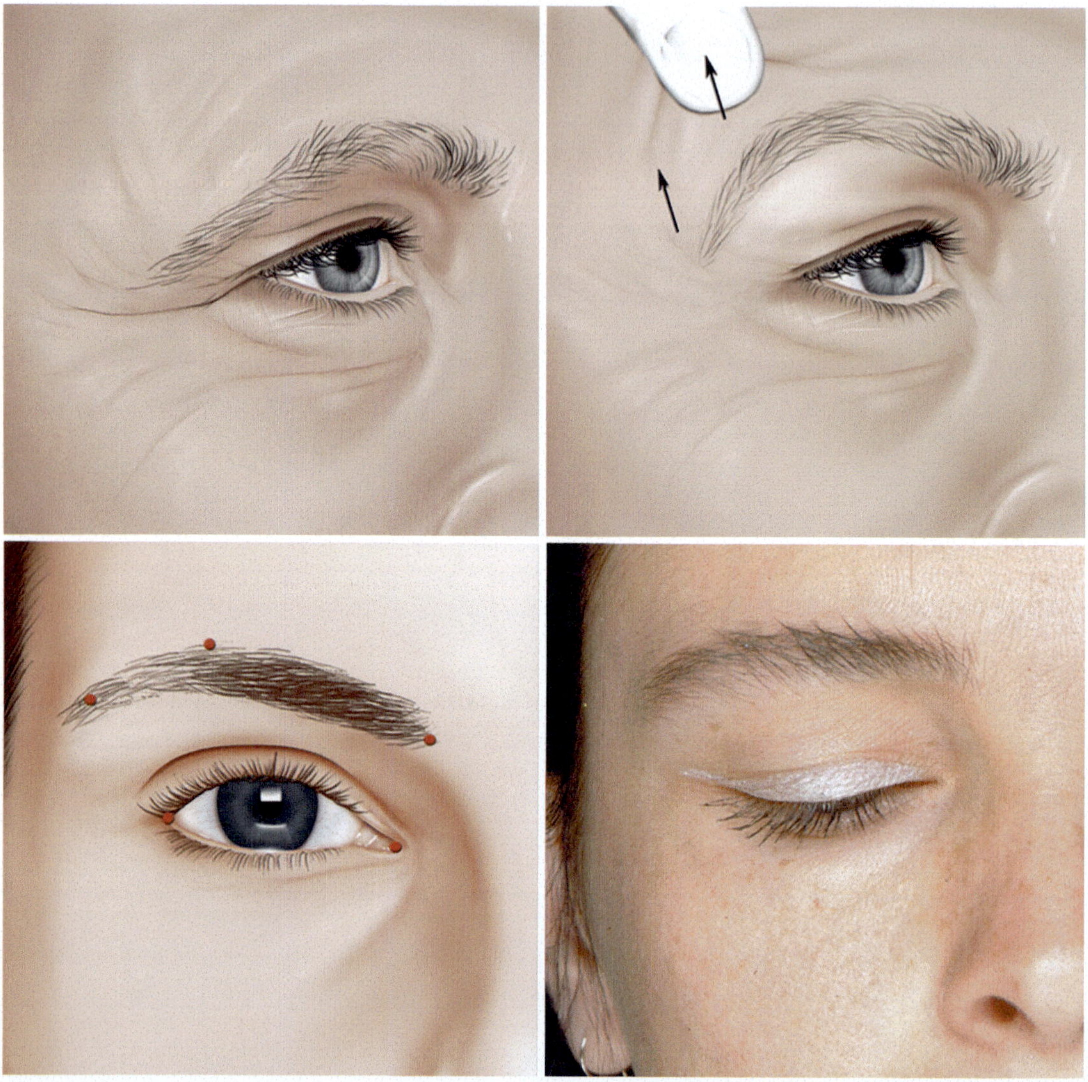

Fig. 13.13 *Above left*: Connell sign. *Above right*: the elevation of lateral brow correction or amelioration of the Connell sign. *Below left*: normal shape and orientation of female eyebrow. *Bottom right*: right eye view looking downward

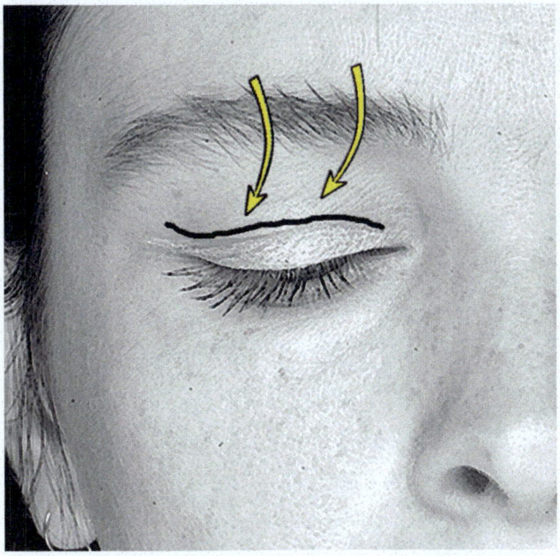

Fig. 13.14 Examples of upper eyelid incision line

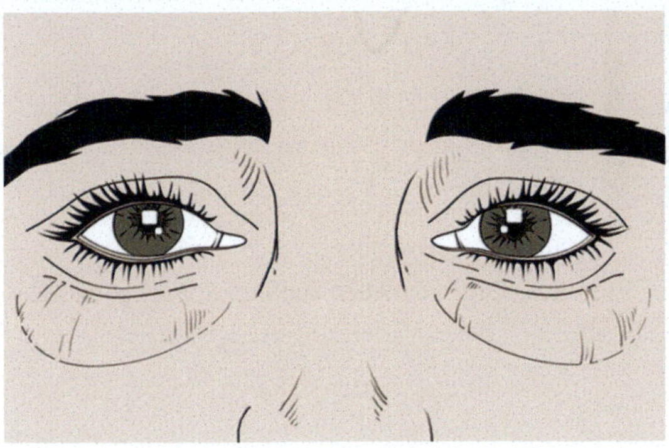

Fig. 13.15 Baggy area of lower lids

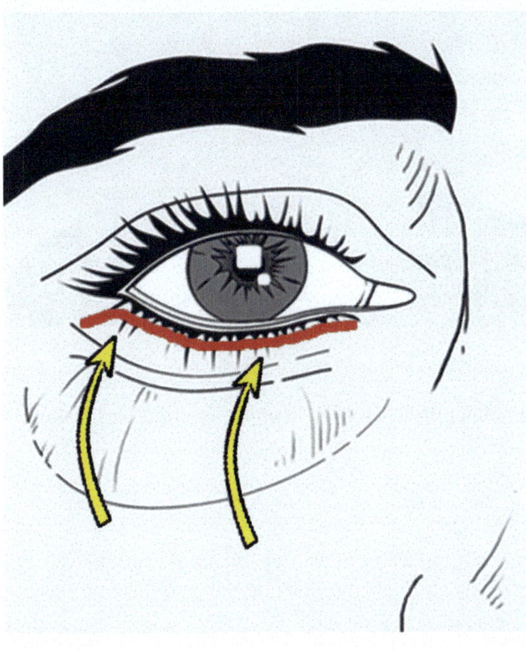

Fig. 13.16 Example of lower lid subciliar incision

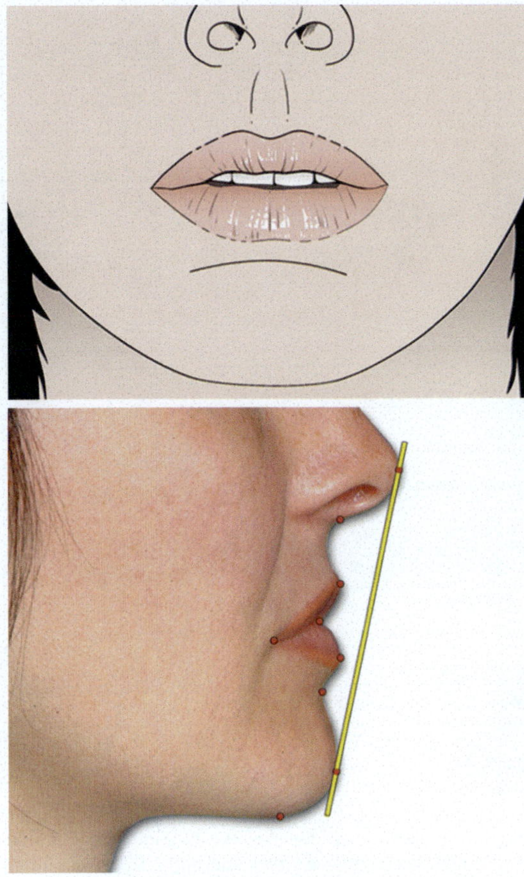

Fig. 13.17 *Above*: normal youthful lips from a frontal view. *Below*: lower-third facial profile view with aesthetic line

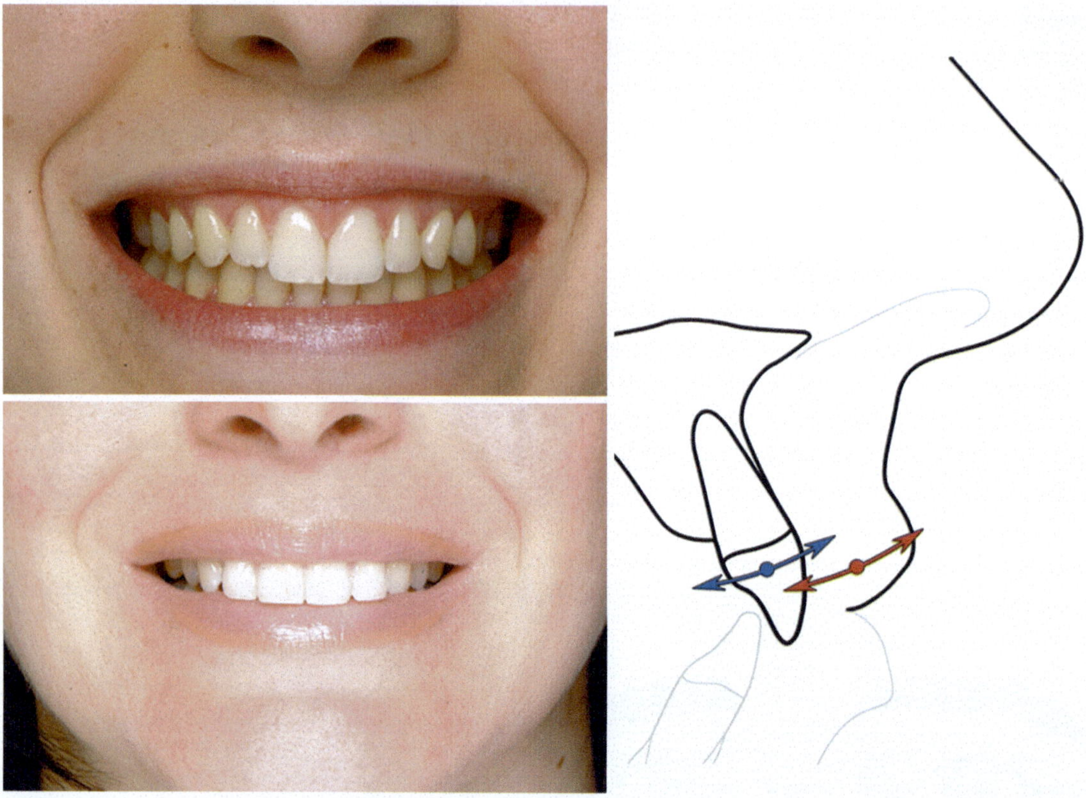

Fig. 13.18 *Left* (*above* and *below*): two examples of upper incision line illustrated when smiling. *Right*: spatial relationship between upper incisors and upper lip

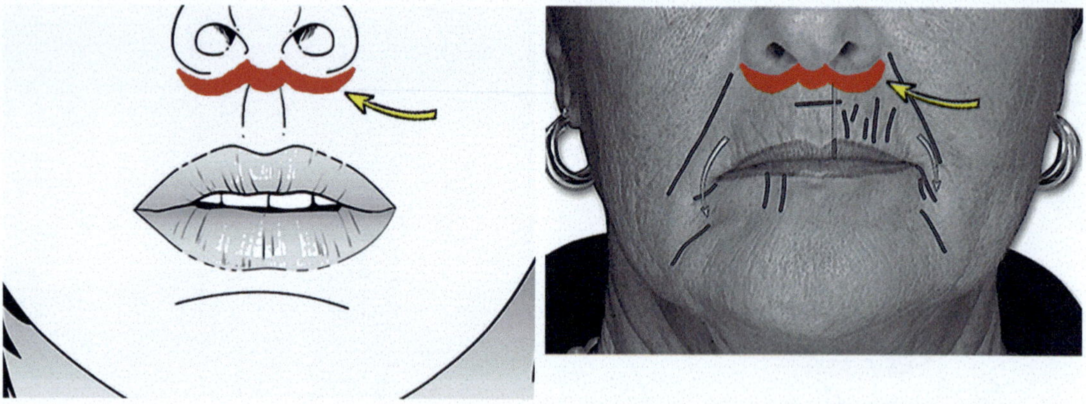

Fig. 13.19 *Left* and *right*: position of skin incision lines and amount of skin excision in upper lip lifting procedures

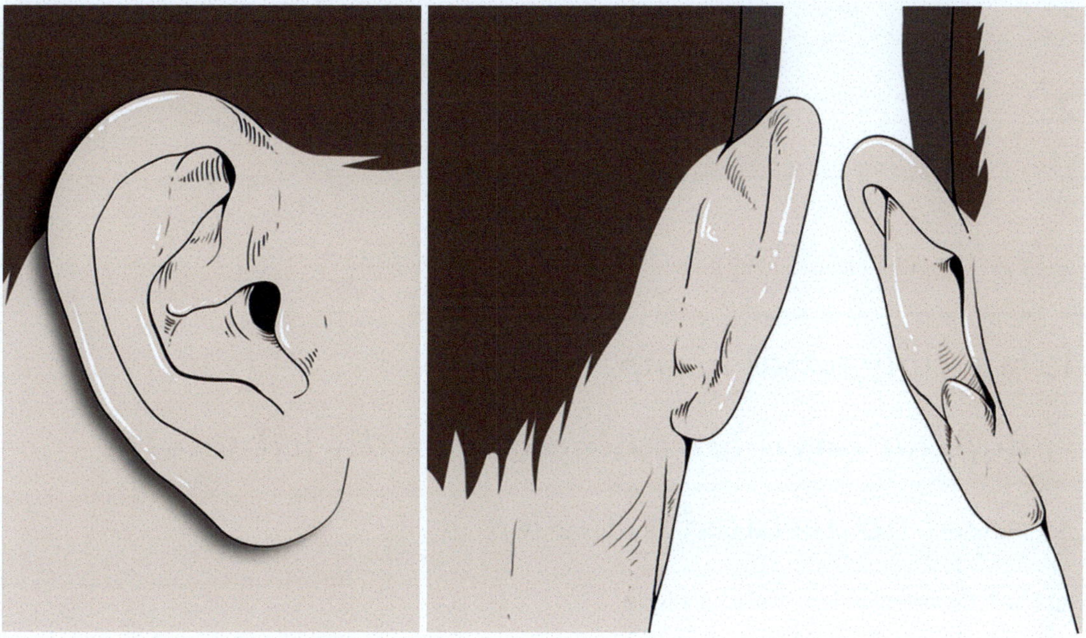

Fig. 13.20 Lateral, rear, and frontal ear projections

Surname................................First..................................Middle.................................

Date of Birth........................Place.........................
Address...
E-mail...
Data Protection Code..

Home Telephone...
Business Telephone..
Mobile Number..
Referred by..☐

Fig. 13.21 Data box for special notes

.... Home Telephone...
.... Business Telephone..
.... Mobile Number...
....
Referred by..Cathy and John Smith..☒

Fig. 13.22 The person who refers the patient is noted in the bottom right-hand corner. The tick in the small box means that the doctor has thanked him

1.

2.

3.

Fig. 13.23 The patient's initial priority list box

1. *big, ugly nasal hump*

2. *difficult nasal breathing (especially left side)*

3. *nasal tip deviated to the left*

Fig. 13.24 Example of patient's initial priority list

Question A: Yes☐ No☐ Question B: Yes☐ No☐

Fig. 13.25 Question A and question B box

Fitzpatrick scale (I to VI) … Glogau scale (I to IV) … Skeletonization/fullness Scale (I to VII) …
Degree of Laxity – Ptosis Scale (I to V) … Spontaneous Musculature Activity Scale (I to V) …

☐ Prolonged bleeding when cut
☐ High blood pressure
☐ Heart disease or attack
☐ Allergies no☐ yes☐ …
☐ Other significant illnesses no☐ yes☐ …
☐ Past surgical history
☐ Past hospital admissions
☐ Current medication (including aspirin and birth control)
☐ Aspirin intake past two weeks (avoid aspirin for two week prior to surgery)
☐ Reaction to local anesthetics in the past no☐ yes☐ …
☐ Skin diseases (herpes, acne, …)
☐ Excessive or unsatisfactory scarring in the past no☐ yes☐ …
☐ Smoking no☐ in the past☐ … yes☐ …
☐ Alcohol drinking no☐ yes☐ …
☐ Any other drugs or medications no☐ yes☐ …
☐ Pregnancy? no☐ yes☐ …
☐ Family History

☐ Patient Information & Informed Consent Sheet – Delivered on … / … / … Signed on … / … / …
☐ Preoperative Laboratory Studies – Requested on … / … / … Checked on … / … / …
☐ Preoperative Radiographic Imaging --______________ – Requested on … / … / … Checked on … / … / …
☐ Preoperative Electrocardiogram – Requested on … / … / … Checked on … / … / …
☐ Preoperative Cardiac Evaluation – Requested on … / … / … Checked on … / … / …
☐ Preoperative ______________ Evaluation – Requested on … / … / … Checked on … / … / …
☐ Pre- & Postoperative Medication Sheet – Delivered on … / … / …

Fig. 13.26 Clinical facial soft tissue evaluation, basic medical history, patient's clinical report requested, and preoperative sheet delivered

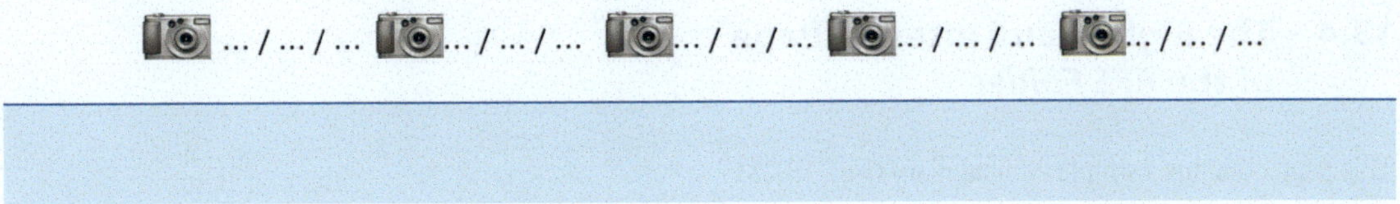

Fig. 13.27 Clinical photography diary

Question A: Does this patient want aesthetic surgery in order to satisfy a personal, innermost desire?

Question B: Has the wish for a better facial appearance via surgical procedure matured over a suitable period of time?

A person can sometimes be convinced by a friend or family member that his nose is too big or his face has aged. The decision to undergo aesthetic surgical intervention can sometimes be made far too recently. In both cases, the answer to questions A and B are no, and this indicates a poor candidate for facial aesthetic surgery, with little probability of postoperative satisfaction.[2]

Another part of the left-hand side inside page of the *AFS Case Sheet* is dedicated to the evaluation of the patient's facial soft tissue, as reported in Chap. 5 of this book, and basic medical history with some aspects that are important for facial surgery, such as high blood pressure, prolonged bleeding in the past, aspirin intake, tobacco smoking, excessive or unsatisfactory scarring, and skin disease (Fig. 13.26).The patient is reminded in this section of some important steps regarding the preoperative phase:

- Patient information and informed consent sheet
- Preoperative laboratory studies
- Preoperative radiographic imaging
- Preoperative electrocardiogram
- Preoperative cardiac evaluation
- Other preoperative evaluations
- Pre- and postoperative medical sheet

Finally, in the bottom left-hand area of the left-hand inside page, a series of drawings resembling a camera report each date in which the patient is documented for clinical facial photography (Fig. 13.27). Again, extensive, repeated patient documentation is strongly recommended and recorded in this and other sections of the *AFS Case Sheet*.

[2] Also see Sect. 15.1.

13.4 The Right-Hand Internal Page of the *AFS Folder*

This page contains a simple clinical diary (Fig. 13.28).

Date	Clinical Diary

Fig. 13.28 Clinical diary box

Exercises in Clinical Photography and Analysis

14

Contents

It is our intention that this chapter should be a sort of final test and a way for the reader to understand and review one more time the elements and techniques previously presented. Many of the materials needed for these four exercises are available on Springer Extra Materials (etras.springer.com), but a complete session of documentation and analysis is best done with a real patient or with a cooperative friend.

14.1 Exercise 1: Orientate the Face in the Natural Head Position

The great majority of clinical photographs and direct clinical examination steps require the natural head position (NHP); this position is also used for the cephalometric analysis. The simplest way to obtain the NHP is to instruct the patient to look straight ahead at a point at eye level on the wall in front of him. Another way to orientate the face in the NHP is to ask the patient to look at his eyes in a large mirror hung on the wall in front of him.

Sometimes the orientation obtained seems unnatural to the examiner, but on asking the patient to tilt the head upward and downward and then return to looking straight ahead to the point at eye level, we can note that the final spatial orientation is very similar to the initial one.

To appreciate more deeply the value of NHP, I suggest taking six or seven photographs of the subject in profile view, requesting small differences in head tilt from down to up. It is amazing how different the relationships between the neck,

F. Meneghini, P. Biondi, *Clinical Facial Analysis*,
DOI 10.1007/978-3-642-27228-8_14, © Springer-Verlag Berlin Heidelberg 2012

chin, nose, and forehead appear to the observer by minimally changing the head position!

14.2 Exercise 2: Perform a Complete Session of Clinical Facial Photography

This practical exercise should be done utilizing, as a guide, the printed version of the poster "Views of clinical facial photography"[1] or the figures reported in Chap. 3. After all the pictures have been taken and printed, the results can be analyzed critically, evaluating these points:

- Subject cooperation
- Subject positioning
- Subject framing
- Unwanted shadows and reflexes over the face
- Background shadows
- Readability of facial features

14.3 Exercise 3: Find and Compare the Facial Points of Interest in Two Different Subjects

Finding the facial points of interest, reported in Chap. 4 helps us in a free activity of clinical evaluation and analysis. As you remember, the facial points of interest can be classified as follows:

- The angular facial point of interest (i.e., the medial canthus point)
- The maximal curvature point on a curve, either a concave or a convex curve (i.e., the nasal radix and the nasal tip points)
- The point when a concavity turns into a convexity (i.e., the subnasal point)

Select and print two clinical case photographs from Sect. 4 on Springer Extra Materials (extras.springer.com), and try to find the facial points of interest of all the views; compare the differences between the two cases.

14.4 Exercise 4: Perform a Systematic, Step-by-Step Facial Analysis

This exercise should be done utilizing the checklists for clinical analysis presented in Chaps. 5, 6, 7, 8, 9, and 10, and using one of the clinical cases in Sect. 4 on Springer Extra Materials (extras.springer.com).

Once the questions in the checklists have been answered, the final and fundamental step of the exercise is the organization of the data collected in order of importance to create the "doctor priority list."

[1] Sect. 1 on Springer Extra Materials (extras.springer.com).

15 Suggested Reading

Contents

This chapter reports a list of international articles and books in which I found many valuable suggestions and help for writing this book. All the arguments are briefly presented and commented on in the same order of appearance as in the previous chapters. The reader is strongly recommended to select from this list to take a closer look at facial analysis or to study other related arguments, which are treated marginally in this book.

I want to express my personal gratitude to these authors, many of whom are international leaders in their fields. They were and still are an immense fount of knowledge and source of inspiration for me.

15.1 Errors in Patient Selection

Errors occur when a patient is too interested in a small detail of his face and cannot see the entire picture, when a woman decides to rejuvenate herself surgically to satisfy her husband's request, when a boy wants Brad Pitt's nose, etc.

Every moment during the initial consultation and the successive preoperative meetings with a patient is a perfect occasion to ask yourself the two questions cited by Rollin K. Daniel: "Will the planned surgery make a significant improvement in this patient?" and "Do I want this person in my practice?" If the answer is no to either question, he suggests not doing their surgery.

Daniel RK (2002) Rhinoplasty. An atlas of surgical techniques. Springer, Berlin, Heidelberg,

F. Meneghini, P. Biondi, *Clinical Facial Analysis*,
DOI 10.1007/978-3-642-27228-8_15, © Springer-Verlag Berlin Heidelberg 2012

New York (Consultation and patient management, pp 280–281)

Further information on errors in patient selection is also available in Chap. 3 of the book by M. Eugene Tardy and J. Regan Thomas.

Tardy ME, Thomas JR, Brown RJ (1995) Facial aesthetic surgery. Mosby – Year Book, Inc, St. Louis

15.2 Enhance Preoperative, Intraoperative, and Postoperative Patient Care

To study further the entire process of patient care, from the call for a consultation to the late follow-up return visit after one year, Edward D. Buckingham and coworkers have written a very interesting text. In particular, the role of the physician's staff in helping and instructing a cosmetic facial surgery patient is debated.

Buckingham ED, Lam SM, Williams EF (2004) An effective strategy for patient care. In: Williams EF, Lam SM (eds) Comprehensive facial rejuvenation. Lippincott Williams & Wilkins, Philadelphia

15.3 The Normal-Average Face and the Beautiful Face

A facial analysis exploring the differences between "unattractive," "average," "attractive," and "beautiful" faces utilizing artistic and scientific approaches was produced and published by Dr. Steven M. Hoefflin. He identifies and evaluates seven facial angles and seven volumetric highlights that, in a beautiful face, have a particularly pleasing orientation, degree, shape, and proportion.

Hoefflin SM (2002) The beautiful face: the first mathematical definition, classification, and creation of true facial beauty. Santa Monica, ISBN 0–9713445–0–7

15.4 Forehead Aesthetics and Preoperative Assessment

Timothy J. Marten and David M. Knize wrote one of the best descriptions on forehead aesthetics and how to recognize the aging process in the upper third of the face. This book also reports the anatomical work and the personal surgical technique of Dr. Knize for the rejuvenation of this facial region.

Marten TJ, Knize DM (2001) Forehead aesthetics and preoperative assessment of the forehead plasty patient. In: Knize DM (ed) The forehead and temporal fossa. Anatomy and technique. Lippincott Williams & Wilkins, Philadelphia, pp 91–99

15.5 Eyelid Aesthetics and Preoperative Assessment

The goals, the applied anatomy, and the preoperative assessment of eyelid aesthetic surgery can be found in Chaps. 2, 3, and 4 of the book by Francis G. Wolfort and William R. Kanter.

Wolfort FG, Kanter WR (1995) Aesthetic blepharoplasty. Little, Brown and Company, Boston

15.6 Understanding the Nasal Airway

Every facial analysis, whether the patient requests a nasal procedure or not, must include a careful nasal medical history and examination. For beginners or doctors working in other specialities, I suggest, as the first step in this argument, the article of Brian K. Howard and Rod J. Rohrich.

Howard BK, Rohrich RJ (2002) Understanding the nasal airways: principles and practice. Plast Reconstr Surg 109:1128–1144

15.7 Planning Rhinoplasty

For every surgeon who is approaching the analysis and planning of rhinoplasty patients, I recommend the articles written by Dr. Guyuron in the journal Plastic and Reconstructive Surgery.

Guyuron B (1988) Precision rhinoplasty. Part I: the role of life-size photographs and soft-tissue cephalometric analysis. Plast Reconstr Surg 81:489–499 Guyuron B (1988) Precision rhinoplasty. Part II: prediction. Plast Reconstr Surg 81:500–505

Guyuron B (1991) Dynamics of rhinoplasty. Plast Reconstr Surg 88:970–978

15.8 From Nasal Analysis to Nasal Surgery

The close relationships between nasal analysis and planning, as well as between planning and surgical maneuvers in rhinoplasty, are well described in the recent and innovative book of Rollin K. Daniel.

Daniel RK (2002) Rhinoplasty. An atlas of surgical techniques. Springer, Berlin, Heidelberg, New York

15.9 The Six Keys to Optimal Dental Occlusion

An in-depth analysis of dental occlusion requires knowledge of the indicators of optimal occlusion described by Lawrence F. Andrews:

- Key I: Interarch relationship
- Key II: Crown angulation
- Key III: Crown inclination
- Key IV: Teeth rotation
- Key V: Tight teeth contacts
- Key VI: Curve of Spee

Andrews LF (1972) The six keys to normal occlusion. Am J Orthod 62:671–690

Andrews LF (1989) Straight wire. The concept and the appliance. L.A. Wells, San Diego

15.10 The Smile Analysis: An Orthodontic Point of View

The shape, size, and position of the incisors; the amount of gingival display; and the transverse dimension of the dental arches are all important factors in smile analysis. The articles presented by M.B. Ackerman and J.L. Ackerman and by D.M. Sarver enrich the recent orthodontic literature on this topic.

Ackerman JL, Ackerman MB, Brensinger CM, Landis JR (1998) A morphometric analysis of the posed smile. Clin Orthod Res 1:2–11

Sarver DM (2001) The importance of incisor positioning in the esthetic smile: the smile arc. Am J Orthod Dentofacial Orthop 120:98–111

Ackerman MB, Ackerman JL (2002) Smile analysis and design in the digital era. J Clin Orthod 36:221–236

15.11 Clinical Cephalometric Analysis

My favorite book on radiographic cephalometry is the one that is edited by Alexander Jacobson. In this text, the radiographic cephalometric technique, the tracing techniques and identification of landmarks, as well as the principal modern cephalometric analysis are presented. Some chapters, like the one dedicated to soft tissue cephalometric analysis, are of great general interest for all specialists dealing with facial aesthetics.

Jacobson A (ed) (1995) Radiographic cephalometry. From basics to videoimaging. Quintessence, Chicago

15.12 Clinical Analysis of Dentofacial Deformities

A modern way to analyze the face for orthodontic and orthognathic surgery diagnosis and planning was published by G. William Arnett and Robert T. Bergman in 1993. In their organized and comprehensive method, 19 key facial traits are considered and examined clinically.

Arnett GW, Bergman RT (1993) Facial keys to orthodontic diagnosis and treatment planning. Part I. Am J Orthod Dentofacial Orthop 103:299–312

Arnett GW, Bergman RT (1993) Facial keys to orthodontic diagnosis and treatment planning. Part II. Am J Orthod Dentofacial Orthop 103:395–411

15.13 Proportion and Disproportion in Dentofacial Deformity

Normalizing the jaw relationship according to the cephalometric standards does not guarantee favorable outcomes. As Harvey M. Rosen of Philadelphia has pointed out in his book, better aesthetic results in cases of dentofacial deformity are sometimes achieved by moving the jaws toward a skeletal disproportion in order to assure an adequate support to the facial soft tissue envelope.

Rosen HM (1999) Aesthetic perspective in jaw surgery. Springer, Berlin, Heidelberg, New York

15.14 How the Skin Ages

The processes of skin aging, its causes, as well the prevention and treatment of age-related lesions are of great interest. The chapters of this recent book by Leslie Baumann on cosmetic dermatology dedicated to excessive sun exposure, smoking habits, hormones, and skin pigmentation are useful in analyzing the "quality" of facial soft tissue.

Baumann L (2002) Cosmetic dermatology: principle and practice. McGraw Hill, New York

15.15 How the Face Ages

The mechanisms involved in the process of facial aging are gravity, skin actinic damage, the drop of estrogen level at the onset of menopause, any change in basal metabolism, fat atrophy and/or increase in fat, progressive fascial and ligamentous laxity, and many others. A chapter dedicated to the theories of aging can be found in the recent book written by Gregory LaTrenta.

LaTrenta GS (2004) Atlas of aesthetic face and neck surgery, Chap. 2. Saunders, Philadelphia

Surround Yourself with Experts (and Other Important Advice for a Constructive and Creative Surgical Practice)

16

Contents

Clinical facial analysis is vital in planning the treatment, evaluating the outcomes, comparing different strategies, and developing new techniques. In this light, we want to enrich our work with a collection of ideas and suggestions taken from different experiences and lectures, which, as clinical facial analysis undoubtedly is, could be useful for your daily practice. One of the best is "surround yourself with experts."

16.1 Surround Yourself with Experts

This precious piece of advice came from Richard Carlson. We have tested it many times and have found that it works exceptionally well.

Many are intimidated by successful people and think that they will not be willing to spend time or share their ideas with us. "Nothing could be farther from the truth," wrote Richard Carlson. "The reality is, accomplished people love it when someone takes an interest in their success; they love to share their wisdom, good ideas, or business secrets. It makes them feel wanted and needed [1]."

Early in our practice, I mailed a small questionnaire about the treatment of a particular facial malformation to five internationally renowned plastic surgeons. All kindly responded and one of them summarized his ideas and guidelines in a few-page syllabus, which we still use.

F. Meneghini, P. Biondi, *Clinical Facial Analysis*,
DOI 10.1007/978-3-642-27228-8_16, © Springer-Verlag Berlin Heidelberg 2012

16.2 The Cost of Complexity

If you are not devoted to breaking up the analysis, planning, and operative work into simple elements and consecutive actions, you must accept the negative extra cost of complexity.

16.3 John F. Kennedy on Myth

Myth: an exaggerated or idealized conception of a person or thing [2].

Do not cultivate within yourself the myth of the perfect analysis, the myth of the perfect aesthetic ratio or rule, the myth of the perfect treatment, the myth of the perfect result, and the myth of the perfect surgeon!

Time and time again we recall John F. Kennedy's views on myth:

> The greatest enemy of truth is very often not the lie – deliberate, contrived, and dishonest, but the myth – persistent, persuasive, and unrealistic.
> – John F. Kennedy, Yale University, June 11, 1962

16.4 Jack Sheen: "A Psychiatrist Once Told Me..."

Jack Sheen, in his two-volume book on aesthetic rhinoplasty (a cornerstone in this field!), has reported wonderful advice on the patient/surgeon relationship. Here it is:

> A psychiatrist once told me, 'If you can't elicit a smile from a patient, don't operate [3].'

16.5 The 20 Rules of Surgical Planning (or the "Think in Terms of..." Planning Series)

This is a list of different approaches to facial surgical planning. When you have a written surgical plan for a patient but your inner voice says that something does not work as well as you would like, read the following 20 "think in terms of…" points:

1. Think in terms of angles.
2. Think in terms of millimeters.
3. Think in terms of vectors.
4. Think in terms of volume (gain or loss of volume in one or more particular facial areas).
5. Think in terms of shapes.
6. Think in terms of proportions (avoid or correct any disproportion).
7. Think in terms of disproportions (enhance or produce a specific disproportion).
8. Think in terms of surgical feasibility.
9. Think in terms of surgical preferences.
10. Think in terms of male/female differences.
11. Think in terms of simplicity/complexity of the treatment.
12. Think in terms of minimally invasive surgery.
13. Think in terms of the patient's desire (seek insight into the patient's true desire – principle number six of D. Ralph Millard [4]).
14. Think in terms of convenience for the patient.
15. Think in terms of the patient's psychological status.
16. Think in terms of long-/short-term results (gain stability!).
17. Think in terms of maximizing functional or esthetic outcome.
18. Think in terms of avoiding surgical stigmata (natural, not-operated look).
19. Think in terms of avoiding postoperative complications or sequels.
20. Think in terms of other specialties (avoid professional loneliness!). I am often quite surprised at the productivity of rethinking a treatment plan, preferably with the aid of a colleague, utilizing the 20 rules of surgical planning.

16.6 David Sarver on "Diagnosis by Procedure"

What happened to the patient who made several consultations with different specialists? As David Sarver wrote in his book, he probably collected several different "diagnoses by procedure [5]." The orthodontist will have focused his problem primarily on the inclination and upper and lower crowding of the anterior teeth; the maxillofacial surgeon, on the small retrognathic mandible and the weak chin; and the plastic surgeon, on the nasal hump and the deviated septum.

The next piece of advice is closely related to David Sarver's statement that we must avoid diagnosis by procedure.

16.7 The Three Most Powerful Treatments

I am convinced that the three most powerful ways to change facial aesthetics are orthodontic treatment, orthognathic surgery, and rhinoplasty. All three are mainly performed on teenagers or young adults, so their lifelong impact is great. All three can be combined with each other, so their power can be enhanced. All three have effects within the central oval of the face, so their visibility is without doubt. All three also have many important functional elements to deal with.

Even if it is a difficult task, for a single professional, to gain competence in all of these three areas, the basic analysis and diagnosis, along with a team-approach philosophy, is mandatory for best serving our younger patients and avoiding any restricted "diagnosis by procedure."

16.8 The Priority List and the 80/20 Rule (Pareto's Law)

I want to draw your attention once again to the goals of treatment. The most important objective of clinical facial analysis and, generally, of all the preoperative processes, lies in the compilation of an itemized list of goals, which is considered to be ideal and personalized to the clinical case and is accepted by the patient as well as the doctor. But in the case of a long, detailed list, for example, a ten-point list itemized in order of importance, is there a method or a principle that effectively guides us in the selection of the treatment plan? Or, in other words, what is the rating of importance given to every point of the list?

I believe that the 80/20 rule, also called Pareto's law, can be helpful.

Vilfredo Pareto (1848–1923), an Italian economist and sociologist, found that the distribution of income and wealth in society exhibits a consistent pattern throughout history, in all parts of the world and in all societies. The distribution of income and wealth follows the ratio of 80/20 because 20% of people hold 80% of wealth or gain 80%t of income. The observation by Pareto stimulated many associated studies and theories in economics, industrial manufacturing, and software development.

The 80/20 rule applied to our preoperative goal list says that obtaining 20% of the goals (the first two or three of the all ten points in the itemized list) is responsible for 80% of the final results. In other words, we can assume that a vital few goals exist and that the outcome is strictly related to them.

16.9 Professional Success Is a Consequence of Interest, Joy, and the Desire for Future Happiness

Finally, I want to suggest that the inner and outer forces that govern the dynamics of professional success are a mixture of interest, joy, and the desire for future happiness, which should be cultivated within you and your team every day.

References

1. Carlson R (1998) Don't worry, make money. Hodder and Stoughton, London
2. (1998) Taken from the New Oxford Dictionary of English. Oxford University Press
3. Sheen JH, Sheen AP (1998) Aesthetic rhinoplasty. Quality Medical, St. Louis, p 131
4. Millard DR Jr (1986) Principlization of plastic surgery. Little Brown, Boston, p 31
5. Sarver DM (1998) Esthetic orthodontics and orthognathic surgery. Mosby – Year Book, St. Louis

Beauty Is Composite By Edoardo Lombardi Vallauri

17

In this book, the terms "physical beauty" or "beautiful face" are never utilized simply because they are inappropriate. Facial surgeons deal preferably with proportion, shape, volume, and the symmetry of a face, as well as function, pain, and patient satisfaction. In order to avoid repeating these terms, we have selected a study that has been carried out from a nonmedical, contemporary point of view of physical beauty by Professor Edoardo Lombardi Vallauri.

"Beauty Is Composite" was presented for the first time during a successful Italian RAI-Radio 3 broadcasting series, *Castelli in Aria* which is a chapter of the book *Semplificare. Micro-filosofie del quotidiano* published in 2010 by Academia Universa Press, Turin, Italy. Professor Lombardi Vallauri teaches Linguistics at Roma 3 University.

Beauty Is Composite

It Is Built, but It Destructs

In this chapter, we shall try to pursue some all too-simple lines of reasoning on a subject of great importance to everyone: *physical beauty*. Where does the beauty of a person lie? Is it a purely anatomical characteristic? More precisely, does the beauty of a face depend only on lineaments, on physical features, or do good looks actually derive from something else?

After answering questions of this kind, we shall ask whether this attribute which a person may possess, which everyone possesses to some extent at a given moment in life, is lasting. How much of our beauty is preserved in time? With advancing age, to what degree can we talk about beauty? There are conflicting opinions on this, and we shall be expressing an unpopular one that people tend to repress because it is bothersome and hard to accept.

So where does the beauty of a person lie? In particular, when and under what conditions does it come natural to say *of a face* that it is beautiful? Many are led to believe that physical beauty is above all an anatomical fact which depends on material form, physical contours, on the *boundary* that the body identifies between itself and surrounding space. Thus, if a face has cheekbones that are too pronounced, it is no longer considered beautiful; if it is too long or too wide and the eyes are closer together than we might expect, it is less beautiful. If one lip is far fleshier than the other, or if it hangs down, and so on. These are all anatomical characteristics. Perhaps this is proof that the commonly held opinion is true: that there are indeed anatomical traits which automatically make it difficult to classify a face as beautiful.

But although this anatomical criterion (regularity of lineaments, correspondence of facial anatomy to the canons of harmony) may be an almost *necessary* condition of beauty, it is not a *sufficient* condition.

Let us take the case of an anatomically regular face that comes under the canons of standard beauty but is *stupid*. In my opinion (once more simplifying a little), we may distinguish two basic types of stupid expressions. The first is the *passive*

F. Meneghini, P. Biondi, *Clinical Facial Analysis*,
DOI 10.1007/978-3-642-27228-8_17,

expression: eyes with the lids typically at half-mast, eyes that are not looking, that are in a position of inertia. The sensation of passivity is given by the fact that the eyelids are rather less open than would be necessary in order to look, while the mouth is slightly open and, in all likelihood, with the corners turned downward, which is to say with the facial muscles in a state of relaxation.

In general, the passive expression is one in which all the facial traits have been neglected, are somewhat sagging. The muscles are not activated because there is no will tautening them, putting them under tension, or driving them to some purpose: they are neglected because they are doing nothing. The passive stupid face is an *abandoned face*. I hope the reader has got a pretty realistic picture of it.

The other stupid face is the "etymological" one. The word *stupid* derives from the Latin *stupor* which means *amazement*: the stupid person is someone who understands so little that whatever she or he sees elicits obtuse amazement. So the "etymological" stupid face is the *face forever caught unawares*: eyebrows raised, mouth protruding (the spout mouth), which tends to form an *oh*! of amazement. Try to imagine or to actually make this face by imitating the description. It is the face of someone who – whatever she or he sees, whatever she or he comes across – expresses amazement, meaning an inability to understand. In brief, lack of intelligence in the etymological sense of the Latin word *intelligo*, "I understand."

What do these two faces have in common, the wholly neglected one and the one "caught unawares" by everything? They are faces behind which *no thought is going on*. Although anatomically perfect, a face that betrays no thought but on the contrary reveals a state of neglect or total inability to understand transmits a sensation of the unbeautiful. It is very difficult to find a face beautiful, for all its regularity, if it bears one of these two expressions, which is to say if it shows no sign of thought.

So our first attempt at simplification is that anatomy is important in determining beauty but that thought must be at work behind this lucky anatomy. A face must be rendered alive, active, and meaningful by the fact that behind it, we see thought in action. If there is no thought, if there is neglect, if there is emptiness, then the face will not be perceived as beautiful. Therefore, beauty is not only the product of anatomical regularity but also of an *internal quality*, if we may so define the intelligence that emanates from a face.

Then it must be said that over and above the established canons of beauty in general, under which we may also include intelligence, the relationship we have with a face is above all *existential*. After we have known a face for some time, it ceases to be beautiful or ugly because it becomes simply the thing by which we identify a person. We no longer associate that face with an aesthetic judgement but with someone's identity. It is no longer a question of beautiful/ugly; if anything, it becomes a question of *I like/I don't like*. And this kind of judgement we may make of a face is actually no longer separate from our saying "I like" or "I don't like" the entire person. So if we like many other aspects of a person, the fact that her or his face may seem ugly to an outsider becomes irrelevant to us since her or his face is no longer either beautiful or ugly but simply the face of that person.

So the beautiful/ugly category is replaced by a different one, linked to our experience of the other and therefore of an existential and affective nature, and the feelings that the face transmits depend on our overall perception of the person. It may happen that after a while a face which at first seemed ugly no longer seems so since it belongs to someone we have learned to appreciate. Maybe it is not so nice to look at, but the concept of *ugly mug* is no longer applicable because it is now the face of Francesca or Giovanni.

I believe this goes more for the face than for the body. It seems to me that when we get to know a person well, her or his body can still appear ugly, if it is in effect a body in decline, but not her or his face. Because the face is so closely bound to the *personality* of the other that if our perception of her or his personality is positive our perception of her or his face will also be positive. Conversely, if our perception of her or his personality is negative, our perception of her or his appearance will be too, even if she or he has a very attractive face.

The beauty of a face, then, is primarily the fruit of a personality. This fits in perfectly with the fact that intelligence, animating a face, renders it beautiful. And it also applies to strangers. But in the case of a person we know, it becomes even truer that the beauty of the face depends on personality. If a face exudes deep and solid thought that we can understand, or an authoritative personality, or is simply the face of someone we love or appreciate, then it is pleasing and *in this sense* we can say it is "beautiful."

In actual fact, we find a face pleasing because *the person* is witty, penetrating or because we know she or he has a great critical spirit, or is wise, or is tranquil: whatever this person might be, her or his face expresses it, and therefore, automatically, is pleasing to us. And rooted in this pleasing, there is some reason for saying that *in our view*, this is a beautiful face.

Even maliciousness, wickedness, can be beautiful. A malicious face may be a face that fascinates us. On one condition: that it is good quality malice. Often, in many things, quality counts more than sign (i.e., positive or negative orientation). Both in a positive and in a negative direction, both toward evil and toward good; if there is high quality, we are fascinated by it.

So if there is wickedness in a face but we feel there is intelligence behind it, meaning an ability to embrace and understand reality, we are struck by it and perceive it favorably. A commanding mind renders a face beautiful, even if it is a wicked mind: if the eyes, the set of the jaw muscles, and, in general, the lineaments of a face express mastery and not mediocrity, we are pleased to look at it.

There are certain well-known faces, part of the collective imagination worldwide, which confirm this argument. For example, the American actor Jack Nicholson is considered by many women to be a very handsome man. Indeed, to put it better, an extremely fascinating man. A desirable man then, in spite of being nothing special from the anatomical point of view. This is because he has a magnetic personality, and this personality is certainly more in the order of the wicked than the order of the good. The roles Jack Nicholson plays in his films are usually diabolic roles (sometimes quite literally in the sense that he plays a character comparable to the devil himself). The superhumanly diabolic wickedness that Jack Nicholson can express in his face makes it pleasing in the sense described above. Or at any rate fascinating.

Another actor who often plays bad guy roles (very different from Nicholson's), and who does not have the anatomical traits of the typical Adonis, is John Malkovich. He is an extremely attractive man because of his type of wickedness, meaning the malice expressed in his face. It is the type of malice that I would call sophisticated, often underhand: here too there is full command, total mastery. Perhaps his major role from this point of view is the Vicomte de Valmont in Stephen Frears' *Dangerous Liaisons* from the novel by Choderlos de Laclos. In his Valmont, there is full mastery of the situation, bent to his purposes, and total contempt for others. Well, this is certainly wickedness, but of such a high level that we are fascinated by it. And John Malkovich is therefore a man supremely capable of pleasing.

Perhaps not so well known, another face that is handsome yet wicked is Gary Oldman's, the actor who among other things played the bad guy in *Léon*, Luc Besson's film with Jean Reno and the very young Natalie Portman. Gary Oldman's malice in this film is a *darkly unbridled* malice. He does not have a particularly handsome face, but we sense that he is capable of absolute brutality. He can (or at least so it seems) abandon himself to limitless cruelty and enjoy it intensely. There is in him a capacity to go beyond normal human faculties. And this capacity, albeit in a wicked direction, certainly generates fascination. We are set before a face that we cannot stop watching.

Then there is beauty's relationship with time. In the first place with "short-term" time: the way the features are set, the active tension behind a face that expresses intelligence, is not the only thing that counts since there is also the *rhythm* with which they move. If a face gives a delayed, slow reaction to external stimuli, the impression is one of stupidity. Rhythm is important. If reactions are fast, if there is synchronicity with reality, if we note rapidity and not delay in response to what is happening, we get an impression of intelligence. And therefore of beauty.

But there should be no uncontrolled outbursts. In some mental or nervous pathologies, rapid movements of the facial muscles occur which however are not harmonious reactions to external stimuli but simply the incoherent emergence of something disordered within. So we have no sensation of either intelligence or beauty. Indeed, a mental disorder often renders a face unpleasing.

What is more interesting is beauty's relationship with long-term time. Time destroys physical beauty. Intellectual beauty usually remains or even increases with age, but people's physical desirability diminishes. We all feel this instinctively, and I believe it should be faced with courage, even in an explicit manner, whereas it usually tends to be swept somewhat under the carpet because we prefer not to see it.

I remember a large billboard in Piazza Venezia, Rome. In the foreground, there was a photo of an old woman's face and the slogan: *You can be beautiful even at eighty. When will the world understand?* I think it was an advertisement for cosmetics. I found the rhetoric behind it irritating. Firstly, she was not 80 but, at the most, about 70. Moreover, she was the most beautiful septuagenarian you could imagine, and the photo had definitely been retouched. So it was decidedly outside the canons of the realistic. Even with all this, the physical attraction which that beautiful septuagenarian could exert was zero. She had *lost all her powers of attraction.* Whereas the advertisement, with its rhetorical question (*When will the world understand?*), aimed at giving credence to the idea that beauty can be saved regardless of the passing of time. That billboard in Piazza Venezia was claiming that people can be attractive in old age in the same way as when they were young.

The truth is that the best example of beauty is found in young women. This is the *bitter* truth. Bitter because, unfortunately, young womanhood does not last long. Of course, the same holds true for young men: we are talking about women here both because the advertisement was directed at them and because all of these questions are usually perceived as being more important to women, a subject which may deserve to be discussed separately. Young people physically are made of better stuff. And although we have argued that beauty consists of many things, there is no denying that *physical desirability*, since it depends on the quality of the physical material we are made of, is closely related to age. We like fresh tissue best: we respond biologically, our hormones respond better to extremely *healthy* and therefore essentially *young* tissue.

Speaking in favor of beauty as of a grouping of different parameters in which the anatomical is only one among many, we should not repress (under the carpets of consciousness) the fact that the physical attractiveness which our bodies exert diminishes after a certain age. So when we speak of that special aspect of beauty which is *desirability*, we cannot consider it a mental question. The mammal in us has a precise instinct that says, *mate with an individual particularly suited to reproduction*: meaning a woman who is still *perfectly* fertile or a man who can best carry out his reproductive functions. This naturally results in an asymmetry between males and females because male reproductive capacity lasts longer, so men retain their sex appeal longer than women.

This is an extremely unpopular argument, but since it is true, we must say it just the same; indeed, precisely because it is unpopular, we need to make even greater efforts in order to face reality instead of pretending that things are different. We will probably live better if we know how things stand, if we admit the truth to ourselves. Our civilization in general tends to repress a whole series of unpleasant things. For example, it tends to repress the idea of death: it is something relegated to the outskirts of public communication, something we all seek to avoid. There have been epochs in our civilization when death could be talked about far more openly, epochs in which people actually *had to* talk about death, whereas nowadays, it is a repressed topic.

Side by side with death there is decay. Old age. People pretend that this too does not exist: old folk are always depicted as substantially young. The old, however, are old. It is better to shout out loud and clear that youth is more beautiful than old age: not subjectively or existentially (I am not saying that young people are happier than old people) but organoleptically, meaning the way our senses grasp it. In others and ourselves, our senses perceive youth as beautiful and old age as ugly. Let us admit this and then face up to the idea of our old age, aware that we cannot place much hope on that plane.

The advertisement with the beautiful "oc togenarian" was misleading because it gave the idea that people can aspire to a kind of exterior beauty even at an advanced age. I believe that the right attitude as a person gradually approaches old age is not to aspire to physical beauty but to accept that physical beauty is no longer there and to go for other types of beauty, or more radically for other types of satisfaction. To tell ourselves the truth about our old age, our faded beauty, helps us toward a more decisive pursuit of other satisfactions. These are certainly not lacking, but we risk missing them when the time comes if we have not prepared for them throughout our lives, for example, by relying on cosmetic art in order to stay eternally young. That really is a dreadful own goal risked by those who repress and seek to ignore the fact that beauty fades with time.

Facing reality in this field means acknowledging that beauty is *first and foremost* a matter of anatomy, *but not only*: it is also largely a matter of character and personality. That anatomical and physical beauty is closely linked to our reproductive instinct and that we all therefore find more beauty in a person who is younger, more adapted to reproduction, healthier, and with fresher tissue. So we should not hide from the fact that we become uglier as we get older. To do so is decidedly disadvantageous.

It is worth repeating: *we become uglier as we get older*. Let us face up to it, take no heed of cosmetics advertisements, and accept the idea that little can be done to avoid it. Let us try to become increasingly interesting within ourselves, increasingly satisfied. Let us spend our life well by fighting the real battle, the inner one, and not fighting cosmetic battles.

Our discourse on beauty has become one on *decay*. Decay is inherent in us and after an initial phase of development it leads to our deterioration, right on down to complete loss. Our body decays to such an extent that at a certain point it can take no more and we die. Matters of this kind are systematically repressed in our civilization; above all, many of the main sources of communication seek to conceal them. In public communication of private origin (typically in advertising), there is a tendency to present the whole subject of decay and old age as a story with a happy ending. As if beauty and youth were everlasting. Old people in advertisements look great and are super-supple in their movements, merrymaking, and surrounded by young people. Well, this is trickery: in particular, physical beauty fades.

Fortunately, there are other kinds of beauty, and even physical beauty without intellectual beauty, without the animation of thought that we mentioned at the start, is of no use to anyone. Indeed it does not, cannot exist: a perfect face with a stupid expression can never be pleasing. So what we have inside is very important. We should go for this, because gambling on the lastingness of a face without wrinkles is simply a losing bet.

Index

F. Meneghini, P. Biondi, *Clinical Facial Analysis*,
DOI 10.1007/978-3-642-27228-8, © Springer-Verlag Berlin Heidelberg 2012